# THE MACHINE AT THE BEDSIDE

# THE MACHINE AT THE BEDSIDE

## Strategies for using technology in patient care

Edited by

**STANLEY JOEL REISER**
University of Texas Health Science Center, Houston

**MICHAEL ANBAR**
State University of New York at Buffalo

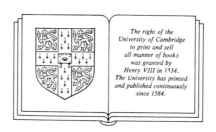

The right of the
University of Cambridge
to print and sell
all manner of books
was granted by
Henry VIII in 1534.
The University has printed
and published continuously
since 1584.

CAMBRIDGE UNIVERSITY PRESS
Cambridge
London   New York   New Rochelle
Melbourne   Sydney

Published by the Press Syndicate of the University of Cambridge
The Pitt Building, Trumpington Street, Cambridge CB2 1RP
32 East 57th Street, New York, NY 10022, USA
296 Beaconsfield Parade, Middle Park, Melbourne 3206, Australia

First published 1984

Printed in the United States of America

*Library of Congress Cataloging in Publication Data*
Main entry under title:
The machine at the bedside.
1. Medical innovations – United States – Evaluation.
2. Medical care – United States – Evaluation. I. Reiser,
Stanley Joel. II. Anbar, Michael.
R856.M284   1984   362.1′042   84–5852
ISBN 0 521 26718 8 hard covers
ISBN 0 521 31832 7 paperback

# CONTENTS

List of contributors                                                                  *page* ix

Foreword                                                                                    xv
*Seymour Perry*

Preface                                                                                   xvii

### PART I. OVERVIEW

1 The machine at the bedside: technological transformations of
  practices and values                                                                       3
  *Stanley Joel Reiser*

### PART II. SCIENTIFIC DIMENSIONS
### OF TECHNOLOGY

2 Penetrating the black box: physical principles behind
  health care technology                                                                    23
  *Michael Anbar*

3 Biological bullets: side effects of health care technology                                35
  *Michael Anbar*

### PART III. CREATION AND DISSEMINATION
### OF TECHNOLOGY

4 The engineering–industrial accord: inventing the technology
  of health care                                                                            49
  *Murray Eden*

5 Embracing or rejecting innovations: clinical diffusion of
  health care technology                                                                    65
  *H. David Banta*

## PART IV. ORGANIZING TECHNOLOGY IN CLINICAL SETTINGS

6 Technology's front line: the intensive care unit      95
*James J. Hassett*

7 Action with dispatch: technology in the emergency department      105
*Michael Eliastam*

## PART V. APPLYING TECHNOLOGY IN CLINICAL PRACTICE

8 The unwanted suitor: law and the use of health care technology      119
*William J. Curran*

9 The machine and the marketplace: economic considerations in applying health care technology      135
*Warren Butt and Duncan Neuhauser*

10 The technological strategist: employing techniques of clinical decision making      153
*Mark J. Young, Sankey V. Williams, and John M. Eisenberg*

11 The technological target: involving the patient in clinical choices      177
*Harold J. Bursztajn, Robert M. Hamm, and Thomas G. Gutheil*

12 Does technology work? judging the validity of clinical evidence      193
*Ralph I. Horwitz, Alvan R. Feinstein, William B. Credé, and John D. Clemens*

## CASE STUDIES

### SECTION A. DILEMMAS OF INTENSIVE CARE

1 The patient who wants to fight      213
*Robert Baker*

2 The triage decision      221
*Albert G. Mulley, Jr.*

3 Survival of the staff      227
*Theodore A. Stern*

## SECTION B. TECHNOLOGY AND THE HOSPITAL

4 Coming to terms with the computer     235
*Edward H. Shortliffe*

5 Resource allocations and imaging of the body     241
*Ann A. Jones and Robert M. Heyssel*

6 Considering an artificial heart program     247
*Deborah P. Lubeck and John P. Bunker*

## SECTION C. TECHNOLOGY AND THE SCREENING AND PREVENTION OF DISEASE

7 The prenatal state: screening and treating neural tube defects     255
*John C. Fletcher*

8 Costs and benefits of preventive strategies: containing hepatitis     261
*Jeffrey P. Koplan*

## SECTION D. TECHNOLOGY AND DIAGNOSTIC EVALUATION

9 The test of the laboratory versus the test of time     267
*Harold C. Sox, Jr.*

10 The penalties of excessive inquisitiveness     279
*Michael Anbar*

11 Reimbursement incentives and clinical strategies     283
*Steven A. Schroeder and Bernard Lo*

12 The cost of the routine order     287
*Philip Greenland and Paul F. Griner*

13 Prospects and dilemmas of the consultant:
the medical imaging specialist     291
*A. Everette James, Jr., Alan C. Winfield, Jeremy J. Kaye,
Frank A. Sloan, Ronald R. Price, C. Leon Partain,
W. Hoyt Stephens, Raleigh J. Hamilton, and
Henry P. Pendergrass*

14 The patient's perception of risk     297
*Keith I. Marton*

## SECTION E. TECHNOLOGY AND SPECIALIZED HEALTH CARE

15 Birth: electronic fetal monitoring 303
   *Miriam D. Orleans and Albert D. Haverkamp*

16 The premature infant: prognostic dilemmas for
   parents and practitioners 307
   *I. David Todres*

17 Neurological disorders: decision analysis and the
   patient's workup 311
   *Arthur S. Elstein, John I. Balla, Marilyn L. Rothert,
   and David R. Rovner*

18 Respiratory failure: technological care in the home and hospital 321
   *Kathleen A. McCormick and Faye G. Abdellah*

19 Heart disease: the ethical quandaries of treating the aged 327
   *Eric J. Cassell*

20 Rehabilitation: the decision to replace a human function
   with a machine 333
   *Ruth B. Purtilo*

21 Multiple injury: burns and heroic measures 337
   *Janet A. Marvin*

22 Gastrointestinal illness: the hunger for certainty 341
   *Howard M. Spiro*

23 Kidney disease: the dialysis–transplantation dilemma 349
   *Patricia L. Schaffer, J. Michael Lazarus, and Stanley Joel Reiser*

Index 355

# CONTRIBUTORS

*Faye G. Abdellah*, Ed.D., Sc.D., LL.D., R.N., F.A.A.N.; Deputy Surgeon General; Chief Nurse Officer; United States Public Health Service; 5600 Fishers Lane; Rockville, Maryland 20857

*Michael Anbar*, Ph.D.; Chairman; Department of Biophysical Sciences; State University of New York; 118 Cary Hall; Buffalo, New York 14214

*Robert Baker*, Ph.D.; Associate Professor; Department of Philosophy; Union College; Schenectady, New York 12308

*John I. Balla*, F.R.A.C.P., M.A.; Prince Henry's Hospital; St. Kilda Road; Melbourne, Australia 3004

*H. David Banta*, M.D., M.P.H.; Deputy Director; Pan American Health Organization; Pan American Sanitary Bureau; Regional Office of the World Health Organization; 525 Twenty-Third Street, N.W.; Washington, D.C. 20037

*John P. Bunker*, M.D.; Professor of Anesthesia and Family, Community and Preventive Medicine; Department of Family, Community and Preventive Medicine; Stanford University Medical Center; Health Research Policy Building, Room 7; Stanford, California 94305

*Harold J. Bursztajn*, M.D.; Clinical Instructor; Harvard Medical School; Massachusetts Mental Health Center; 74 Fenwood Road; Boston, Massachusetts 02115

*Warren Butt*, M.D.; Resident; Department of Internal Medicine; Cleveland Metropolitan General Hospital; 3395 Scranton Road; Cleveland, Ohio 44109

*Eric J. Cassell*, M.D.; Clinical Professor of Public Health; Cornell University Medical College; Director; Cornell Program for the Study of Ethics and Values in Medicine; The New York Hospital-Cornell Medical Center; 525 East 68th Street; New York, New York 10021

*John D. Clemens*, M.D.; Assistant Professor of Medicine; Yale University School of Medicine; 333 Cedar Street; New Haven, Connecticut 06510

*William B. Credé*, M.D.; Assistant Professor of Medicine; Yale University School of Medicine; 333 Cedar Street; New Haven, Connecticut 06510

*William J. Curran*, J.D., LL.M., S.M. Hyg.; Frances Glessner Lee Professor of Legal Medicine; Department of Health Policy and Management; Harvard School of Public Health; 677 Huntington Avenue; Boston, Massachusetts 02115

*Murray Eden*, Ph.D.; Chief; Biomedical Engineering and Instrumentation Branch; Building 13, Room 3W13; National Institutes of Health; 9000 Rockville Pike; Bethesda, Maryland 20205

*John M. Eisenberg*, M.D.; Sol Katz Associate Professor of General Medicine; Chief; Section of General Medicine; Hospital of the University of Pennsylvania; 3400 Spruce Street; Philadelphia, Pennsylvania 19104

*Michael Eliastam*, M.D., M.P.A., M.P.P.; Assistant Professor of Medicine and Surgery; Department of Medicine and Surgery; Stanford University Medical Center; Room P1016; 300 Pasteur Drive; Stanford, California 94305

*Arthur S. Elstein*, Ph.D.; Professor, Center for Educational Development; University of Illinois at Chicago; 808 Southwood; Chicago, Illinois 60612

*Alvan R. Feinstein*, M.D.; Professor of Epidemiology and Director; Robert Wood Johnson Clinical Scholars Program; Yale University School of Medicine; 333 Cedar Street; New Haven, Connecticut 06510

*John C. Fletcher*, Ph.D.; Assistant for Bioethics Clinical Center; National Institutes of Health; 9000 Rockville Pike, Building 10-1C150; Bethesda, Maryland 20205

*Philip Greenland*, M.D.; Assistant Professor of Medicine; Department of Medicine; School of Medicine and Dentistry; The University of Rochester; Rochester, New York 14620

*Paul F. Griner*, M.D.; Samuel E. Durand Professor of Medicine; Department of Medicine; School of Medicine and Dentistry; The University of Rochester; Rochester, New York 14620

*Thomas G. Gutheil*, M.D.; Associate Professor of Psychiatry; Harvard Medical School; Director of Medical Student Training; Massachusetts Mental Health Center; 74 Fenwood Road; Boston, Massachusetts 02115

*Raleigh J. Hamilton*, M.B.A.; Administrative Officer; Department of Radiology and Radiological Sciences; School of Medicine; Vanderbilt University; Nashville, Tennessee 37232

*Robert M. Hamm*, Ph.D.; Senior Research Associate; The Center for Research on Judgement and Policy; University of Colorado; P.O. Box 344; Boulder, Colorado 80309

*James J. Hassett*, M.D.; Assistant Professor of Surgery and Biophysics; Department of Surgery; Erie County Medical Center; 462 Grider Street; Buffalo, New York 14215

*Albert D. Haverkamp*, M.D.; Associate Professor of Obstetrics and Gynecology; Director of Perinatal Research; Denver General Hospital; Denver, Colorado 80262

*Robert M. Heyssel*, M.D.; President; The Johns Hopkins Hospital; Baltimore, Maryland 21205

*Ralph I. Horwitz*, M.D.; Associate Professor of Medicine and Assistant Director; Robert Wood Johnson Clinical Scholars program; Yale University School of Medicine; 333 Cedar Street; New Haven, Connecticut 06510

*A. Everette James, Jr.*, Sc.M., J.D., M.D.; Professor and Chairman; Department of Radiology and Radiological Sciences; School of Medicine; Vanderbilt University; Nashville, Tennessee 37232

*Ann A. Jones*, Ph.D.; Vice President; Planning and Development; The Johns Hopkins Hospital; Baltimore, Maryland 21205

*Jeremy J. Kaye*, M.D.; Professor of Radiology; Department of Radiology and Radiological Sciences; School of Medicine; Vanderbilt University; Nashville, Tennessee 37232

*Jeffrey P. Koplan*, M.D., M.P.H.; Assistant Director for Public Health Practice; Department of Health and Human Services; Center for Disease Control; Atlanta, Georgia 30333

*J. Michael Lazarus*, M.D.; Associate Professor of Medicine; Harvard Medical School; Director; End Stage Renal Disease Program; Brigham and Women's Hospital; 75 Francis Street; Boston, Massachusetts 02115

*Bernard Lo*, M.D.; Assistant Professor of Medicine; Division of General Internal Medicine; School of Medicine; University of California at San Francisco; 400 Parnassus, Room A405; San Francisco, California 94143

*Deborah P. Lubeck*, Ph.D.; Senior Health Care Analyst; SysteMetrics; 104 West Anapamu Street; Santa Barbara, California 93101

*Kathleen A. McCormick*, Ph.D., R.N.; Research Nurse; National Institutes of Health–National Institute of Aging; Laboratory of Behavioral Sciences; Gerontology Research Center; Baltimore City Hospital; 4900 Eastern Avenue; Baltimore, Maryland 21224

*Keith I. Marton*, M.D.; Assistant Professor of Medicine; Department of Medicine; Stanford Medical School; Stanford, California 94305

*Janet A. Marvin*, R.N., M.N.; Associate Professor; Department of Surgery, Department of Physiological Nursing; University of Washington; Medical School, and School of Nursing; VA-16; Harborview Medical Center; Seattle, Washington 98104

*Albert G. Mulley, Jr.*, M.D.; Assistant Professor of Medicine; Harvard Medical School; Chief, General Internal Medicine Unit; Division of Internal Medicine; Associate Director of Medical Practices Evaluation Unit; Massachusetts General Hospital; 5555 Fruit Street; Boston, Massachusetts 02114

*Duncan Neuhauser*, Ph.D.; Professor of Epidemiology and Community Health; School of Medicine; Case Western Reserve University; 2119 Abington Road; Cleveland, Ohio 44106

*Miriam D. Orleans*, Ph.D.; Professor of Preventive Medicine and Biometrics; Department of Preventive Medicine and Biometrics; Health Sciences Center; University of Colorado; Campus Box C245; 4200 East Ninth Street; Denver, Colorado 80262

*C. Leon Partain*, Ph.D., M.D.; Associate Professor of Radiology; Director of Nuclear Medicine; Department of Radiology and Radiological Sciences; School of Medicine; Vanderbilt University; Nashville, Tennessee 37232

*Henry P. Pendergrass*, M.P.H., M.D.; Professor of Radiology; Department of Radiology and Radiological Sciences; School of Medicine; Vanderbilt University; Nashville, Tennessee 37232

*Seymour Perry*, M.D.; Deputy Director; Institute for Health Policy Analysis; Georgetown University Medical Center; 2233 Wisconsin Avenue; Suite 324; Washington, D.C. 20007

*Ronald R. Price*, Ph.D.; Associate Professor of Radiology; Director of Radiological Sciences; Department of Radiology and Radiological Sciences; School of Medicine; Vanderbilt University; Nashville, Tennessee 37232

*Ruth B. Purtilo*, R.P.T., Ph.D.; Associate Professor of Medical Jurisprudence and Humanities; The University of Nebraska Medical Center; 42nd and Dewey Avenue; Omaha, Nebraska 68105

*Stanley Joel Reiser*, M.D., Ph.D.; Griff T. Ross Professor of Humanities and Technology in Health Care; The University of Texas; Health Science Center at Houston; P.O. Box 20708; 6431 Fannin, Suite 1.500; Houston, Texas 77225

*Marilyn L. Rothert*, R.N., Ph.D.; Associate Professor of Medical Education; Office of Medical Education, Research, and Development; College of Human Medicine; Director of Lifelong Education for Nursing; College of Nursing; Michigan State University; A 202 East Fee Hall; East Lansing, Michigan 48824

*David R. Rovner*, M.D.; Professor of Medicine; Chief of Endocrinology and Metabolism; Department of Medicine; College of Human Medicine; Michigan State University; B 234 Life Sciences Building; East Lansing, Michigan 48824

*Patricia L. Schaffer*; Medical Student; Harvard Medical School; 25 Shattuck Street; Boston, Massachusetts 02115

*Steven A. Schroeder*, M.D.; Professor of Medicine; Chief, Division of General Internal Medicine; Member of Institute for Health Policy Studies; School of Medicine; University of California at San Francisco; 400 Parnassus, Room A405; San Francisco, California 94143

*Edward H. Shortliffe*, M.D., Ph.D.; Assistant Professor of Medicine and Computer Science; Department of Medicine; Stanford University; Stanford, California 94305

*Frank A. Sloan*, Ph.D.; Senior Research Associate; Health Policy Center; Institute for Public Policy Study; Box 1503, Station B; Vanderbilt University; Nashville, Tennessee 37232

*Harold C. Sox, Jr.*, M.D.; Associate Professor of General Internal Medicine; Department of Medicine; Stanford University Medical Center; Stanford, California 94305

*Howard M. Spiro*, M.D.; Professor of Medicine; Department of Medicine; Yale University School of Medicine; 333 Cedar Street; New Haven, Connecticut 06510

*Col. W. Hoyt Stephens*, M.S.; Director of Center for Medical Imaging Research; Department of Radiology and Radiological Sciences; School of Medicine; Vanderbilt University; Nashville, Tennessee 37232

*Theodore A. Stern*, M.D.; Assistant Professor; Department of Psychiatry; Harvard Medical School; Staff Psychiatrist; Psychiatric Consultation Service; Massachusetts General Hospital; 5555 Fruit Street; Boston, Massachusetts 02114

*I. David Todres*, M.D.; Associate Professor of Anaesthesia (Paediatrics); Harvard Medical School; Director of Neonatal and Pediatric Intensive Care Units; Massachusetts General Hospital; 5555 Fruit Street; Boston, Massachusetts 02114

*Sankey V. Williams*, M.D.; Henry J. Kaiser Foundation Faculty Scholar; Assistant Professor of Medicine; Section of General Medicine; Hospital of the

University of Pennsylvania; 3400 Spruce Street; Philadelphia, Pennsylvania 19104

*Alan C. Winfield*, M.D.; Associate Professor of Radiology; Department of Radiology and Radiological Sciences; School of Medicine; Vanderbilt University; Nashville, Tennessee 37232

*Mark J. Young*, M.D.; Assistant Professor of Internal Medicine; General Medicine Division; University of Michigan; The Medical Professional Building, 5111; University Hospital; Ann Arbor, Michigan 48109

# FOREWORD

Technological advances in medicine have greatly enhanced the capacity of health care providers to prevent, detect, diagnose, and treat disease; to rehabilitate those with physical or other handicaps; and to promote health. In only a few years, these innovations have remarkably altered the character of health care and its delivery in the hospital, clinic, office, and home. They have changed the relationships among physicians, nurses, and patients, and have led to the establishment of technology-focused units to provide complex, specialized, and intensive care for serious medical conditions. The technologies have generated a whole array of specialized practitioners among physicians, nurses, and allied health personnel. Unfortunately, they have also brought with them unprecedented problems concerning risk and benefit, costs and effectiveness, and ethical and legal implications for patients, clinicians, and society.

Within the past several years, efforts were mounted by governmental agencies, particularly the National Center for Health Care Technology, and by a number of medical professional societies to address these problems through the process of technology assessment. However, institutions responsible for the education and training of physicians, nurses, and allied health professionals have not taken steps to prepare their students to deal with complex issues associated with technologies when they leave the academic setting and enter the health care delivery system. In the course of their education, students encounter many of the technologies they will subsequently apply, but they are rarely, if ever, exposed to a consideration of the problems these technologies engender in practice. This book is designed to stimulate and facilitate the development of academic studies to fill this void and to provide useful concepts and strategies for those interested in the use of technology from the viewpoints of practice, policy, and graduate work. This volume is an enormously important effort in this era of technological innovation, one that promises even greater technological achievements.

Seymour Perry, M.D.

Former Director
National Center for Health Care Technology
Currently Deputy Director
Institute for Health Policy Analysis
Georgetown University Medical Center

# PREFACE

This book is about the technology of health care – its creation, dissemination, and use – and is written to give health care providers and decision makers, patients included, a view of how this technology affects us. It deals principally with that aspect of technology embodied by instruments and machines, creations in the vanguard of developments that are shaping this modern era of health care.

The technological revolution in health care is a significant feature of modern life and one of our greatest achievements. However, the power technology gives us makes it necessary to ensure that we apply it humanely and efficiently. Health care providers who are not adequately trained may either use technology with insufficient understanding or delegate its application to specialists, who themselves may apply it unwisely. The results, in either case, are a suboptimal use of these powerful tools. Such misuse may not only raise the cost of health care but can harm the patient. The occurrence of iatrogenic diseases has increased since the the introduction of powerful technology-dependent procedures. This book attempts to delineate views and approaches to meet these critical deficiencies so that the promise of improved health that our technological creations offer can be more fully realized.

Technology poses another type of challenge even to the practitioner who masters it technically. It not only offers the means to improve dramatically the patient's quality of life, but also allows us to sustain life under conditions of great suffering. The appropriate use of technology, therefore, involves not only a mastery of science and engineering tools and concepts, but also the ability to cope with a difficult set of ethical and economic issues and with choices whose complexity requires a more methodical approach to the subject of clinical decision making. This book addresses these ramifications of modern technology.

Health care providers also face significant problems in adapting to the introduction of new technology. Innovations play a central role in altering the responsibilities and the status of medical staff. The introduction of the x-ray and later imaging techniques of the lungs and heart, for example, reduced the standing of clinicians whose position was principally dependent on their skill in the physical examination of the chest. The computer, by the same token, alters the status of nurses in relation to physicians when the nurses using the computer acquire greater responsibilities for developing and interpreting the clinical data base. Allied health personnel, many of whose functions are technologically created and determined, face the problem of being distanced from patients by their technology, and are often unclear about the nature of their technologically influenced responsibilities to patients. They also are threatened, like others in health care, by obsolescence as technology changes.

This book is composed of chapters and case studies. The chapters provide a general view of the facets of modern knowledge necessary to understand and use health care technology wisely – from its bases in physical principles to the process of its invention and diffusion to the role of law, ethics, economics, and strategies of decision making and choice in determining and facilitating its application. The case studies discuss the chief technological issues of our times. Each case is accompanied by a bibliography, which provides essential background material for those who wish to treat the subject of the case comprehensively.

It is our hope that this volume will serve the needs of educators, practitioners, and social decision makers, allowing them to address comprehensively the central problems in this technological era of health care.

The editors wish to acknowledge their gratitude to all those at the National Center for Health Care Technology whose belief in and support of this volume enabled it to come into being. We thank especially Dr. Seymour Perry, its former director, whose abiding confidence in the necessity for this work stirred in us the dedication to pursue it.

SJR
MA

PART I

# OVERVIEW

# CHAPTER 1

# THE MACHINE AT THE BEDSIDE: TECHNOLOGICAL TRANSFORMATIONS OF PRACTICES AND VALUES

STANLEY JOEL REISER

The landscape of modern health care is filled with machines. Its features are marked by their angles and metallic surfaces and enveloped by an atmosphere of mechanical bleeps and clicks, which denote a vital presence at the same time reassuring and distracting.

A technological dominance of health care has developed in the twentieth century, although some of its key ideological and pragmatic goals reach back in time to the Renaissance and the scientific revolution, which transformed the reigning view of medicine that had been shaped by the ancient Greeks.

The Greek physicians, steeped in the learning of the Hippocratic school, saw the natural world as an environment to live with and adapt to, rather than to conquer and dominate. Their theory of illness, the humoral theory, concerned an equilibrium that existed among the four basic constituents of the body (humors), which in turn were connected with environmental elements (physical, social, and personal) that surrounded and interacted with the humors and determined health and illness.

According to this view, illness occurred when one or more of the four humors became excessive or deficient and upset the equilibrium in which they existed. The resulting imbalance produced symptoms related to the particular humoral dysfunction. The idea that disruption of one aspect of this biological system would affect all connecting parts implied that illness involved the whole person, not just a segment of the body. Diagnosis consisted in specifying which of the humors had changed, and this meant making detailed analyses of the environmental factors likely to have produced the dysfunctional humoral state.

Seasons and humors were intimately connected. The season whose climate was closest in quality to a given humor was likely to be responsible for a given humoral imbalance. The humor blood, for example, with qualities of warmth and moistness, was most likely to be affected in the spring, whose climate had these characteristics. The humor phlegm, being cold and moist, was particularly

3

vulnerable to the season marked by these traits, winter (Jones 1923). Accordingly, in this theory, the microcosm of one's biological makeup and the macrocosm of the physical world in which one lived were intimately linked.

Therapeutics were modest, in keeping with the power the Hippocratic Greeks attributed to nature and their recognition of how little they truly knew, or could do, to influence directly the course of events. Physicians viewed their task as assisting the natural powers of recovery by intervening at strategic and critical times in the course of illness. The ability to detect these moments was a central feature of Greek medical learning. To treat with harsh remedies in an attempt to overpower nature, and thereby to disregard the rational limits of one's therapeutic means, was to expose the practitioner to accusations of arrogance and to threaten the social standing of medicine. This approach to illness is epitomized in the Hippocratic essay "The Art" (Jones 1923, vol. 2):

> For if a man demand from an art a power over what does not belong to the art, or from nature a power over what does not belong to nature, his ignorance is more allied to madness than to lack of knowledge. For in cases where we may have the mastery through the means afforded by a natural constitution or by an art, there we may be craftsmen, but nowhere else. Whenever therefore a man suffers from an ill which is too strong for the means at the disposal of medicine, surely he must not expect that it can be overcome by medicine.

This point of view about nature began to be challenged in the sixteenth century. In biology, nature was assaulted first by the scalpel. Until this time, analysis of human anatomy had occurred basically through textual study. Professors read from the books of the learned ancients, usually Galen (A.D. 130–200). When the infrequent dissection of cadavers took place, students were supposed to see in the body what the book said was there. Nature was not interrogated during such lessons. Its form, in this case the body's, was thought to be inscribed in authoritative texts whose truths were accepted on faith. Medievalists did not believe that they could essentially improve on the views of revered, seemingly authoritative ancient geniuses. Although the Hippocratic Greeks had freely acknowledged their ignorance, they were committed to continual explorations of disease, mainly by bedside observation of the response of patients to illness. This spirit of inquiry became dulled in the Middle Ages, when scholars accepted as true what the ancients had written.

The Italian anatomist Andreas Vesalius challenged this medieval perspective. In a work published in 1543, *De corporis humani fabrica*, he demonstrated, by innovative dissection, over 200 errors in the accepted structure of the human body described by Galen. He proclaimed the necessity of studying nature by directly encountering and manipulating it, not by memorizing and memorializing existing texts. His words and actions penetrated and intermingled with the views of other scientists, who began actively to explore the natural world, seeking its truths by directly examining it (O'Malley 1965).

The metaphor of dissection, of separating wholes into parts in order to understand their working, became a central if not the most significant method of exploration as the scientific revolution took hold.

At the turn of the sixteenth century, the newly invented microscope provided a tool for such efforts. An innovative user of this instrument, Robert Hooke, curator of experiments and member of the Royal Society of London, described in 1665 his examination of cork and the discovery of the cellular composition of living matter (Hooke 1665):

> I took a good clear piece of cork, and with a pen-knife sharpened as keen as a razor, I cut a piece off.... Examining it very diligently with a *Microscope* ... I could exceedingly plainly perceive it to be all perforated and porous, much like a honey-comb.... [I] found that there were usually about three score of these small cells placed end-ways in the eighteenth part of an inch in length ... more that a thousand in the length of an inch and therefore in a square inch above a million, or 1166400, and in a cubick inch, about twelve hundred millions, or 1259712000, a thing almost incredible, did not our *Microscope* assure us of it by ocular demonstration.

It was the breaking down of complex matter, or analysis, that was for Isaac Newton the cornerstone of scientific investigation. He wrote in *Opticks*, published in 1687 (Newton 1952):

> As in Mathematics, so in Natural Philosophy, the investigation of difficult things by the Method of Analysis, ought even to precede the method of composition. This analysis consists in making experiments and observations, and in drawing general conclusions from them by instruction, and admitting of no objections against the conclusions, but such as are taken from experiments, or certain truths. For hypotheses are not to be regarded in experimental philosophy. And although the arguing from experiments and observations by induction be no demonstration of general conclusions, yet it is the best way of arguing which the nature of things admits of....
> By this way of analysis we may proceed from compounds to ingredients, and from motions to the forces producing them; and in general, from effects to their causes.

By this time, the idea was developing that nature was not merely to be lived with; it could be dominated by humans, who learned its secrets by the new experimental and analytic techniques of science.

Along with the ethos of dominance, the analytic, anatomic perspective generated a view of illness that segregated disease and disorder to specific places in the body. This concept replaced the ancient Greek notion of illness as a dynamic process involving place and lifestyle and affecting the whole person. It has become the prevailing concept of the nature of illness, and has influenced greatly the development and adoption of health care technology.

This view received its most comprehensive and influential formulation in the

1761 work of the Italian anatomist J. B. Morgagni, *The Seats and Causes of Diseases Investigated by Anatomy* (Morgagni 1960). This book synthesized concepts of structural changes produced by disease in parts of the body that had developed since the interest in the study of anatomy stirred two centuries before by Vesalius. Morgagni argued, as the title of his book states, that each disease had a seat, or anatomic resting place, in the body. The structural changes created by the disease in this place were unique, like fingerprints, and allowed those who inspected them to determine which sickness had affected the patient in life. They also explained the reason for the symptoms experienced by the patient.

Morgagni argued that these alterations were not merely of interest to the researcher seeking to understand disease processes, but critical for the learning and practice of clinicians. Only by examining changes in the body after death could those who worked at the bedside establish with certainty the veracity of their diagnostic conclusions. Morgagni advocated clinicopathologic correlation as a cornerstone of clinical education and evaluation. The clinicopathologic conference, now ubiquitous in health care, is one legacy of this view.

Anatomists developed a new perspective on Disease: It was a disorder of a bodily structure localized in a site. A small change in a vital part could result in serious damage to an otherwise normal body. Anatomists thus isolated diseases in places, and introduced into the discourse of health care what has become the principal question in the evaluation of patients: Where is the disease?

This concept is fundamentally different from the humoral-physiologic view of illness it replaced: that illness was the disruption of a balance among the basic constituents of the body, as well as with the total environment, and was thus a condition affecting the whole person. With the rise of anatomical thinking, illness became an event that basically affected an aspect of the body.

As the nineteenth century progressed, the acceptance of these views by clinicians paved the way for the modern specialization of health care. The rise of anatomical thinking and specialization are events inextricably bound. Specialization elevates the status of those who develop great knowledge about an aspect of things. Specialization of medical function did not begin with the acceptance of anatomy; it had existed since the earliest days of medicine. Specialists in the first half of the nineteenth century were largely informally trained people – midwives, bone setters, and so on. Those with a formal medical training, who so narrowed their practice, were looked down upon by their colleagues. The sage Philadelphia physician S. Weir Mitchell wrote that such doctors at this time, who practiced as specialists rather than generalists, were thought to be odd and misguided: "I can remember when older physicians refused to recognize socially a man who devoted himself to the eye alone" (Mitchell 1892).

But the logical justification for specialism, offered by an anatomically influenced perspective that isolated illness in specific bodily places, and the practical justification for specialism based on a need to create and master technology in order to detect and treat anatomical disruptions, combined to initiate the growth and acceptance of specialization in orthodox medicine during the nineteenth century. At this time the place of technology in practice became established, along with the multiple justifications for its use.

When the nineteenth century began, technology was not a part of diagnosis. In addition, its use in therapeutics was basically confined to the cutting instruments of surgery, a discipline not practiced by most university-trained physicians. This antitechnological bias in medicine can be traced to the thirteenth century, when the medieval universities, which were just beginning, became the locus of formal medical training. Learning their skills alongside theologians and lawyers in graduate faculties of the university, physicians came to accept and adopt the belief of these disciplines that the use of tools and manipulation lowered the esteem and social standing of scholars and physicians. Learning in the university was book learning. In pursuing their activities, scholars could not act like tradesmen, with whom the use of instruments was associated. This prejudice caused surgery to become disconnected from medicine. Surgeons were forced to set up their own schools outside of the framework of the university. Those physicians who lowered themselves to establish manual contact with patients were derisively labeled ''body physicians.''

This antitechnological, antimanual tradition was one Vesalius had to combat when he launched his campaign urging students and physicians who wanted to learn about the body to engage it actively. He decried physicians who, ''despising the use of the hands,'' delegated to others ''those things which had to be done manually for their patients and to stand over them like architects'' (O'Malley 1965).

With the acceptance of the importance to research and practice of dissecting the dead body, through the work between the sixteenth and eighteenth centuries of anatomists such as Vesalius and Morgagni, a crucial blow was dealt to the bias against technology and manual contact with patients. Dissection involved both touching patients and using tools for the clearly important purpose of locating and understanding the nature of structural changes caused by disease. In the nineteenth century, the desire to evaluate and treat such structural changes in the living overwhelmed the antitechnological, antimanual bias and transformed medicine.

In diagnosis, techniques were introduced such as percussion of the chest, together with instruments such as the stethoscope, laryngoscope, and ophthalmoscope, which established the first half of the nineteenth century as the age of physical diagnosis. Physicians, using these simple tools, attempted to perceive the living body's interior. Indeed, they became so enraptured by the evidence produced by applying their own senses to the evaluation of illness that they increasingly disregarded the sensations experienced and described by the patient as unreliable, unconfirmable, and inferior by comparison.

The decision to accept manipulation reintegrated the surgical approach to illness into the armory of practice. However, the rise of surgery to its modern status was dependent on two discoveries of the mid-nineteenth century. The first was proof by the dentist William Morton in 1846 that ether could eliminate operative pain. This was followed by the development of a technique to reduce infection by the surgeon Joseph Lister, who introduced sterile operating procedures (antisepsis) in the mid-1860s. These discoveries, and the possibility they carried of greatly improving surgical success, achieved real acceptance only when Robert Koch and others in the 1880s demonstrated the causal role of bacteria in disease. The germs in the air and on the wound that Lister insisted be eliminated were now shown to have a real effect on infection.

The great interest in identifying the nature of the different bacterial agents now implicated in disease causation led to the development of sophisticated instruments for the visual and chemical analysis of body fluids and tissues. Microscopes, incubators, staining agents, colorimeters, and other such devices were gathered together to form the diagnostic laboratory. This institution depended increasingly on technicians with the time and skill to apply the new techniques. Physicians, impressed with the connection of these instruments and techniques to science, and thinking of themselves as practicing scientifically by using them, increasingly turned from the judgments of their own senses and the techniques of physical diagnosis to the impressive data of the laboratory.

This change was in keeping with the original emphasis of the scientific revolution of the seventeenth century. One of its tenets was to place inquiry on an objective basis. In the investigation of nature, it sought to eliminate evidence influenced by human values or bias. It attempted to establish a rigorous set of methodologies to establish facts, such as experimentation, and to describe the facts wherever possible in objective ways, such as through the use of numbers.

Developments in medicine in the second half of the nineteenth century had made possible the statement of medical facts in objective forms. The chemical tests coming out of the diagnostic laboratory often expressed results in numbers. Further, instruments being invented in this period such as the sphygmograph, spirograph, and electrocardiograph made it possible to depict the motions of muscles, nerves, and blood in a graphic format. With such evidence, many physicians hoped that they could now take their place among the men and women of science. As the twentieth century began, the mathematician and philosopher Karl Pearson, in his well-known book *The Grammar of Science* (1900), called on the scientist "above all things to strive at self-elimination in his judgments, to provide an argument which is as true for each individual mind as for his own." He insisted that judging facts "unbiased by personal feeling is characteristic of what may be termed the scientific frame of mind." Doctors strove to establish this image.

The nineteenth century ended with technology firmly linked to diagnosis, and with surgery reunited with medicine, enjoying an enhanced status and forming the vanguard of therapeutics. However, these developments created three crucial problems for the twentieth century: first, how to organize rationally this growing technologic armory; second, how to distribute its goods among the increasing number of patients whom it would benefit; and third, how to construct a fruitful relationship among patients, practitioners, and medical technology.

The first major twentieth-century issue was to organize specialized personnel, technology, and patients to treat illness. The hospitals became the key agents to accomplish this integration and, accordingly, greatly increased in number and significance. Statistics tell the story: In 1875, the number of hospitals in the United States was between 200 and 600. By 1909, there were over 4,000; by 1928, almost 7,000.

The growth of hospitals was accompanied and influenced by medical specialization. The decline of the generalist approach to health care in this century is epitomized in the 1912 comment of William Mayo, a founder of the Rochester, Minnesota, clinic bearing his name: "So vast is the extent of knowledge to be gained of disease that no one man can hope to accomplish more than a small share during his lifetime. The old-time family practitioner has passed away and with him has passed individualism in medicine."

This prediction would soon be realized. By 1930, one physician in four in the United States was a specialist; by 1980, more than four in five. Specialism has been growing not only within medicine but also within other health care disciplines. At the start of the twentieth century, for example, there were about 345,000 health care providers, of whom about one in three were physicians. Most of the others were nurses. But gradually, as the century progressed, the demand for the expeditious performance of specialized tasks introduced into health care a new cadre of people to run the burgeoning technology and to perform new tasks generated by the acquisition of knowledge. In the mid-1960s, this heterogeneous group of individuals became called *allied health personnel*; by the mid-1970s, their number in the United States had reached some 1.8 million. Included within their ranks were 152 different specialists – such as cytotechnologist, health physics technician, dietitian, and rehabilitation therapist. The health care force at this time numbered about 5.1 million people, of whom only 1 in 13 was a physician (National Commission on Allied Health Education 1982). If one now adds the 152 allied health specialties to the 23 major specialties among physicians and the 8 among dentists, and then takes account of the specialties of nursing, optometry, and other health professions, one finds that there exist today over 200 specializations (Wilson and Neuhauser 1980), whose practitioners must somehow focus on the object of this whole enterprise – the patient.

How to marshall the expertise of this array of technology and people to meet the needs of an individual, not only efficiently but also humanely, is a central problem of modern health care. A significant issue in meeting this challenge is an organizational one: What is the best arrangement of personnel and machines? The main response of the twentieth century has been the hospital, which has gradually assumed the major role in Western societies to provide health care. Whereas in the United States, as the century began, the vast majority of births and deaths occurred outside of the hospital, they now occur mostly within its walls. The offices of physicians at the turn of this century, spread throughout cities and towns, are now largely located in or near hospitals. Insurance companies are more likely to pay for therapy programs conducted within rather than outside of hospitals. And not surprisingly, the cost of hospital care now represents the major portion of medical expenditures: In 1981 it was approximately $118 billion, or 41.2 percent of the total.

The hospital thus is a crucial means of integrating and centralizing health services. The hospital is the place in which agents of health care, their technology, and their patients meet; the hospital is the locus of medical care. But the organization of medical services requires something more. It is critical that the hospital provide a means of linking the separate medical interventions of diverse people. This is the function of the medical record.

If the hospital is the geographic locus, the record is the information locus of medical care. In an age of specialization, the record becomes central to organization. How else can the myriad actions the patient experiences daily be evaluated and altered unless an accurate and orderly account of them exists? Hospital records were somewhat randomly kept and unevenly supervised in the United States until reforms were initiated by the newly organized American College of Surgeons in the second decade of this century. This group inaugurated an annual inspection of hospitals and began to publish yearly lists of those that met agreed-upon standards. Certification by the college gradually became a mark of distinction, and failure to gain it a stigma. A significant aspect of its certification review was the state of the medical record. Through the work of the College of Surgeons and that of others, the medical record steadily improved. However, this improvement has been inadequate to meet the burdens it must bear. Its handwritten format, bulkiness, and general disorder, which make it difficult to find and at times to read data, tend to dishearten clinicians and encumber care.

The hospital and its system of integrating staff and medical data replaced a decentralized system of care. Before the twentieth century, medical care took place mainly in the home. Hospitals were for the poor, who could not afford home attendance and maintenance. Technology, which helped the hospital to rise to its present status, now makes possible the reinstitution of home care for many patients. During this century, we have developed increasingly sophisticated forms of communication, which permit detailed monitoring of most body functions at a distance. This capacity began with Alexander Graham Bell's invention in 1876 of the telephone, which linked doctors to patients' homes. It was furthered when Willem Einthoven, inventor of the modern electrocardiograph, developed in 1905 a technique of sending these electric records of heart actions a distance of 1.5 km between his laboratory and the local hospital; he called these transmissions *telecardiograms*.

Today we possess capabilities of transmitting over distance virtually every form of visual representation of illness, such as the interior of the retina, an x-ray film of the chest, and the actions of the heart expressed as numbers and graphs. We can monitor the physiological activities of the body as it changes over time, and transmit the physical examination findings of doctors and nurses to distant places. As electronic communication becomes an acceptable substitute for face-to-face meetings, crucial medical encounters need not take place solely in an institution developed to facilitate communication between specialized personnel and patients – which the hospital represents.

What applies to the monitoring of patient functions applies also to therapeutics. Respirators to maintain breathing and kidney dialysis technologies are now commonly used in the home. Parenteral nutrition, a technique of intravenous feeding for patients who cannot take in or digest food, has recently become a major home care activity. An example of this last advance is a 27-year-old man who developed a narrowing of his esophagus after surgery. He was fed intravenously in the hospital at the beginning, but then decided to try therapy at home. A company that specialized in the home use of parenteral therapy taught him how to use the pump that sent nutrients into his body, and how to hook up and unhook himself from it during the 8-hour period at night when it was on. This schedule allowed him to participate in activities and work during the day. A nurse made periodic visits to draw blood for chemical analysis and to check on his condition. Intravenous fluids were delivered weekly. A 1983 survey put home care expenditures in the United States at over $5 billion. They are expected to reach $16 billion by the end of the decade, increased by the growth of medical technology, the costs of hospital care, and an aging population (Kleinfield 1983).

These factors imply that a changing role for hospitals is possible. This institution might increasingly evolve into an arena in which acute critical care takes place, and in which specialized teams exist that can evaluate and respond as consultants to monitored information and wired medical data relayed from the apparatus at the bedside of a distant patient or the office of distant physician.

Clearly, a large cadre of health care providers becomes necessary to maintain patients at home; they are as important to such decentralized care as the machines. What should be appreciated is that the centralization of medical care in hospitals occurred as a result of the need to bring patients, providers, and technology together in a single place. New technological advances will provide opportunities for returning certain health care functions to the home and the community, with all of the advantages such settings can bring to patients, but also with the economic and organization problems of creating efficient patterns of delivery.

The possibilities of a more decentralized health care system make even more acute the integration of information about what patients experience and what medical actions are taken. The medical record, as presently constructed, does not provide effective integration.

When computers were introduced into clinical care at the start of the 1960s, one of the earliest hopes for them was to bring order to the collection, storage, and analysis of patient data. Computers introduced into hospitals could better integrate the activities of health care providers. But the use of this technology has proved difficult, not only for reasons of technical design but also of human response. Technology has a great capacity to change hierarchical arrangements, status, and power. This was illustrated by the reaction of hospital staff at the

Medical Center Hospital of Vermont in the 1970s to the introduction of a computerized information storage and retrieval system on a 19-bed general medical ward. The system was designed to encourage the systematic collection of critical data in a manner that revealed the logic of medical actions (which could then be subject to audit), to reduce the dependence of health providers on memory, and to improve communication between staff members. The effort was not successful. Formal evaluation of it revealed that a key group, consisting of interns and attending physicians on the medical staff, resented having to change their style of data recording and clinical actions in accordance with the system, and worried about encroachment by other staff members on their prerogatives as decision makers. In contrast, nurses were enthusiastic, for the new system encouraged greater participation in data acquisition and clinical decision making. Pharmacists welcomed the system for the same reasons, as did radiologists, who now had access to the complete patient record on demand, making x-ray reading easier (Fisher et al. 1980).

The development of better computer tools and the more widespread use of computerized data and records is crucial if the technological possibilities of decentralization are to be realized and if hospital staff are to keep pace with the growing number of medical interventions performed. The importance of the medical record as an organizing focus and a crucial mechanism of modern health care has not been widely appreciated. Attention to its form, substance, and use has been the concern of far too few.

The use of an organization to bring together health care services during the twentieth century was not confined to hospitals. By the early 1930s, the concept of group practice was growing; it has since attracted large numbers of providers. It assumes many forms, ranging from a legally constituted arrangement of physicians and sometimes other health care providers working together, sharing equipment, space, and earnings, to less formally integrated specialists referring patients to each other. By 1980, more than 25 percent of physicians were practicing in formal group settings. This outcome was meant to justify a policy that reduced the number of generalists. Specialists practicing in coordinated settings both inside and outside the hospital, it was felt, could integrate a patient's health care needs and provide, at the same time, up-to-date, specialized knowledge about the illness.

By the mid-1960s, in reaction to the fragmentation of care that this specialized system often created, the primary care and family care movements began. Their purpose was to create generalists who were able to integrate, more adequately than group practitioners, the new knowledge and technology of modern health care. The ideology that underlay the training of such people was to take responsibility. These practitioners did not see themselves as "traffic cops," evaluating patients only enough to know to which specialist to refer them. They saw their role as evaluation with the aim of treating the majority of routine illnesses to which the population was susceptible.

Whether single physicians can still care for the basic needs of patients, or whether groups of doctors only can fulfill this function is in effect now being tested. Technology in the future, particularly the computer, will play an increasing role in this test. The challenge will be to see if computers can be programmed to provide individual doctors with enough of the information held by specialists to allow them to function with increasing confidence and efficiency when physically separated from collegial groups. Such a possibility, in conjunction with more sophisticated forms of telecommunication with hospitals and specialists, could make individuals in health care more capable of performing wider patient care functions and revive an era of generalism.

The organization of health care services raises issues not only of allocating technologic tasks among providers but also of sharing the benefits of technology equitably among patients and finding the money to pay for it all. In the early 1950s, the ability of medicine to maintain the functions of critically damaged vital organs began to grow dramatically. It was initiated by the development of techniques to sustain polio victims through the use of improved ventilation technology and resuscitation techniques, brought to the clinic from the operating room by anesthesiologists (Pontoppidan et al. 1977). By the late 1950s, the success of such respiratory care had brought with it unanticipated ethical problems. One of the earliest formulations of these issues was a discussion published in 1958 by Pope Pius XII about the moral justifications of removing patients from mechanical ventilators. The essay was a response to a letter received by the pope from a Viennese anesthesiologist, who was perplexed about what to do when his technology permitted patients in coma to survive what before would have been a fatal injury, but whose condition had become static, whose prognosis for recovery seemed hopeless, and whose life was sustained only by the respiratory apparatus. On what moral grounds, he asked the pope, should doctors, patients, families, and society reach judgments when issues of suffering versus maintaining life functions were raised? Should the quality of a patient's life determine whether it should be sustained? And who is to judge this quality, if it is to be a factor in decision making? Families, physicians, the patient, society?

Such questions became increasingly significant in formulating medical decisions during the 1960s and 1970s. Ethics, a discipline that examines the right-making and wrong-making characteristics of actions, entered the clinic to an extent never before experienced. The importance of analyzing the ethical values held by the people and institutions involved in making clinical choices, and of the possible outcomes of maximizing some values over others, was now recognized.

Discussions about the dilemma of resuscitation led to an attempt in 1966 to restructure the concept of death to meet the capabilities of the new technology. If machines could sustain for long periods such vital functions as respiration, then the natural failure of vital physiological systems could not be used as the basis for defining death. Thus, the centuries-old standards that used respiratory and cardiac cessation as the hallmarks of death were replaced by a set of criteria focused on brain function. These criteria included, among other things, a flat electroencephalogram for a 24-hour period ("A definition of irreversible coma" 1968).

In the mid-1970s a case appeared, centered on the issue of respiratory resuscitation, that involved many ethical dilemmas caused by the introduction of advanced technology into health care. Karen Ann Quinlan, a 21-year old woman, collapsed and ceased breathing for at least two 15-minute periods during a party in April 1975. She was rushed to a hospital, and immediately placed on a respirator to maintain breathing. As weeks went by, her condition remained basically static: Her brain was able to maintain a number of essential physiologic functions, but she was not aware of anyone or anything around her. She continued to require a respirator to breathe, was fed by a gastric tube, and her arms, legs, and other related muscles and joints were becoming rigid and deformed. Despite severe brain damage and coma, she was not considered brain dead by the 1966 criteria. After months had passed with no improvement, Karen's parents requested doctors to remove the respirator, for its use seemed to them futile.

This led to heated ethical controversy involving the parents, hospital staff, courts, and other institutions about whether this request should be granted. The debate centered on the patient's right to forsake the possibility of further life with therapy that prolongs suffering and dying, and the ability and trustworthiness of parents or other surrogates to decide such questions for patients when they cannot decide for themselves. It raised questions about the obligation of physicians and other health care practitioners to sustain life and relieve suffering, and about what to do when these two obligations conflicted. It asked all of those involved to ponder which is the greater good: conferring a benefit, or preventing harm to a patient. To answer such questions, decision makers referred to ethical values embedded in the traditions and codes of the health professions, society, and religion, and to discussions of these issues in the growing literature of medical ethics.

In this debate, the respirator became a symbol of both the advanced technology of modern health care and the ambivalence toward it that many were coming to feel. Once turned on, the respirator seemed autonomous, its power to save life matched by its power to torment life. The absence of dependable ethical criteria that could be applied to justify its withdrawal threatened to imperil the decision to initiate its use. It was a machine that showed that in health care, the creation of technological capacities must be matched by the development and use of ethical canons of direction.

In the end, the respirator was removed. Karen was able to breathe without it, and to the time of this writing nearly a decade after her illness began, has lived in a nursing home, still in a coma.

Also in the 1960s, following the success of assisting threatened respiratory function, a significant advance occurred in treating renal failure: The Seattle Artificial Kidney Center opened its doors. It became the first major clinical center to apply a machine to replace kidney function. The device had been developed by the physician Willem Kolff in the Netherlands during the early 1940s. The machine was not long in use before it became apparent that the ethical dilemmas of providing access to it were as significant and difficult to resolve as the technical problems of clinical application. Candidates generally had kidney failure that threatened to end their lives. The decision about who to place in the machine and who to bypass dealt with the continuance of life.

The persons charged with making these judgments recognized their gravity and did their best to construct a system of allocation that balanced conflicting moral and social interests. An advisory committee was empaneled by the center, composed of laymen and physicians who were to represent the public interest. The committee functioned under a set of guidelines to facilitate patient selection that contained biological, psychological, monetary, geographic, ethical, and social criteria. Controversy arose over the use of these standards and the application of guidelines and standards per se, as opposed to a process of random selection that did not require a choice of one human life over another (Haviland 1966). The issue forced upon American society in the 1960s recognition of a problem that would become increasingly acute in the 1970s and 1980s – that medical science was creating more therapeutic agents than it had the capacity to give to those who might benefit from them.

This problem was complicated in the mid-1960s by the passage in the United States of legislation giving persons over age 65 and persons with low incomes government subsidies to pay for a substantial portion of their medical needs. This legislation was the culmination of a century-long controversy concerning the obligation of society to care for the health needs of its citizens. On the obligation of governments to provide these benefits and the corresponding right of people to have them, a consensus had been reached in post–World War II Europe that such a right should be acknowledged. In the mid-1960s, for at least a portion of its people, a similar consensus emerged in the United States.

The notion that health is a right raises for those societies holding this view several basic questions: What does this right entail? What sacrifices should be made to meet it? In the United States, the historical coincidence of the clinical use of artificial kidneys and the emergence of a modern right to health care made the idea of limiting access to a lifesaving procedure through an allocation process difficult to bear. Thus, it was not surprising that in 1972 the U.S. Congress passed legislation under which the federal government became responsible for paying the medical costs of virtually all patients, regardless of age or income, who required therapy with an artificial kidney or a kidney transplantation.[1]

Whether patients with kidney disease should have a right to such resources, given their dire need, would not be a great problem were not great financial costs involved. When this legislation was passed in 1972, it was estimated that expenditures would level off at about $200 million a year. By 1975, however, the annual cost was over $300 million, 50 percent more than expected; in 1982 it totaled about $2 billion.

The modern escalation of health care costs began in the early 1960s, coinciding with the introduction of numerous increasingly expensive medical technologies that were not only costly as hardware but also required an increased number of skilled and unskilled personnel to maintain and use. Such technology, for example, became incorporated into the intensive care and coronary care units, which became ubiquitous features of hospitals in the early 1960s. As these expenses have grown, the concern in the 1960s about an equitable distribution of medical resources in the United States and other countries turned in the 1970s and 1980s to a concern about cost (in the United States in 1982, about 10 percent of the gross national product, over $300 billion, was spent on health care).

Efforts to control health care costs in the United States have focused essentially on creating policies to reduce the use of current medical resources. The latest innovations are regulations that no longer permit hospitals to charge government insurance programs for the cost of patient care after it is provided. Rather, the government now applies a fixed fee schedule to given procedures, forcing hospitals to absorb cost overruns and operate prospectively within tighter budgets. However, efforts to reduce costs through policies designed to encourage more efficient use of available technology do not solve the problem caused by the dynamics of technological innovation and growth. This is because in the foreseeable future, it is unlikely (though certainly desirable) that illness will be treated by quick fixes stemming from basic causal knowledge about disease processes and simple remedies that follow from it. It is unlikely that the prime example of such a fix – treating bacterial illness with penicillin – will be replicated in the near future to deal with the spectrum of chronic illnesses and the degenerative changes of an aging population. A more likely prospect for the immediate future is the use of an increasingly complex and generally more expensive technology for a growing array of health problems.

Although continuing our efforts to improve efficiency through economic policy, we must recognize that this, by itself, will be inadequate to deal with the technological dynamic. Thus, we need to develop better prognostic indices and clinical decision-making strategies to state, and to determine more clearly for patients and providers, the outcomes of interventions, and to develop carefully thought-out ethical positions that will help patients, families, providers, and society to balance justly limited resources and patient needs. Even with all of these efforts, it is likely that the total percentage of our economic resources devoted to meeting health needs will grow, though not as rapidly as it would without these measures.

The difficult problems of choice raised by the need to provide technological benefits with limited resources give even more importance to the human association we call the medical relationship. In treating illness, a single provider of health care ultimately encounters a single patient. In the specialized system that modern health care has become, these encounters are numerous; but each meeting is contained, personal.

Technology has altered significantly the form and meaning of the medical relationship. It allows us to direct our vision and attention to variables singled out by it as significant. Thus, stethoscopes increase the significance of chest sounds, x-rays of anatomic shadows, electrocardiograms of waves on a graph, computers of printouts, dialysis machines of chemical balances, and so forth. Such evidence is important for diagnosis and therapy, and the more precisely it can be stated, the more valuable it becomes. In comparison, evidence given by patients, and altered by its passage through the prism of their experience and personality, has seemed to the technological age of the past two centuries less substantive, accurate, and meaningful as a basis for clinical decision-making and actions. Increasingly, practitioners encounter patients for relatively brief and intermittent periods – such as the consultant visiting a hospitalized patient whom he or she has never before met. In such visits the technical aspects often dominate, for there is no time or prior relationship to determine much about who the patient is, or what the patient thinks about the illness or the needs it engenders. And even in medical relationships that are not so discontinuous, technological measurements and measures tend to crowd out other dimensions of evaluation and therapeutics.

To speak so of the attention focused on the technological features of practice does not diminish their great significance and benefit. Rather, it points out that they do not encompass all critical aspects of diagnosis or treatment. In diagnosis, we seek to place a patient into a category with earlier patients who exhibited similar manifestations of illness. The similarity of the pattern or symptoms between one patient and another does not make them identical. That which is unique in a patient's illness can often be learned best by nontechnological inquiries based mainly on dialogue. Such inquiries deal with the patient's sensations and perceptions, with the values held by the patient that are relevant to treating the illness. An illness is not only a physical disturbance of the body's structure and function; it is an experience by the patient, who invests the illness with meaning. Knowing what this personal response involves is crucial information for therapy. Therapeutics is successful to the extent that it meets not only the needs of the disease but also the needs of the patient, who modifies and feels the effects of the disease in a unique way.

Dialogue, a means to retrieve and understand the experiential dimensions of illness, is critical. To the extent that inordinate fixation on the technical aspects of medicine diminishes the possibilities for or the importance of person-to-person dialogue, we become less effective in meeting illness. The triadic relationship of practitioners, patients, and machines is one of the most difficult of all associations to master in health care.

Machines programmed to question patients about illness and monitor physiological functions, and to analyze the data generated by these activities, are here, and their use will become ubiquitous in the future. More and more medical activities now performed by humans will be possible to capture and simulate using machines. How should we distribute responsibilities among human and nonhuman elements, and what might be the outcome? Machines can liberate human senses from the fatigue of acquiring facts and human memory from the burden of retaining them. They can supplement or replace human analyses of facts, and simplify or automate therapeutic actions. They can make it possible for a provider or a patient to evaluate independently and care for an illness. They can coordinate the activities of teams of providers where teams are needed, and provide the synthesis so crucial in a specialized environment.

These great gains are possible, but require a corresponding effort by those who use machines never to abrogate responsibility for the consequences of their use. Practitioners must not hide behind the programmed answers of machines in order to seek escape from the obligations to benefit and not harm imposed on us by our relationship with patients. Only by accepting this moral duty can we assure a medical future in which technological and humanistic values converge. To assume such responsibility implies that critical knowledge about the world of machines be continually sought and strengthened in the course of a practitioner's life. Accepting this burden of responsibility is the ethical anodyne to the false sense of security into which machines can lull us.

From the beginning of their introduction in the mid-nineteenth century, automated machines that generated results in objective formats such as graphs and numbers were thought capable of purging from health care the distortions of subjective human opinion. They were supposed to produce facts free of personal bias, and thus to reduce the uncertainty associated with human choice. This view, held by both practitioners and patients, stimulated the intense use of these devices, sometimes to excess. This excess has been characterized by overreliance on technologically depicted features of illness, inadequate understanding of the capabilities and limits of machines and the information they generate, and relative inattention to those aspects of medicine learned by inquiry into the patient's experiences and views. Machines can seem so accurate, so right. They can make us forget who made them, and who designed into them – with all the possibilities of human frailty and error – the programs that dictate their function. They can make us forget the hands and minds behind their creation; they can make us forget ourselves.

NOTE

**1** Historically, the U.S. government has generally provided health benefits to populations (a) whose illness has created a threat to others or (b) posed a significant, long-term burden on them and their families or (c) whose circumstances made it difficult for them to obtain medical care. Smallpox hospitals and quarantine stations exemplify category 1, mental hospitals category 2, and public hospitals for the poor category 3. In general, health care in the United States has been viewed as a basic need that, like food and housing, should be earned by personal labor. Thus, the institution of Medicare for the population over 65 and Medicaid for the poor was a traditional approach to the social provision of medical benefits, as represented by category 3. The poor and the elderly are well-defined populations with special health needs and clear deprivations. On this point, see O. D. Anderson, *The Uneasy Equilibrium* (New Haven, Conn.: College and University Press, 1968).

SELECTED BIBLIOGRAPHY

A definition of irreversible coma: report of the Ad Hoc Committee of the Harvard Medical School to examine the definition of brain death. (1968). *J.A.M.A. 205*:337–40.

Fisher, P. J., Stratmann, W. C., Lundsgaarde, H. P. et al. (1980). User reaction to PROMIS: issues related to acceptability of medical innovations. In *Proceedings: Fourth Annual Symposium on Computer Applications in Medical Care*. IEEE, vol. 3, pp. 1722–30.

Haviland, J. W. (1966). Experiences in establishing a community artificial kidney center. *Trans. Am. Clin. and Climatol. Assoc. 77*:133–4.

Hooke, R. (1665). *Micrographia*. Cited in *Moments of Discovery: The Development of Modern Science* (G. Schwartz and P. W. Bishop, eds.). New York: Basic Books, 1958, pp. 534–7.

Jones, W. H. S. (trans.) (1923). *Hippocrates*, Airs waters places, vol. 1, Cambridge, Mass.: Harvard University Press, pp. 71–137.

Jones, W. H. S. (trans.) (1923). *Hippocrates*, The art, vol. 2, pp. 203, 205.

Kleinfield, N. R. (1983). The home health care boom, *The New York Times*, June 30, pp. 27, 30.

Mayo, W. J. (1912). Contributions of the nineteenth century to a living pathology. *Boston Med. Surg. J. 167*:754.

Mitchell, S. W. (1892). *The Early History of Instrumental Precision in Medicine*. New Haven: Tuttle, Morehouse and Taylor, p. 3.

Morgagni, J. B. (1960). *The Seats and Causes of Diseases Investigated by Anatomy*. Trans. Benjamin Alexander, with a Preface, Introduction, and new translations of five letters by Paul Klemperer. New York: MacMillan Hafner Press.

National Commission on Allied Health Education. (1980). *The Future of Allied Health Education*. San Francisco: Jossey-Bass, pp. 2, 18, 234–55.

Newton, I. (1952). *Opticks: A Treatise of the Reflections, Refractions, Inflections and Colours of Light*, 4th ed. New York: Dover Press, p. 4011.

O'Malley, C. D. (1965). *Andreas Vesalius of Brussels: 1514–1564*. Berkeley: University of California Press, p. 318.

Pearson, K. (1900). *The Grammar of Science*, 2nd ed. London: Adam and Charles Black, p. 6.

Pontoppidan, II., Wilson, R., Rie, M. A. et al. (1977). Respiratory intensive care. *Anesthesiology 47*:96–116.

Pope Pius XII. (1958). The prolongation of life. In *Ethics in Medicine: Historical Perspectives and Contemporary Concerns* (S. J. Reiser, A. J. Dyck, and W. J. Curran, eds.). Cambridge, Mass.: MIT Press, 1977, pp. 501–4.

Reiser, S.J. (1978). *Medicine and the Reign of Technology*. New York: Cambridge University Press, pp. 23–69.

Rorem, C. R. (1930). *Capital Investment in Hospitals*. Washington: Committee on the Costs of Medical Care, p. 9.

Wilson, F. A., and Neuhauser, D. (eds.) (1982). *Health Services in the United States*, 2nd ed. Cambridge, Mass.: Ballinger, pp. 61–98.

PART II

# SCIENTIFIC DIMENSIONS OF TECHNOLOGY

# PENETRATING THE BLACK BOX: PHYSICAL PRINCIPLES BEHIND HEALTH CARE TECHNOLOGY

MICHAEL ANBAR

## TECHNOLOGY AND ITS ROLE IN MODERN HEALTH CARE

Health care depends more and more on technology to meet its large variety of needs. It uses technology to gather information necessary for appropriate diagnosis; to process this information and present it in comprehensible forms; to treat disorders effectively when diagnosed; to monitor treatment and evaluate its efficacy; and, last but not least, to prevent disease. There is practically no step in the sequence of medical actions that is not dependent on technology (Figure 1).

Health care technology, viewed from the perspective of devices, involves practically all types of technology – mechanical and acoustic, electrical and electronic, chemical and physicochemical, electromagnetic and optical (Figure 2). It includes not only small, simple devices such as the thermometer, the stethoscope, or corrective eyeglasses, but also highly sophisticated combinations of electrical, mechanical, and electronic systems such as computerized x-ray or ultrasonic tomographs and computerized radiation treatment units. To understand the function of such technological systems, which are outstanding examples of the fruits of interdisciplinary efforts, one needs a background in a diversity of disciplines (Figure 3).

Projections into the future predict an even greater role for technology in medical practice, especially in the applications of computers. Pattern recognition of complex physical phenomena, as provided by the electrocardiogram (ECG) or electroencephalogram (EEG), is today almost within the state of the art, and computerized recognition of two-dimensional or three-dimensional images will probably be achieved before the end of this century. Computerized diagnosis and decision analysis are not science fiction, nor are computerized monitoring of patients and automated treatment systems. These techniques are now in the

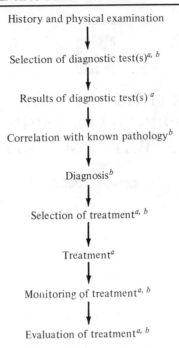

History and physical examination

↓

Selection of diagnostic test(s)[a, b]

↓

Results of diagnostic test(s) [a]

↓

Correlation with known pathology[b]

↓

Diagnosis[b]

↓

Selection of treatment[a, b]

↓

Treatment[a]

↓

Monitoring of treatment[a, b]

↓

Evaluation of treatment[a, b]

[a]Understanding of health care technology required.
[b]Computerization desirable.

Figure 1. Sequence of actions in medical practice.

experimental stage, and they will probably be deployed within the next decade, at least at the level of tertiary care.

Today's practitioners cannot afford, therefore, to ignore technology; they will have to control it and use it effectively. The practitioner of the 1980s has to understand the underlying principles of health care technology and be able to assess its scope and limitations. This is especially important because a clinician is now required to choose, from among many available alternatives, an appropriate technological solution to a given medical problem.

Understanding health care technology includes understanding how it evolves, what its physical or physicochemical principles are, and how it interacts with and affects the biological system. This chapter is limited to a generic description of the needs of health care and their fulfillment by technological means; Chapter 3 discusses the potential detrimental consequences of the uses of technology.

## HOW DOES HEALTH CARE TECHNOLOGY EVOLVE?

There are two principal pathways in its evolution: (1) the development of a new and better technological solution to an existing medical problem; and (2) the

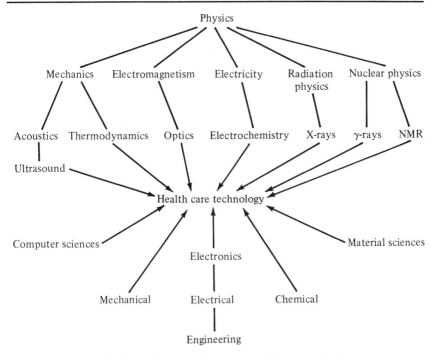

Figure 2. Disciplines contributing to health care technology.

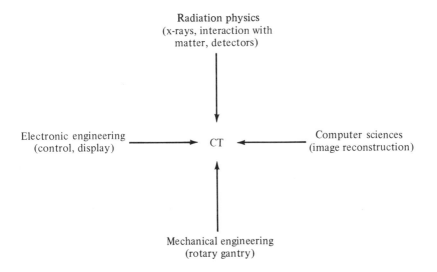

Figure 3. Disciplines contributing to computerized x-ray tomography.

identification of a medical problem for which an existing technology can offer a new or better solution. The stethoscope and the phonocardiograph are examples of the first pathway. They offer an improvement in auscultation of the heart, replacing direct auscultation, which required putting the physician's ear to the patient's chest. The ECG and the recently developed computerized ECG are additional examples of the same pathway, extracting meaningful quantitative diagnostic information from the dynamic electrophysiological behavior of the heart muscle. X-ray radiography is an example of the other pathway, in which discovery of the penetrating power of x-rays prompted their use in imaging internal organs in a noninvasive manner. The clinical uses of ultrasonics and the more recent application of nuclear magnetic resonance (NMR) for diagnostic imaging are other examples of the second pathway.

The practicing clinician does not care how a certain diagnostic or therapeutic instrument developed, as long as it is useful; x-ray imaging and the ECG are probably the two most widely used diagnostic techniques in current practice. However, when considering a *new* technological solution to a given medical problem, it may be very important to know whether this new device was developed in response to a definite medical need or in an effort to find new uses for a given technology. In the first case, it is necessary only to assess whether the new solution to the medical problem is better than the existing solution or solutions; in the second case, it is imperative to find out first whether the proposed medical need actually exists or was invented by the proponents of the given technology. Even if the latter situation exists, the newly discovered medical need may be real and very important, as it was in the case of x-ray radiography. Caution should be exercised, however, to avoid unnecessary expenditure of resources to meet trivial medical needs just because an appropriate technological solution is available.

WHAT NEEDS OF DIAGNOSIS CAN TECHNOLOGY MEET?

Among the critical needs of medicine are two: (1) the need for information on the state of the patient and (2) the need to alleviate the patient's physical or physiological disorders. The different roles of technology in practice are summarized schematically in Figure 4.

The state of the patient can be considered in one of two modes: static or dynamic. In the static mode, we are interested in the patient's condition, for example, anatomic shape or biochemical status at a given instant. Occasionally, we may want to know if the patient's state is stationary or changing over a period of time. We will then repeat the static test and compare the findings. In the dynamic mode of diagnosis, on the other hand, we are interested in the actual *rate* of anatomical or physiological changes. Technology facilitates the acquisition of both static and dynamic information on different organ systems by monitoring different physical or chemical properties.

Static diagnostic information includes extracorporal and intracorporal imaging,

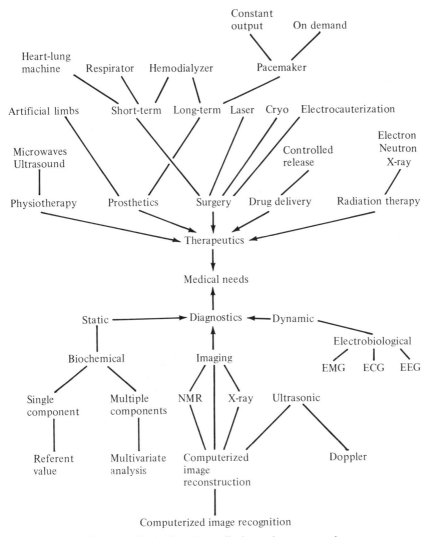

Figure 4. Technology in medical practice: an overview.

data on the concentration of metabolites in biologic fluids, and microscopic morphologic information on blood and other tissues. Dynamic diagnostic information includes data on the function of organs, for example, neurological function, neuromuscular action, the responses of sensory organs, rates of blood flow or pulmonary gas exchange, or rates of biochemical interconversion of metabolites.

We may acquire extracorporal morphological information by monitoring the selective light absorption and reflection of organs and tissues. We can do this with our eyes without any technological assistance, but frequently we have to augment the capability of our eyes by magnification (microscopy), by observing behind obstructions using artificial illumination or mirrors on light pipes (enteroscopy), and by observing subtle changes in emissions or reflections, especially in the infrared region of the spectrum (photography through filters and thermography).

Next, we can acquire morphological information on internal organs and tissues by using more energetic electromagnetic radiation (x-rays). This radiation, which is more penetrating than light, allows us to distinguish differences in tissue densities rather than differences in the electronic structure of their constituents. Alternatively, we can use ultrasonic radiation to interrogate internal structures, monitoring the reflections from interfaces between tissues. The effectiveness of reflection depends on the differences in density *and* speed of sound in different tissues. We can also obtain diagnostic information from the absorption and scattering of ultrasound, which depend on the internal structure of tissues. Using NMR, we can obtain images of tissues and organs (zeugmatography), depending on their hydrogen content and their intrinsic viscosities. In the foreseeable future, the content of other elements, especially carbon and phosphorus, will enable us to characterize tissues using another independent parameter, producing another mode of imaging by NMR.

From the technological standpont, ultrasonic reflective imaging has been made possible by accurate measurement of time intervals, a procedure developed originally for radar and sonar technologies. NMR imaging required highly sensitive and precise radiofrequency technology (originally developed for radar), the design of large superconductive magnets, and computerized image reconstruction, which was originally developed for the reconstruction of x-ray images. These two examples show the interrelations among technologies required to generate a new technological solution to a given medical problem.

In brief, when we wish to obtain morphological information, we select a measurable physical probe – light, sound, x-ray, NMR – that is affected by a certain property of tissue – its density, elemental composition, elasticity, viscosity, temperature, or the electronic structure of individual materials (color) – and use the appropriate techniques to detect and display the image. For detection and display, we may use a physicochemical process such as photography or purely physical processes such as piezoelectricity, electron multiplication, or radiofrequency resonance detection. We then use the modulation of these properties at different points on the surface of or inside the interrogated object (patient), and at different times, to obtain an image that is visually displayed on a cathode ray tube (CRT). This image can then be photographed to obtain a stationary permanent record.

The next step in the diagnostic imaging process is psychological. We view the displayed image, the photographic plate, or the CRT and make the diagnostic decision based on our knowledge of the normal anatomy and/or normal properties of the interrogated tissues. This psychological subjective phase in diagnosis may in the foreseeable future be replaced by computerized image-processing procedures that will detect abnormalities and report them in terms of the probability of certain diseases.

The same imaging techniques that provide us with static morphological information may also be used to obtain dynamic physiological information, because the response time of the detection systems is generally fast in comparison with the physiological morphological changes. X-ray cinematography (e.g., angiography) is an excellent example of this approach, as is real-time ultrasonic B-scanning or the modern, rapid computerized x-ray tomography. Ultrasound provides us with the additional option of Doppler imaging. This technique, which measures the velocity of motion of objects, is being used to obtain images of the vascular system (by virtue of the motion of the erythrocytes), and it will soon be used to obtain information on blood flow velocity in capillary beds.

A different set of technologies has been applied to obtain static information about the chemical composition of biological fluids. These technologies involve many different physicochemical measuring techniques including calorimetry, spectrophotometry, fluorometry, coulometry, potentiometry, and scintillation counting. To deal with the complex composition of biologic fluids, different separation techniques are being utilized, including chromatographic (thin layer chromatography, high-performance liquid chromatography or HPLC, gas–liquid chromatography or GLC) and electrophoretic (thin layer and gel electrophoresis) techniques. Alternatively, highly specific enzymatic and immunological (e.g., radioimmunoassay) procedures are being applied to assay quantitatively minute amounts of certain metabolites, with minimal interference from the thousands of other constituents of plasma, urine, or cerebrospinal fluid.

Any of these different analytical techniques provides the clinician with a certain value – the concentration of the constituent of interest. It is then up to the clinician to determine the diagnostic value of the information – whether or not it indicates disease. This decision depends on the *referent value* that separates normality from disorder. This value is by and large arbitrary, since there is no test that is 100 percent *sensitive* (assigning correctly 100 percent of the pathological cases) and, at the same time, 100 percent *specific* (assigning correctly 100 percent of the nonpathological cases).

There is an increasing tendency to look for correlations between abnormal values of *several* clinical tests and a certain disease – in other words, to look for a *pattern* or profile associated with specific disorder. Such a pattern can be evaluated better with the aid of a computer that analyzes all the clinical information, identifies the independent variables, and recognizes a characteristic pathological biochemical pattern.

The clinical laboratory has become automated and computerized in recent years, a trend that will continue for the foreseeable future. Single analyzing systems that quantitatively analyze 20 or more constituents are now common. Quantitative chromatography, GLC, and HPLC, especially in conjunction with mass spectrometry, are capable of providing quantitative information on hundreds of constituents in a single analysis. The handling of such enormous amounts of analytical data has to be left exclusively to computers, which also identify diagnostic patterns and provide the clinician with a tentative diagnosis. In this respect, the clinical laboratory may be one of the first systems that makes diagnostic decisions instead of providing data for diagnostic evaluation by the clinician.

To summarize, diagnostic information derived from an abnormal concentration of metabolites in biological fluids is being obtained by chemical or physiochemical techniques. In all cases, the concentration is determined by a physical instrument, and the measured value is generally picked up by a microprocessor or computer to assess its diagnostic significance. There is an increasing tendency to use computerized multivariate analysis to detect a specific diagnostic pattern associated with a given disorder. Technology thus prevails in the collection and evaluation of chemical information, as it does in the collection of diagnostic morphological information.

The same physical techniques can be applied to obtain dynamic biochemical information by monitoring rapid changes in the concentration of metabolites. In this case, however, more sophisticated equipment is needed, because preseparation techniques cannot be performed in real time. The techniques of choice for dynamic biochemical monitoring are electrochemical, using rapidly responding electrodes, and direct mass spectrometric measurements, which have become routine for performing gas composition studies (e.g., for anesthesia control). In the foreseeable future, mass spectrometry may be applied to monitor volatile metabolites released through the skin, and NMR may be applied to obtain real-time information on the concentration of specific metabolites in circulating blood or in muscle (e.g., a finger or earlobe).

Electrophysiology offers a third sizable group of diagnostic tests, the most popular ones being ECG and EEG. Here we are monitoring a physiologic change in real time, and it is the change itself that is of diagnostic value. The diagnosis of aberrations in the performance of the heart muscle is best diagnosed by ECG. Other neuromuscular disorders can be diagnosed by electromyography (EMG), the neurological response of the eye by electroretinography (ERG), and certain central nervous disorders by EEG.

In all of these techniques, the electrical potential difference between two points is measured on the surface of the patient as a function of time. The pattern of these changes, whether intrinsic or externally stimulated, is of substantial diagnostic value. Computerized pattern analysis is being applied to these complex temporal changes to gain more reliable information than can be obtained by trained personnel. Although at present the computerized pattern recognition of, say, ECG is limited to the simpler types of aberrations, it is conceivable that within the next decade the computerized technique will supersede the performance of the clinician, who will be happy to receive a tentative diagnosis of a disorder rather than search for it in the intricacies of complex electrical potential-time displays.

To summarize, from the standpoint of diagnosis, we are interested in the propagation of action potentials in nerves and muscles, in the efficacy of the neuromuscular interface, and in the effectiveness of sensory transduction. The measurement of electrical potential as a function of time provides this information, which is ready to be processed by a computer and eventually to produce a tentative diagnosis of neurological or neuromuscular disorders.

These three examples of different types of diagnostic areas – morphologic imaging, biochemical analysis, and electrophysiological monitoring – offer a good representation of diagnostic tests and their dependence on technology. Without technology, we would be left, in addition to history taking (the value of which is unfortunately underestimated these days), with visual observation of the patient (which unfortunately has been neglected with the advent of technology), direct auscultation, and a number of simple physical and chemical tests of biological fluids. In brief, a large proportion of the diagnostic information we use today is produced by modern medical technology, and in the near future, much of this information will be processed and interpreted by computers.

What should we expect to occur in the future? With the exception of magnetism and electron spin resonance (ESR), probably the next physical values to be used, there is hardly a physical property of matter that has not been applied to clinical diagnosis. Still, I believe that we are witnessing only the beginning of technological diagnosis. In the past 10 years, we have seen ultrasonics evolve from a laboratory curiosity to a routine imaging technique, with a resolution approaching that of x-rays and with potential diagnostic applications exceeding by far those of diagnostic x-ray technology. We have also witnessed the revolutionizing of x-ray radiology by the advent of computerized tomography, which is now achieving fast response times that will allow real-time computerized imaging, a feat that would have seemed utterly unattainable just 5 years ago. Computerized ECG is gaining popularity among clinicians, and pattern recognition of biochemical aberrations is not far behind. We may expect NMR and ESR, as well as nondispersive infrared analysis, to be much more widely applied than they are today. Further, there are foreseeable major technological developments in the pattern recognition of electrophysiologic phenomena, ECG and EEG in particular.

Multivariate analysis offers a most exciting diagnostic approach that has not yet been exploited – the early diagnosis of disorders that are undetectable today because of the uncertainties of the referent values. A number of test values, each of which may be within the normal range of their referent values, may constitute a pattern characteristic of an incipient disorder. Alternatively, a number of pathologic test findings may constitute a pattern that will provide the clinician with an unambiguous differential diagnosis.

In brief, I believe that the contribution of technology to clinical diagnosis has not yet reached its climax. This climax will be approached with the advent of microprocessors and minicomputers, interfaced with large central computerized data banks, to generate reliable diagnostic patterns based on a large number of simple, noninvasive physical measurements.

## WHAT NEEDS OF PATIENT MANAGEMENT AND TREATMENT DOES TECHNOLOGY MEET?

Diagnosis is just the first step in patient management. A key purpose of health care is therapy – treating the disorder in a manner that will restore the patient to health or at least to a state in which the patient can live normally.

Technology has revolutionized therapy to no less extent than it has diagnosis, even if we exclude from consideration the nineteenth-century technologies that have supported classic chemotherapy, surgery, ophthalmology, and orthopedics.

The advent of technology has produced an unprecedented number of new and effective prosthetic devices. These include not only hard and soft contact lenses, hearing aids, cardiac or diaphragm pacemakers, and artificial limbs of unsurpassed precision and dexterity, but also short-term prosthetics such as respirators, hemodialyzers, and heart–lung machines, which have dramatically changed the probability of survival in severely ill patients.

Generically, each of these prosthetic devices is a "brute force" solution or a crude imitation of the natural organ it replaces, but as time goes on, technology becomes more refined and the similarity between the organ and the prosthetic device increases. Just as a wooden block tied to an amputated leg has been replaced by a prosthesis that simulates normal leg function to an amazing extent, and just as the modern hearing aid is no longer an indiscriminant broad-band amplifier, so are other prosthetic devices being increasingly refined. The cardiac pacemaker, which has no nineteenth-century analog, is a good example of the combination of electrophysiology with electronics and electrochemistry. Modern cardiac pacemakers that provide stimulation only on demand and that can accelerate their stimulation rate when required by the patient's activity, are an excellent example of the rapid advance of therapeutic technology. It is interesting to remember that just over 10 years ago, we were severely limited by the lifetime of implantable batteries and by the size of the logic unit. The culmination of prosthetic devices in this decade is evidently the artificial heart, the construction of which combines chemical, physical, and engineering know-how. It is conceivable that such devices will be used routinely before the end of this century.

Surgery in the broader sense has been the medical specialty most strongly affected by the advent of technology. The scalpel is being replaced by a laser beam, and certain tissues may be destroyed by focused ultrasonic hyperthermia, by electrocauterization, or by cryosurgery, eliminating the need for surgical removal. Radiation therapy, which is a technology in its own right, made substantial progress when it incorporated the computerized control of the energy and position of the irradiating beam. Focused hyperthermia, in conjunction with computer programmed ionizing radiation treatment, is another promising development made available by the combination of a number of technologies (Figure 5). The latter examples show the application of two different physical effects detrimental to living systems for the destruction of undesirable tissue.

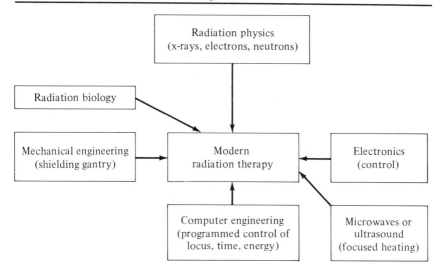

Figure 5. Sciences and technologies contributing to radiation therapy.

A third area in therapeutics that has been substantially changed by the use of technology, although not yet to the same extent as prosthetics and surgery, is controlled chemotherapy. The efficacy of many drugs is diminished by their rapid clearance or metabolization. This requires, on the one hand, overdosing to attain a therapeutic effect and, on the other, reduced doses in the intervals between delivery. The optimal effect of any drug depends on its sustained concentration in the circulation, which can be achieved for most drugs only by slow, constant release. When the demand for a given pharmacologic agent is transient, as in the case of hormone substitution therapy (e.g., insulin), optimal dosing involves drug release on demand. Both of these clinical needs can be met by technology. Constant release can be attained using chemical or physical slow-release devices. The demand-controlled supply calls for more sophisticated technology, which involves an electrochemical sensor of the agent or of its substrate (glucose, in the case of insulin) that controls the release. Devices of the latter type (prosthetic endocrine systems) are under development and are expected to be used within this decade. In the case of diabetes mellitus, this technology is in competition with the transplantation of insulin-producing cells.

The three areas of therapy cited above are just examples of the impact of technology on health care. There are specialties, such as surgery, orthopedics, physiotherapy, or ophthalmology, that are more technology-intensive than others; however, even nontechnological specialties such as psychiatry adopt technology wherever possible (e.g., video cameras and tape recorders). It should also be noted that many diagnostic techniques are being used in therapy to monitor the progress of treatment and thus to optimize the course of therapy.

## SUMMARY

Technology has changed the character of health care. Irrespective of whether a certain device or technique was developed in response to a medical need or was the result of "a solution looking for a problem," the current quality of health care could never be offered without existing technology. The instruments of health care technology are based mainly on physics – on classic physics (mechanics, acoustics, optics, electricity, and magnetism), on the so-called modern physics (the physics of x-rays, nuclear radiations, nuclear and electron spin resonance, lasers), and, last but not least, on computer technology and computer science. In order to utilize technology appropriately, the modern clinician has to understand the physical principles underlying the technology used in a given clinical situation, assess the usefulness of this technological solution in comparison with the alternatives, and be aware of the costs, including potential side effects of the technology in question. The understanding of technological devices in the 1980s is as essential to practice as is the understanding of pharmacology. As in the latter case, the clinician has to choose from among a number of alternatives, each with its own benefits and contraindications. However, unlike pharmacology, technological devices can be applied to both diagnosis and therapeutics, and unlike pharmacology, they are based on a much broader spectrum of underlying principles. It is surprising, therefore, that this technology has not yet achieved an established position in health care education. It seems inevitable that a substantial change in this education will take place in this decade to cope with these new needs of patient care.

## SELECTED BIBLIOGRAPHY

Bergveld, P. (1980). *Electromedical Instrumentation*. New York: Cambridge University Press.

Brown, S. S., Mitchell, S. L., and Young, G. S. (eds.) (1979). *Chemical Diagnosis of Disease*. New York: Elsevier.

Cameron, J. R., and Skofronick, J. G. (1978). *Medical Physics*. New York: Wiley.

D'Crus, I. A. (ed.) (1981). *Primer of Echocardiography*. New York: Grune & Stratton.

Gesses, L. A., and Baker, L. E. (1977). *Principles of Applied Biomedical Instrumentation*. New York: Wiley.

Haber, K. (1980). Diagnostic uses of ultrasonic imaging. In *Imaging for Medicine* (S. Nudelman and D. D. Patton, eds.). New York: Plenum Press.

McAlister, J. M. (1979). *Radionuclide Techniques in Medicine*. New York: Cambridge University Press.

Newton, T. H., and Potts, D. G. (1981). *Technical Aspects of Computed Tomography*. St. Louis: C. V. Mosby.

Preston, K., Taylor, K. J. W., Johnson, S. A. et al., (eds.) (1979). *Medical Imaging Techniques*. New York: Plenum Press.

Pykett, I. L. (1982). NMR imaging in medicine. *Sci. Am. 245*:78.

Van Berger, W. S. (1980). *Obstetric Ultrasound*. Reading, Mass.: Addison-Wesley.

# CHAPTER 3

# BIOLOGICAL BULLETS:
# SIDE EFFECTS OF HEALTH
# CARE TECHNOLOGY

MICHAEL ANBAR

The preceding chapter described different technological inputs to the diagnosis and treatment of disease and illustrated the help offered to medical practice by their use. As in any other enterprise, there is no benefit without cost. The universal adoption of technological solutions to medical problems indicates the general acceptance by the medical community that the benefits outweigh the costs. Nevertheless, we cannot ignore the costs altogether, and in selecting a certain technological solution to a given medical problem, we should always maximize the benefit/cost ratio. The assessment of the costs of health care technology is thus a prerequisite for its optimal utilization.

The costs of health care technology include the monetary cost of the equipment, which itself includes the costs of research and development as well as of design, construction, and marketing; the cost of operation and maintenance; the cost of training personnel; the cost of the patient's time and inconvenience; and last but not least, the cost and risks of detrimental biological side effects to the patient's health. This chapter is limited to a discussion of the costs to the patient's health. Other chapters deal with the non-health-related costs of health care technology. The nature of these biological costs requires careful discussion, because deep and pervasive medical and social concern about their effects, based on incomplete knowledge, has often led to an underestimated or exaggerated view of harm.

Our discussion of the biological effects of health care technology is limited to technologic approaches that involve transfer of energy or materials into the biologic system, as most clinical devices or procedures do. The only category of technology that does not involve this is clinical chemistry, which examines samples removed from the biological system.

When considering energy exchange within biological systems, we have to specify the level of interaction. We must distinguish between macroscopic interactions at the organ or tissue level and microscopic interactions at the cellular, molecular, or atomic level. The forms of energy to be considered include me-

35

chanical energy at the macroscopic, microscopic (ultrasound), and molecular (heat) levels; they also include electric or electrostatic energy at the macroscopic (electrolytic conductance) and molecular (molecular ionization) levels. Finally, there is electromagnetic energy at the molecular level (microwaves, light) and atomic level (x-rays), as well as magnetic energy effects at the molecular level.

When considering the effect of nonbiological materials introduced into the biological system by different devices and procedures (for reasons other than chemotherapy), we should distinguish between intentional macroscopic transfer (e.g., inserting radiological contrast agents into the body), unwarranted micro-transfer (e.g., release of plasticizers or monomers from "inert" polymeric materials, release of trace metals by corrosion), and catalytic effects of surfaces of nonbiological materials that do not involve any material transport.

We also have to distinguish between acute short-term and long-term effects. The acute damage is manifested within seconds to hours following the biological insult, and the damaged tissue may be repaired within days to weeks. If there is no remaining scar (any residual permanent change), we were dealing with a short-term biological effect. There are, however, effects that result in immediately observable, irreparable damage or in latent permanent damage, the detrimental effects of which may be manifested only months or years following the insult. Unlike the short-term effects, these long-term detrimental biological effects are generally cumulative.

Finally, we should consider the potential synergistic effect of two or more forms of insult – for example, the augmentation of radiobiological damage at a higher temperature or the aggravation of a bacterial infection near a cytotoxic surface. Synergistic effects may also exist between drugs and biophysical insults, for example, the potentiation of radiobiological effects by "sensitizing" agents or the aggravation of hypothermia by vasoconstrictors. Relatively little is known about such synergistic effects, which are analogous to drug–drug interactions, but undoubtedly they will become more significant when the use of technology becomes more extensive.


## EFFECTS OF MECHANICAL ENERGY

Detrimental effects of gross mechanical energy include not only the trivial destruction of tissue by severe mechanical impact or bacterial infections following severing of the skin but also the short-term and long-term biological effects of persistent localized pressure on tissue. The latter side effects are a particular problem with mechanical prosthetic devices.

Of greater interest, however, is the potential biological effect of a rapidly varied mechanical impact as used in diagnostic or therapeutic ultrasound. Ultrasonic energy may affect a fluid medium in three principal ways: disruption, cavitation, and heat. The periodic compression and rarefaction process, when of sufficient amplitude and of short duration, may exert sufficient shearing force to disrupt biological membranes, and even chemical bonds in large macromolecules such as DNA.

If the amplitude and frequency are higher, ultrasound may disrupt the continuity of a fluid medium, producing cavitation (miniature bubbles). Once cavitation has been induced, these bublets will expand and contract very rapidly in synchrony with the ultrasonic cycle, resulting in heating of the volatile material, which diffuses into the cavities. The temperature inside the cavities may rise to tens or even hundreds of thousands of degrees Centigrade, resulting in complete decomposition of the volatile constituents of the intracavity gas. The fragments of these volatile materials, many of them free radicals such as H, OH, or $CH_3$, will then diffuse into the bulk of the fluid and react chemically with any constituent of the medium. The chemical changes induced in the latter substances are similar to those produced by free radicals formed by ionizing radiation.

The ultrasonic energy that has not been converted into chemical energy in the shearing of molecules or in the cavitation process is turned into heat. In fact, even under conditions most favorable for sonochemical effects, over 99 percent of the sonic energy is converted into heat.

Three parameters characterize ultrasonics: frequency, amplitude, and intensity. The amplitude, which is critical in the induction of cavitation and the shearing of macromolecules, increases with the square root of intensity for a given frequency, and for a given intensity it decreases with frequency. Consequently, to induce sonochemical effects at the high frequencies ($> 1$ MHz) used for diagnostic imaging, substantially higher intensities are needed than are generally used in diagnosis. Therefore, the only mode of energy conversion in the range of diagnostic ultrasound is heat. But because the power output of diagnostic devices is small, the heating of diagnostic ultrasound is insignificant. Thus, to the best of our understanding and knowledge, diagnostic ultrasound is free of short-term or long-term side effects.

However, when ultrasound is being used for deep heat therapy (e.g., in physiotherapy or in cancer treatment, generally in conjunction with radiation therapy), there may be significant chemical changes associated with the ultrasonic treatment. In cancer therapy, these changes are minor compared with those induced by ionizing radiation. On the other hand, ultrasonic physiotherapy may involve long-term detrimental side effects, that is, sonochemically induced mutagenesis or carcinogenesis. This potential detrimental biological effect of therapeutic ultrasonics might make this treatment less attractive than the local hyperthermia induced by microwaves or radiofrequency radiation.

### EFFECTS OF THERMAL ENERGY

A special type of mechanical effect to be considered here is heat. Heat in subcutaneous tissues may be induced by the absorption of ultrasound, as discussed above, by absorption of microwaves, and by convection or conduction from the skin (e.g., produced by infrared light or an electric heating pad). In addition, very high localized temperatures can be produced by passing an electric current (electrocauterization) or by absorption of intense infrared or visible light (produced by lasers).

The biological effect of heat depends on the temperature level attained. It ranges from enhancing the microcirculation in tissue to changing the relative rates of certain enzymatic processes, and at higher temperatures to the death of cells by denaturation of proteins. In extreme forms, it may result in complete evaporation of the affected cells (laser surgery). Permanent heat damage to the retina is a well-known hazard of laser technology. Yet, lasers can be used under controlled conditions in ophthalmological surgery to arrest the detachment of the retina by heat coagulation of the boundary line surrounding the detached area. When extensive regions of tissue are exposed to excessive heat that kills off the whole stem cell population, the region is irreversibly damaged and the affected cells are replaced by scar tissue. This is definitely an undesirable outcome of any heat treatment. Local hyperthermia has been shown to enhance chemotherapy and radiation therapy of cancer. But by the same token, it may alter the effects of other pharmacological agents on nonmalignant cells and cause undesirable short-term or long-term side effects. Although there is insufficient information on the therapeutic synergistic effects of local mild hyperthermia, there is reason to believe that both beneficial and detrimental effects are associated with hyperthermic treatment.

In brief, certain treatments (e.g., of arthritis and of certain malignancies) are associated with controlled hyperthermia, which can be induced by microwaves or ultrasonics. These treatments are not free of side effects. Localized tissue heating above the denaturation temperature of proteins can be used therapeutically, but we have to be aware that somewhere along the temperature gradient between the superthermal lethal and the normal thermal regions, there will be a hyperthermal region where unpredictable biological effects may occur. The steeper the gradient, the narrower will be this region of undesirable side effects. This makes laser-induced, highly localized heating the preferential superthermal treatment (compared with hot wire coagulation or electrocauterization).

When discussing hyperthermic health care technology, we should also consider hypothermal treatments and their potential side effects. Unlike localized heat, localized cold can be induced only by physical contact from outside the tissue; therefore, it cannot be as well controlled and focused as heat. Certain tissues can be cooled by perfusion with cold blood or another oxygen-carrying fluid, a technique that is being utilized in the preservation of the heart during open heart surgery. Also, organs to be transplanted (e.g., kidney, cornea) are preserved under mild hypothermal conditions above the freezing point. The biochemistry of tissues at low temperatures is not yet fully understood, and in spite of the proven advantages of hypothermic over normal temperature conditions, metabolic aberrations take place in hypothermal tissues. Whether these aberrations are completely reversible has not been established. Until then, there remains the open question of the existence of incipient long-term side effects.

Cooling tissues slowly below the freezing point and then rapidly thawing them results in cell destruction – a phenomenon that is being utilized in cryosurgery. The temperature gradient around the intentionally damaged tissue may interfere with the recovery process, making cryosurgery the method of choice only in very special situations.

In brief, although temporary hypothermic treatment of organs or tissues may be beneficial for their preservation under nonphysiological conditions, the long-term side effects of such a treatment may differ from organ to organ. Further studies are required to establish the optimal conditions for such treatments.

## EFFECTS OF ELECTRICAL ENERGY

Electricity is carried in biological systems by positive and negative ions rather than by electrons, which are the common carriers in electrical metallic conductors. Potential differences of the order of 0.1 V occur physiologically across biological membranes (ion concentration polarization), and the electrolytic currents that are produced under this potential propagate information in nerve fibers and activate muscular contraction. The propagation of the depolarization along a neuron results in a transient change in its membrane potential, called *action potential*. Exogenous currents on the order of milliamperes may override the physiological threshold of the action potential, and result in the impairment of neuromuscular functions. If such a current traverses the heart muscle, it will abolish the normal propagation of the front of the action potential through the muscle and lead to cardiac arrest. The persistence of such a condition for a second or more may not be reversible and would be lethal. On the other hand, a momentary cardiac arrest may overcome heart fibrillation, caused for instance by an acute infarct, and restore the normal propagation of the action potential through the heart. This effect is being used in the cardiac defibrillator, a device that is saving thousands of lives a year. In the cardiac pacemaker, discussed in the previous chapter, a short electric pulse of low intensity is repeatedly applied to an appropriate region of the heart, inducing the desired paced contraction without any side effects. In other words, the duration and intensity of the current determine the biological outcome of an electric cardiac shock.

Potentially one of the most detrimental consequences of modern technology is the pickup of a stray electric potential by a catheterized patient, especially when the catheter reaches into the vicinity of the heart. The catheter used for monitoring blood pressure and for rapid drug delivery is an effective electrical conductor, which may deliver a lethal current to the heart muscle when exposed to a potential difference of a fraction of a volt. This hazard can be minimized by carefully grounding all electrical equipment in hospital rooms of patients who may be catheterized.

Fortunately, the effect of an electric shock is transient, and once the impairment of the neuromuscular interaction relaxes, there are no known long-term side effects. However, if the current passed through the tissue is high enough to generate heat along its path, it may produce slow-healing electrical burns. This latter effect is being utilized in surgery to destroy tissue with minimal bleeding (electrocauterization).

In brief, the flow of exogenous current through tissue is highly hazardous, especially when it affects the heart or the brain, but under controlled conditions it can be used therapeutically. The abundance of electrical instruments and appliances in the vicinity of catheterized patients poses a severe hazard. We see here an example of detrimental effects precipitated by the combination of different tools of health care technology.

A special case of the effect of electromagnetic energy (to be discussed in the next section) on the neuromuscular system is the possible triggering of cardiac pacemakers by external radiofrequency or microwave radiation. This short-term side effect, which has drawn some general public attention, can exist only when the given radiation is present at a very high intensity; and even then, appropriate design of the pacemaker and its electrical leads can eliminate this problem altogether. Here we have an example of a side effect of technology that was discovered after the development and use of the first generation of a new clinical device. This side effect could have been avoided in the first place with proper foresight, and it is now no longer a problem.

### EFFECTS OF ELECTROMAGNETIC ENERGY

Depending on their wavelength (or photon energy), electromagnetic waves can produce heat (microwaves, infrared radiation), molecular excitation (infrared), electronic excitation (light), and ionization of molecules (ultraviolet, x-rays) in tissue. The best-known detrimental biological effect of microwaves (e.g., radar) is the induction of cataracts, probably by protein denaturation. We do not know with certainty whether this effect is cumulative, like some of the radiological effects discussed below, or whether the damage will repair itself as long as it is not excessive. From the mechanistic standpoint, it is conceivable that this biological effect is completely reversible below a certain threshold.

It is well known that electronic excitation, especially ionization, produces permanent chemical changes and therefore induces permanent biological damage. Long-term biological effects are produced by cleavage of bonds in DNA molecules. Most of the radiobiological cellular damage is repaired by a sequence of enzymatic reactions involving recognition of the damaged site, cleavage of the modified strand, excision of the damaged region, buildup of a repaired strand by using the other undamaged strand as a template, and, finally, ligation of the repaired strand to the undamaged segment, forming a repaired DNA molecule. The repair process is, however, not free from errors that may result in point mutations on the repaired DNA. Furthermore, there are situations in which the repair is less effective, especially when both DNA strands have been damaged in nearby regions. Less specific nonenzymatic repairs may also take place by radical–radical reactions between the primary or secondary products of DNA radiolysis. These processes, which are responsible for chromosomal morphological aberrations, are evidently more likely to be mutagenic. Further, DNA constituents may be modified by reaction with small free radicals (e.g., H atoms or OH radicals) to an extent that is unrecognizable by the repair enzymes but that will affect transcription or DNA replication. The irreparable damage to DNA results in the death of the cell because of the loss of either the DNA replication capacity or the ability to produce a critical enzyme.

The death of individual cells is of little biological consequence as long as only a small fraction of the cell population of a given tissue is affected. A much more severe biological problem is created by cells that survive and replicate in spite of being radiobiologically damaged. The modified DNA molecules that can still undergo replication and transcription functions, having been only slightly impaired, are the basis for the long-term detrimental effects of radiation.

The formation of replicating damaged cells, some of which might have lost some of their differentiation ability and been transformed to a malignant form, is the most severe long-term side effect of ionizing radiation. The number of such potentially highly undesirable biological entities is directly proportional to the amount of ionizing radiation energy dissipated per cell or per gram of tissue. This means that even the smallest amount of ionizing radiation energy dissipated in tissue results in a finite probability of radiation-induced cancer.

The energy dissipated per gram of tissue is measured in units called *rads*. A conventional chest x-ray is associated with a dose of about 0.05 rad to the chest; an upper gastrointestinal (GI) x-ray study involves about 1 rad to the stomach; and computerized tomograms of the abdomen involve about 2 to 3 rads to the abdomen. Each rad is associated with a probability of about 1 in 5,000 of inducing cancer in the irradiated tissue. Since different tissues have different susceptibilities to cancer induction, the stated probability should be considered as a rough guideline only. However, this nontrivial probability of cancer induction associates a calculated risk with every x-ray diagnostic examination. Since this radiobiological damage is cumulative, the risk of cancer induction increases with the total dose absorbed by a given tissue.

The radiation doses associated with the diagnostic use of internally administered radioisotopes are generally higher than those associated with diagnostic x-rays. In addition, radiation therapy that involves thousandfold higher doses to the treated malignant tissue deposits substantial doses of radiation in the adjacent tissue and even in remote tissues. Thus, although there is a chance of, say, 90 percent of eradicating a given malignant tumor by radiation, there is a 10 percent risk of producing a new cancer in another tissue. This new cancer, which might be manifested 10 to 30 years following treatment, is of little concern if the patient is 65 years old. But it may be a significant contraindication if the patient is 25. In this case, the long-term side effects of the treatment should be a decisive factor in the choice of the strategy for patient management.

In using diagnostic x-rays, we generally ignore their potential carcinogenic effect, even when a certain organ may be radiographed tens of times over the years. There is, however, a much greater awareness of the teratological and genetic effects of diagnostic radiation, as well as of the potential induction of leukemia in children who have been irradiated in utero. This is the reason for avoidance of diagnostic x-ray radiography in pregnant women, and for the general avoidance of irradiating the ovaries of women before menopause.

The mechanisms of genetic mutations, radiation-induced malformations (somatic mutations) and leukemia, or other forms of cancer induction are probably very similar, involving nonlethal damage to the DNA of different cell lines. All of these effects are cumulative, and all of them seem to have no threshold; in other words, there is no safe dose of radiation below which no detrimental radiobiological effects will occur. The only point of reference we may have in distinguishing between acceptable and unacceptable radiobiological risks is the level of natural background ionizing radiation (from cosmic rays and naturally occurring radioisotopes) to which all of us are exposed. This level amounts to about 0.1 rad per year, or about 6 to 7 rads over a lifetime. Populations living at high altitudes (e.g., in Denver or Mexico City) are exposed to about twice the natural background radiation of those living at sea level. Still, it is hard to demonstrate in these populations an enhanced mutation rate or incidence of cancer. It might be concluded, therefore, that diagnostic radiation doses on the order of 0.1 rad (such as associated with a single chest x-ray) are virtually safe. This conclusion is, however, not completely justified, because the susceptibility of a given patient to cancer induction may be significantly higher than that of an average member of the population. For instance, if we require a cigarette smoker to undergo a chest x-ray twice a year to detect incipient lung cancer, we may in the long run induce lung cancer, especially when computerized image reconstruction and pattern recognition become standard imaging procedures. The current cost of software development will become inconsequential in the future, when thousands of instruments will be used. The cost of computer hardware will also decrease dramatically when the fifth or sixth generation of miniaturized computer hardware is used.

## EFFECT OF MATERIALS USED IN HEALTH CARE TECHNOLOGY

In the previous sections, we discussed the side effects of different forms of energy introduced into the biological system that are incidental to the use of health care technology. Certain clinical techniques and procedures involve the introduction of foreign materials into the biological system, materials that may have side effects of their own.

We shall consider here three examples of foreign materials that come into direct contact with the patient's tissues in conjunction with three different technological procedures: contrast agents in diagnostic x-ray angiography, metallic pins in orthopedics, and elastomers in hemodialysis.

In the first example, we intentionally introduce blood-soluble, iodinated organic chemicals into the circulation. These materials may be antigenic and, in rare cases, may induce anaphylactic shock. They may be hepatotoxic, especially when liver function is compromised, and they may interfere with the function of diseased kidneys. The immunological effect is unpredictable unless a prior test of the patient's immune response has been performed. The latter two effects can be predicted if we know beforehand the status of the liver and kidney. Barring these potential complications, the use of approved iodinated agents is harmless. Even if a patient is allergic to certain agents, an alternative may be acceptable. Moreover, one can apply angiographic contrast agents in the presence of short-term immune suppressants to circumvent the short-term side effect. In other words, all that is necessary for the avoidance of side effects of contrast agents is awareness of the problem.

In a patient with compromised liver or kidney function, angiography can be performed, although with lower resolution, using computerized tomography (CT) instead of photographic radiography. CT requires considerably lower concentrations of contrast agents. As computerized x-ray tomography develops, it will facilitate informative angiographic examinations such as those obtainable by x-ray cinematography, with a much lower risk of side effects from iodinated contrast agents. Here is a situation in which the development of new instrumentation, intended to provide better imaging information, also minimizes one of the side effects of the older technology.

The second example – introduction of metallic structural materials into the patient's body – posed a severe toxicological problem until the development of appropriate alloys (e.g., vitallium) that minimize these effects. The state of the art is not ideal as yet, even though the problem of corrosion has been solved. For one thing, there is always the possibility of forming a galvanic cell out of two parts of the metallic object if these parts are under different stresses or have different temperatures. Although the potentials produced may be on the order of microvolts, they may still induce local electrochemical effects. The development of nonmetallic structural materials might seem to be a good solution to this problem. However, as we shall soon see, organic artificial polymers (cross-linked or elastomers) may pose even more severe toxicological problems than metals.

Elastomers are being used extensively in modern clinical practice, ranging from syringes and whole blood containers to catheters and hemodialyzing membranes. Any of these polymeric materials may contain certain low molecular weight constituents introduced intentionally (e.g., plasticizers) or unintentionally (trace impurities, monomers, residual catalysts, etc.). Many of these low molecular weight contaminants, which may leach out slowly from the elastomer while in contact with blood or tissue, exhibit toxic effects. Polymer technology is improving the quality of polymers designed for clinical use, but this improvement has not yet reached its optimum. Consequently, there are potential side effects from the use of most polymers in intimate contact with tissue. There is an even more severe problem: The surface of many polymeric materials, even when in ultrapure form, may exert a catalytic effect on certain proteins or polypeptides, producing, for instance, the slow release of clotting factors. This may result in a higher titer of these factors in patients who have implanted elastomers or are undergoing chronic hemodialysis. The long-term side effect of this surface activity of polymers is aggravated arteriosclerosis in patients who have this tendency. It has been documented that long-term hemodialysis is associated with severe arteriosclerosis, which may result in myocardial infarction or other vascular complications. The same problem may arise in the use of an artificial heart – especially because recipients of this device, which is composed of elastomers, are very likely to be suffering already from severe arteriosclerosis. It is conceivable that in the foreseeable future, new elastomers or their surface treatment will alleviate this critical side effect. For the time being, however this long-term side effect should be an important factor in the development of a strategy for patient management involving devices that contain elastomers.

These three examples of side effects produced by materials complement the examples of those effects associated with energy input into the biological system. As in the latter cases, there may be ways to circumvent the side effects. However, until they have been found, we should be aware of the problems and take them into consideration in making clinical decisions.

## SUMMARY

Health care technology, like any other technology, is associated with certain risks. Some of them are controllable or avoidable when technology is appropriately applied; others are intrinsic and at best can only be minimized. The hazards of accidental electrocution while under intensive care can be completely eliminated with appropriate attention to technical details; so also can any potentially harmful effects of diagnostic ultrasound. The risks of diagnostic x-ray radiology can be reduced to an insignificant level with appropriate equipment and well-designed procedures. The side effects of foreign materials can be minimized or eliminated completely with further materials research. The risk of hemodialysis may thus be substantially decreased, making this procedure significantly more attractive. However, the side effects of radiation therapy, and possibly those of ultrasonic hyperthermia, cannot be eliminated, and they should not be ignored when comparing alternative strategies of patient management.

Any new instrument or technique may produce a new set of side effects, and occasionally these are discovered long after the technique has been used. It is important, therefore, to follow the current literature on users' experience with a given technique, rather than relying only on the information that convinced clinicians initially to apply the technique as a solution to a given medical problem.

The process of decision making under probabilistic conditions will be discussed in a later chapter. Here we have discussed qualitatively just a few examples of so-called calculated risks. This nonexhaustive list of side effects is intended only to illustrate the potential problems. A better understanding of the incipient side effects will lead to a more effective use of health care technology.

## SELECTED BIBLIOGRAPHY

Alper, T. (1979). *Cellular Radiobiology*. New York: Cambridge University Press.
Andrews, J. R. (1978). *The Radiobiology of Human Cancer: Radiotherapy*. Baltimore: University Park Press.
Brodsky, C., ed. (1982). *CRC Handbook of Radiation Measurement and Protection*. Boca Raton, Fla.: CRC.
Waggener, R. C. (ed.) (1982). *Handbook of Medical Physics*. Boca Raton, Fla.: CRC.
Williams, F. (ed.) (1981). *Fundamental Aspects of Biocompatibility*, vols. 1 and 2. Boca Raton, Fla.: CRC.

# PART III

# CREATION AND DISSEMINATION OF TECHNOLOGY

# THE ENGINEERING–INDUSTRIAL ACCORD: INVENTING THE TECHNOLOGY OF HEALTH CARE

MURRAY EDEN

It is common knowledge that health technologies in many different forms – information processing systems, elaborate diagnostic devices, new modes of therapy – are playing an increasingly larger role in the delivery of health care here and in the other industrialized countries. Although the inroads of technology into a highly labor-intensive sector of society appears to be a new phenomenon, a moment's reflection will show that devices began to be used at more or less the same time that scientific attitudes began to change the direction of progress in medicine. The stethoscope in the early nineteenth century, the thermometer and roentgen rays in the late nineteenth century, the sphygmomanometer and the electrocardiogram (ECG) recorders in the early twentieth century are only a few of the devices introduced in the past two centuries.

### HEALTH CARE TECHNOLOGY AFTER WORLD WAR II

The pace of technological innovation underwent a vast change following World War II. To be sure, sensitive electrical measurements – the sine qua non of virtually every modern device – could be made if their determination were essential, as in the ECG, but the equipment was large and expensive, requiring frequent calibration and constant attention. The only electronic devices in common use were radios and phonographs. Vacuum tubes and the circuits into which they were integrated were not well understood on a theoretical level. Electronics was in large measure an empirical art.

Technological development and the hard sciences underwent a great expansion because of the military needs of World War II. In the years that followed, many of the scientists and engineers who had participated in the war effort turned to more peaceful pursuits; applications of their work to biology and medicine had a particular appeal. A pattern of technology transfer was begun, although not in the form in which it exists today. There is little evidence of any conscious

49

intention to take a device from where it was first used and seek out a lucrative or socially constructive use in medicine or elsewhere. Rather, the physical science, mathematical, and engineering skills that were applied to military problems and the people who had these skills were put to a different use.

The early impact was predominantly on the research laboratory. Physiologists and biochemists tended to be more receptive to the tools and the spirit of the physical sciences than were the practicing physicians of that time. The electron microscope, ultracentrifuge, mass spectrometer, and spectrophotometer were incorporated rapidly into the armamentarium of the research biologist; a new discipline, *biophysics*, began to emerge. A further specialization, *molecular biology*, which was to revolutionize biology, started in the late 1950s. It is worth noting that a remarkably large fraction of the early participants in the new field of molecular biology had begun their careers as physicists.

In medicine the major new ingredient was electronics. The electronic engineers could readily perceive that their techniques might facilitate the kinds of measurement required in medical practice: temperature, blood pressure, pulse rate, and heart sounds.

Entrepreneurs perceived medicine to be a fertile field for exploitation. The medical instrumentation industry included a few large companies, notably those making x-ray equipment, but generally the companies were very small and almost always undercapitalized. Although the newspapers and the fledgling societies of medical electronics, biomedical engineering, and the like foretold rapid growth and a significant impact on health care, the fact was that the market for their potential products had not yet been formed.

Many reasons have been offered to explain the slow growth: Physicians tend to be conservative, are generally unfamiliar with physical science, and distrust measurements that they cannot perform personally; the health care system is too fragmented, and in consequence is a cottage industry; engineers are naive and do not appreciate the complexity of medical problems.

Although all of these factors are relevant, probably the prime explanation is that the scientific basis for medical practice in both therapy and diagnosis was rudimentary. Medicine was still largely empirical. If medicine were to progress toward a more thoroughgoing scientific basis, it was necessary first to understand the processes of normal function and their pathologies at a fundamental level.

Moreover, the evolution of the technological devices intended to address a medical problem involves an interplay between the instrumental design and the state of scientific knowledge of that problem; this evolutionary process takes time.

## EXAMPLES OF TECHNOLOGICAL DEVELOPMENTS

We may consider the development of the artificial kidney as an illustration. Hemodialysis was first demonstrated in 1913. John J. Abel, Leonard G. Rowndtree, and B. B. Turner in the Johns Hopkins Pharmacology Department established in a rabbit model that an extracorporeal device would partially correct chemical imbalances associated with uremia (Abel et al. 1913–14). Their intention was to develop a pharmacological research tool. So far as we know, they were not motivated by a perceived need for a therapeutic device. Indeed, it may not have occurred to them that their device could have a therapeutic application. It remained for Willem J. Kolff, a physician in the Netherlands, to develop the first clinical tool of its kind, popularly referred to as an artificial kidney. His work was carried out during World War II and published in 1944 (Kolff and Berk 1944). In the early devices, the cannulas were made of glass or metal. They were removed after dialysis, and the vessels were ligated. In order to avoid the wholesale destruction of vessels and to enable the treatment to be extended to patients with chronic kidney disease, Allwall, Norvitt, and Steins developed a configuration that included an arteriovenous shunt, indwelling and made of glass (Allwall et al. 1948). It failed because the shunt induced rapid formation of thrombi. Twelve years later, Belding H. Scribner and Wayne E. Quinton, a neurologist and a mechanical engineer, respectively, demonstrated the first arteriovenous shunt appropriate to chronic application (Quinton et al. 1960); Kolff's apparatus was applicable only to acute uremia. The success of their preparation depended crucially on the use of polytetrafluoroethylene (PTFE) as the shunt material. PTFE is a plastic developed originally for quite different industrial uses; under the trade name Teflon it produced commercial success as the nonstick surface of cookware. Scribner and Quinton also managed to diminish further the thrombogenic effects and trauma to the patient by coating the points of the shunt that made contact with tissue with a softer material, silicone rubber, another industrial product. However, in this instance, the technology had already been applied to biomedical problems, and in 1963 a so-called medical grade of silicone rubber was available. About three years later, surgeons began to develop techniques for establishing arteriovenous fistulas using saphenous vein grafts. This further improvement still did not deal with the trauma and pain of repeated needle puncture. In 1979 Golding, Nissenson, and Raible developed a device intended to permit percutaneous access to a vein by introducing another new material as the interface between the external environment and the vascular system (Golding et al. 1979). They used vitrified carbon, a material developed originally for the heat shields for the reentry vehicles of the National Aeronautics and Space Administration. Hemodialysis, as a feasible procedure for patients with chronic renal disease, was perfected by a series of steps over a long period; we have alluded to a few of the major steps. The crucial role of the artificial kidney was quickly recognized. Congress was impelled to act by amending the Social Security Act in 1972 so that the expensive treatment could be guaranteed. Currently there are some 60,000 individuals with kidney failure who are being dialyzed in the United States at a cost of almost $2 billion a year.

Medical practitioners and biologists initiated and developed the artificial kidney. By contrast, automation of laboratory procedures was accomplished by industry. In this instance, the spectrophotometer and its control by electronic means led to the development of a variety of analytical measuring devices in the period following World War II.

The availability of relatively inexpensive data processing equipment enabled the Technicon Corporation to develop a continuous-flow automatic laboratory analyzer, which was introduced in 1957. Clinical laboratory automation has been extended continuously, so that all of the common tests are now carried out by this means.

The most recent innovation in medical technology is the microprocessor, a product of the integrated circuit industry. Driven by competition for mass markets, the integrated circuit manufacturers have developed microprocessors and microcomputers that are tiny (the chip itself is less than 1 cm wide and a fraction of a millimeter thick), inexpensive (a few dollars will suffice to buy almost any of them), and efficient (a tiny battery will keep it running for months). They are the basic elements of digital timepieces, hand calculators, and video games, to name the most common uses. So far as health care is concerned, it is now relatively easy to foresee the construction of complex diagnostic or therapeutic devices that are easily portable, perform a variety of functions, and require little or no attention. They may be especially important for ambulatory patients and for the disabled, but they can also be expected to spur the development of all sorts of "smart" instruments.

Even within this brief anecdotal history of medical technology, it should be possible to discern a pattern for innovation.[1] An esoteric procedure developed for basic research is perceived to be relevant to clinical medicine. In all likelihood, the research tool will have been adapted from a development in the physical sciences, modern biology, or both; modern examples include the electron probe, lasers, nuclear magnetic resonance (NMR) spectrometry, monoclonal antibodies, and gene splicing. A prototype is designed for the new setting. The adaptation will almost certainly be opportunistic in that the technologists carrying it out will draw on modern technology. For example, NMR imaging is a development dependent upon the 25-year history of NMR spectrometry. NMR imaging was first proposed by a physician, Raymond Damadian (1971). The techniques he used for examining biological tissues were regarded by physical scientists working in NMR spectroscopy as methodologically unsound. Nevertheless, to some extent, Damadian's initiative spurred physical scientists to examine the NMR imaging problem in a more rigorous manner. Paul Lauterbur, a physicist at Stony Brook, developed and demonstrated the feasibility of proton NMR imaging on a physically secure basis (Lauterbur 1973). It is now being developed for biology and medicine at a rapid rate, primarily by large industrial concerns. It draws upon magnet design including that of superconducting magnets, electromagnetic theory, radio frequency circuitry, modern computational methods, and multi-dimensional signal processing. Its clinical use reveals problems, shortcomings, and inconvenient modes of operation. The device will be modified, reconfigured, and refined, a process that may go through many stages. Of course, at each step, the engineer and the health practitioner must compare notes to carry the development further. If some group of health practitioners perceives it to satisfy a need, then a consensus of users may establish the device as the standard procedure.

### PHYSICIANS AND TECHNOLOGICAL DEVELOPMENT

How do new developments come about? Logically, the process must begin with the recognition of a need. Consider the stethoscope. Physicians in the early nineteenth century became convinced by its inventor, René Laennec, that auscultation of the chest elicited signs that could closely correlate with structural defects in tissues revealed at autopsy, and thus provide considerable aid in diagnosis. It became common practice for the physician to use this instrument to hear sounds arising within the body, once Laennec had proved their value and generated a need for the instrument.

But today, more faithful sound transmission appears to be of little or no concern to clinical practitioners. Electronic stethoscopes have been manufactured but have had very meager commercial success, although stethoscopes furnished with an electronic microphone and high-quality amplifiers have an excellent frequency response. One must presume that practicing physicians, having invested a good deal of their time in learning how to interpret chest and heart sounds with a stethoscope that filters out high frequencies, are not inclined to relearn this skill unless it can be demonstrated that a better diagnostic result is to be achieved with more faithful sound reproduction. Thus, it would appear that the impulse to innovate must be tempered by an assessment of current practice.

The historical example just given raises the question of physician acceptance or nonacceptance. For patients, insurers, and social or political bodies, the more important issues are those of efficacy and safety. As pointed out in Chapter 5 and discussed elsewhere in this book, careful evaluation does not invariably, or even often, precede research and development.

To cast some light on the forces that drive innovation, we must realize that there are a number of interested parties and that their motivations differ. Physicians seek technology that will improve their performance as diagnosticians or therapists, or to make performance of their services easier or more convenient. Engineers view medicine as an area of application for the products of their profession. Manufacturers search for new products that will have a profitable market or, more frequently, for profitable markets for the products they already know how to make. Insurers, governments that pay for health care, and hospital administrators look for ways to provide services more inexpensively or more expeditiously by substituting capital-intensive automatic devices for human labor. And, of course, patients and their families are always concerned about finding earlier diagnosis, less dangerous diagnostic procedures, more favorable outcomes, and decreased pain and discomfort.

The process of innovation in medical technology differs little from that of any other branch of application. But the complicated interaction of the many interested parties and their varying perceptions of an optimal strategy for innovation make the analysis quite different from, say, that related to the development of military technology, robotics, or agriculture.

The author once participated in the development of a technique for recognizing automatically malarial parasites in blood smears of possible carriers. The intended use was in screening populations during malaria eradication campaigns in developing countries. Ultimately, this technique would have been similar to devices currently marketed for differential white cell counting by pattern recognition algorithms (Eden et al. 1973).

Although the technique itself is feasible in the sense that the plasmodia causing malaria could be recognized with relatively high reliability by machine, the procedure was wildly inappropriate to the application. Consider some of the economic factors. The modern device costs about $100,000. It requires an operator with technical training, a regulated source of power, an air-conditioned environment, and relatively careful handling. The current manual method uses a simple microscope, is illuminated by the sun or an alcohol lamp, and is operated by a technician who receives about $50 a month in the poorer countries, and not much more in many of the other countries where the incidence of malaria justifies the cost of an intensive screening program.

In many if not most instances, the impetus to improve medical care comes from a physician who recognizes a particular diagnostic or therapeutic need. Thus, Kolff conceived of the need for an artificial kidney and began a line of development that continues to this day. Current versions of the artificial kidney are eminently practical, but research continues on ways to decrease its cost by using less expensive components and more easily prepared dialysis solutions; to increase its convenience – smaller size, ease of cleaning, simpler procedures for dialysis in the home; to decrease trauma; and so on.

Another example of the physician's role in a chain of developments is to be found in the current interest in interventional radiography. Once radiologists demonstrated that catheters can be inserted safely into many parts of the vascular system, many potential therapeutic uses were perceived. Radiologists are now experimenting with the delivery of embolizing agents to seal off aneurysms, thrombolytic agents such as streptokinase to clear vessels of clots, chemotherapeutic agents that can be introduced in high concentrations into the arterial supply of inoperable tumors, and catheters that dilate so as to compress atherosclerotic plaques. It is clear that the recognition of a particular need in this instance is the domain of the clinical specialist. But it is also part of a closely knit sequence of invention, development, and use that depends on knowledge of and familiarity with prior technological achievements: catheters, the modern fluoroscope, contrast agents, and therapeutic chemicals. Furthermore, recognition of the *potentiality* to act in a new way on the pathological condition calls forth new technological needs. Thus recognition that treatment can be affected locally from within the vasculature emphasizes the requirement for getting the catheter to the pathological area. Simply put, one must steer the catheter to the site; hence the need for *steerable* catheters. In all likelihood the steerable catheter

– not yet a reality – represents an innovation that will result from the efforts and ingenuity of engineers or materials scientists who are made aware of the relevance of the need.

### ENGINEERS AND TECHNOLOGICAL DEVELOPMENT

The engineer, like the physician, is an interested party. In most cases, engineers will have only a nodding acquaintance with the biomedical details of the problem. In this sense, their role is complementary to that of the physician, who, on the other hand, is not likely to know the details of existing relevant technology and is even less likely to have the requisite physics or mathematics. Nevertheless, there are instances in which an engineer will attempt to produce biomedical innovations.

There appear to be two different motivations. The engineer may become aware of a personal need – his or her own illness or that of a relative. Of course, in such instances, the need is no different from that of any patient or family member, but the engineer may feel that his or her special competence can be put to good use, especially when the existing technology is – from a personal viewpoint – inadequate and old-fashioned. Although I am unaware of any device in general use today that was originated in this way, there are many examples of special sensory aids and modifications of prostheses designed for a particular patient. For example, the physicist Leo Szilard designed a special shield to minimize damage to himself as a part of a course of radiation therapy for his own malignancy.

A more common motivation for engineers is the desire to use the technology of their speciality in a medical application of which they have become aware. This can be characterized as a technology in pursuit of a new application. Because the medical need may be poorly understood by the engineer, many of the initiatives will result in a device that has no real use, is of only marginal value, is not in a form acceptable to practitioners, or is too expensive. The electronic stethoscope cited earlier is an example.

Notwithstanding the occasional naiveté of the engineer–inventor, many important technologies originated with precisely such ideas. Computerized tomography (CT) scanning, whose history is sketched by Banta in Chapter 5, seems to be a case in point. Cormack, who first developed the theory of image reconstruction, is a physicist; Hounsfield, who directed the development of the first commercial scanner, is an engineer.

The history of the CT scanner is instructive in another sense as well: It illustrates the importance of the entrepreneur in the process of innovation. Cormack produced his results with virtually no reference to practical applications (Cormack 1963). Of course, the technology of computers and image processing at that time was inadequate for the task of producing a practical device. But in addition, it seems that no manufacturer was sufficiently interested to explore the possibilities. In contrast, Hounsfield had the resources of EMI to draw upon (Hounsfield et al. 1973). It is worth noting that EMI was not known primarily as a manufacturer of x-ray equipment. Thus, Cormack's results, which were unused by industry, were largely forgotten, only to be recalled after the explosive success of CT scanners 15 years later.

## INDUSTRY AND TECHNOLOGICAL DEVELOPMENT

Obviously, the commercial firm, as an interested party, is motivated first and foremost by the potential for profit. In countries with a predominantly capitalist economy, technological novelties relevant to medical care must reach the health service provider through the offices of a concern that regards the product as financially gainful.

A company contemplating the introduction of a biomedical technical innovation has a number of factors to consider. As with the introduction of any other product, the company must estimate the market size and the costs of penetrating the market – advertising and the like. It must estimate the cost of manufacture and sale, the profit margin it can hope to sustain, and the expected competition from products in the same technology, as well as from products addressing the same market but based in other technologies. But entrepreneurs in medical technology have special problems. They must demonstrate the safety and efficacy of the product by passing it through a sequence of steps prescribed by federal regulation, particularly the FDA. Aside from the risk that the proposed product cannot satisfy the regulatory requirements, there is inevitably the high cost associated with demonstrating safety and efficacy as defined by the regulatory process.

But initially, there is the cost associated with the research and development of a new technology. Money for research and development must be spent first, long before a product can begin to provide a return on investment and – as with the issues of safety and efficacy – with no certainty that a product can be developed successfully.

This element of risk is related to the level of novelty of the proposed innovation; the greater the novelty, the greater the risk. It is no surprise to find that most development activity in medical technology focuses on the improvement of existing techniques and products. The *Medical Devices Report*, a weekly newsletter for the medical instrumentation industry, publishes the titles of the U.S. Patent Office grants issued on medical and surgical products. The report of September 30, 1982, cites 26 patents ("Patent news" 1982). Although only the titles are given, it is clear that virtually all of them are minor modifications of devices on the market. A few examples are a "structure for preventing the breakage of end portions of a protective covering for the adjustable bend section of an endoscope," a "cardiac pacer having quick-disconnect lead terminals," a "direct water coupling device for ultrasound breast scanning in a supine position," and a "heart beat sensor holding device."

Even when the need is obvious to the health professional and the entrepreneur's market is large and potentially profitable, the research requirement is a great inhibitor. *The Economist* of October 9, 1982, discusses the problem of cryopreservation:

> Chemists studying cell membranes believe that, with a modest push in the right direction, they could lick most of the outstanding problems associated with preserving living organisms. The results would provide an enormous benefit to industry. Some, however, fear that it would also lead to (possibly unpatentable) laboratory techniques which would then benefit their competitors. Few biotechnology firms are therefore enthusiastic about splashing out on much research. This is precisely the sort of work that needs to attract industry-wide (or even international) support. The British government, keen to set up a project, has been talking about the possibility with the West Germans.

### GOVERNMENT AND TECHNOLOGICAL DEVELOPMENT

This brings us to the role of government, which must weigh the needs and desires of industry, the health deliverers, and, most of all, the electorate, who in this context are the end users of medical care. The government intervenes in the innovation process in several important ways. Earlier, we alluded to government as a regulator and referee in the determination of efficacy and safety for both drugs and devices.

A priori, regulation for safety and efficacy is neutral in terms of stimulating or inhibiting innovation. But more often than not, manufacturers find adherence to the regulations, for example, premarket clearance, to be costly and onerous. Not a few innovators, including physicians and technologists, find restrictions on the clinical use of experimental prototypes to be inhibitory, absurdly over-cautious – a frozen brake on progress. At the same time, the government's ideological commitment to efficacy and safety is a reflection of the electorate's strong feelings, especially regarding safety, and should encourage innovators in the belief that government will be on their side whenever a new design concept serves a particular health need and is safe as well.

A second role is alluded to in *The Economist's* previously stated comments on cryopreservation. When development is too costly or too risky, the government is the primary or even the sole source of funding. As far as basic research[2] is concerned, by its very definition it is too risky. Most basic biomedical research in the United States is funded by the federal government – principally by the National Institutes of Health, with smaller amounts from the National Science Foundation and other agencies and additional support from nonprofit foundations. Conversely, industry, including the medical technology industry, the health insurers, and health providers, such as hospitals, provide virtually no support for basic research. These sectors support some applied research and prototype development, but most of their financial resources go to product development.

Basic research, applied research, prototype development, and product development are activities that have vague and overlapping definitions. A *basic research* project is defined as one undertaken with no idea that the facts discovered have any direct bearing on a nonscientific (i.e., practical or applied) problem. *Applied research* shares with basic research the quality that new facts about nature are to be discovered, but these facts have a direct bearing on a goal outside the system of science itself. *Prototype development* refers to the process of preparing a device, technique, or system that demonstrates the feasibility of a particular solution to a perceived social problem. In general, prototypes are operated only by their creators or by others who understand the technology of the device. Finally, *product development* denotes the part of the innovative process that takes a prototype and shapes it to the needs of the ultimate user. The delicate controls are put inside the box and out of harm's way, the operating format is tailored to the user, and the package is designed for the environment in which it will fit. It is believed that a physician need know as little about the construction of an electrocardiograph as a typist knows about that of a word processor.

Industrial innovation is limited largely to the development of modifications and improvements in technologies whose principles and practice are already fairly well understood. Even the big companies do not make money on expensive fundamental research unless it is funded by governmental contract. The British government provided financial support for three research groups that were developing the idea of NMR imaging. The first NMR scanner installed in a clinical setting was developed by EMI using money provided largely by the United Kingdom's Ministry of Health. Even so, EMI divested itself of this project by sale to Picker International.

Every year, the editorial advisory board of the magazine *Industrial Research and Development* selects 100 significant new products on the basis of "importance, uniqueness and usefulness from a technical standpoint" (*I.R.* 1982). The selection is made from a list of products entered in the competition by their developers. In 1982, average development costs were about $890,000. Almost two-thirds of the winners were products of industrial development; U.S. governmental agencies had 21 awards; foreign government-sponsored groups, 4 awards; universities, 4 awards; and independent research laboratories, 6 awards. In the past 3 years, the federal government has supported, in whole or in part, approximately 35 percent of the products developed. Obviously, federal government support is a very significant factor even in product development, let alone basic research and prototype development.

Only eight of the 1982 awards are included in the category "biomedical tools and materials." This is somewhat misleading, however, because many of the other devices on the list are designed to perform physical or chemical manipulations or analyses related to biomedicine, for example, spectrometers, a high-performance liquid chromatography system, a curve tracer, a superconducting magnet, a digital correlator, and a laboratory information system. A number of the descriptions cite medical or pharmacological applications for the equipment.

One interesting example reverses the usual direction of technology transfer: A new Perkin-Elmer integrating sphere was "originally developed for detecting changes in lumen skin color as an aid to diagnosis and research. It is also useful for measuring color on surfaces of such items as textiles, ceramics, paper, food, and coatings."

### INNOVATION AND PROFIT

Thus, the decision to innovate or not, and which innovation a company chooses to spend its research and development budget on, is modulated by the need to make money from the sale of medical technology. A company may occasionally decide to risk some money and time on a development that is likely to be only marginally profitable, but will provide some other form of reward: entry into a new field, good public relations, or prestige. As a general rule, no company will invest research and development resources in an unprofitable product. Conversely, the greater the potential financial reward, the more enthusiastic is the pursuit of innovation. An Office of Technology Assessment report notes that in 1982 total industry sales were an estimated $14 billion, more than three times the 1972 level and eleven times that spent in 1958 in current dollars. The greatest growth occurred among technologies whose use was likely to be covered by health insurance (Office of Technology Assessment, in press).

The converse must also be true; when a device has only a small market – perhaps for use in the therapy of a relatively rare disease – it is not likely to be developed. If the need as perceived by the public and the decision makers is sufficiently great, its development will be subsidized. We have already cited the case of the artificial kidney; the treatment is so costly and the need so obvious that both development and therapy are almost completely underwritten by the federal government.

When government funds are not available to alter the free market, the company's decisions about biomedical technological products can be no different from its decisions about any other products.

The magazine *High Technology*, in its November/December 1982 issue, discusses the future of medical imaging. Its business editor, Irving Geller, comments on the business outlook for medical imaging:

> The $2 billion recession-proof medical imaging field is growing rapidly. Digital x-ray, nuclear magnetic resonance (NMR) and real-time ultrasound systems offer the highest growth potential. Lower growth products include standard x-rays and computerized tomography (CT) scanners. Positron emission tomography (PET) scanners are not expected to have a commercial future.

The logic behind Geller's forecast bears directly on the issue of the market. Note that for these costly systems, the market is restricted to hospitals.

Digital radiography, the fastest growing segment, is in commercial use, while NMR has only reached the late development stage. Nevertheless, NMR's long run impact and growth should be greater because of its potential to transform medical diagnosis.

Ultrasound has undergone steady expansion and technological innovation over the past five years; it should continue as a good growth market.

Digital radiography, which uses computers to enhance x-ray images, emerged as a separate market in 1981, sales are expected to skyrocket to $80 million this year, $120 million in 1983, and $1.2 billion in 1986.

The ultrasound market should total $275 million in 1982 and expand 15 percent annually.

Cardiology is the fastest growing ultrasound segment, at thirty percent annually. Radiology follows, growing fifteen percent per year. Real-time computerized ultrasound units for cardiology and radiology cost more than $60,000 each and account for sixty-seven percent of sales. The remainder divides evenly between the obstetrics/gynecology and ophthalmology markets. About sixty percent of the units will be placed in hospitals, and the remainder in physicians' private offices.

Although NMRs are still undergoing clinical evaluation, encouraging results have led hospitals to place orders. A long waiting list already exists. Despite high prices – either $1 million or $1.5 million, depending on the type of magnet used – NMRs should be cost effective. An angiogram, for example, may require a two-to-three day hospital stay; NMR is an outpatient procedure.

From this year's 20–25 NMR units valued at $24 -$30 million, shipments should rise to 250–350 units worth $380–$530 million by 1985. In 1990, the market should reach 750–1000 machines valued at $1.5–$2.5 billion, predicts Jack W. Lasersohn, analyst at F. Eberstadt & Co.

Except for Diasonics, the companies offering complete NMR systems are all large conglomerates or their subsidiaries. Technicare and Picker International lead the other companies including Siemens, Phillips, Toshiba, Hitachi, and CGR, a French firm.

NMR will begin cutting into the CT scanner market by 1984. CT sales will plateau and decline twenty percent as early as 1986.

But CT scanner sales will continue. Firms expect to install 2440 units costing $600,000 each (a total of $1.5 billion) in 1982 through 1985. The major market will be hospitals of 200 to 400 beds; only 40 percent now have CT units.

Because GE leads the world in CT manufacture, the company will probably become a major competitor in the NMR market. GE's interest in protecting its CT market would indicate that it may move quite slowly.

Geller is quite pessimistic about the future of PET scanners.

No one sees any commercial future for positron emission tomography. These systems will be limited to research laboratories and used for diagnosing brain or psychiatric disorders. Scientists do not fully understand the information produced by the machines; and it will take years to develop data. A PET system must include a cyclotron, which produces high amounts of radiation and requires extensive shielding and skilled operators. Few hospitals are likely to accept the risks.

It seems fair to conclude that the profits from the diagnosis of brain or psychiatric disorders are not very high. If we compare the companies in NMR imaging and PET scanning, we find some corroboration for this view. As indicated previously, the companies in the NMR market are giants; the five or six firms in the PET market are very small by comparison, except for EGG, which bought Ortek, one of the small companies first in the field.

## CONCLUSION ABOUT THE INNOVATION PROCESS

Some tentative conclusions may be drawn regarding innovations in biomedical technology. The risk of undertaking major technological innovations can be borne only by big companies. Being large, these companies will enter only those technologies that have the promise of large markets. Small companies must generally be content with innovating in product markets that are more highly specialized as well as smaller.

It should be clear by now that technological innovation in medicine is an intricate process, one that rarely proceeds in a straight developmental line. Nonetheless, we can outline the general guidelines and steps that the development of every product must take, even though more often than not, orderly progression is likely to be honored in the breach.

One begins with the recognition of a need. The clinician, as the principal health provider, is the person most likely to recognize the need and to state the problem in the medically appropriate context. Consider the example of a patient who has recovered after an intestinal resection. The patient perceives discomfort and inconvenience, but is not likely to explain the nature of the problem. On the other hand, the clinician may theorize that the symptomatology is consistent with the discontinuity in the peristaltic phase induced by the surgery. Thus, the perception of a need is followed by a more precise statement of the problem. The clinician is also in a position to assess current practice – an essential step, because existing practices will influence heavily the likelihood of a successful introduction of a substitute method.

In the interests of careful definition of the problem, it is useful to attempt to model the pathological process. Undoubtedly, there is a physiological theory that describes the pulsatory and phase-coherent movement of intestinal smooth muscle. It may even be useful at this juncture to add to the development team an expert in biological control theory to solidify the model.

At this juncture, one can begin to think of potential alternative approaches to a solution. In our example, one might suggest possible modifications or tests of peristaltic motion to be made as part of the initial surgery. Another alternative might be corrective action, the design of a prosthetic device, or perhaps an externally actuated phasing device to assure a smooth peristaltic wave. This might be called choosing a design concept or the "brainstorming" component of the design process.

Once a specific approach has been agreed upon, the project's development must be organized. What kinds of competencies are required? The search for collaborators is a common problem for innovators, whether the initial impetus comes from a physician or a technologist. The "two cultures" problem is well known. It has been remarked that communication between medical practitioners and engineers is made doubly difficult because each thinks he or she is speaking English, whereas in reality each is using a different language. Some familiarity with the vocabulary and modes of thought of one's collaborator is essential for all of the professionals involved.

Work can now begin on validating the technological proposal and searching for funds. Some elements of validation can be accomplished through mathematical analysis, computer simulation, animal model studies, and the like. Ultimate validation occurs only after the prototype is made and tested. This phase of the project is largely the domain of the engineer, since it lies within his or her principal area of competence.

At the same time, the variety of business considerations that enter into a company's calculations needs to be made. However, even if development is being conducted in a noncommercial setting, the project participants would be well advised to spend some time evaluating the market, the likelihood of physician acceptability, the range of cost, and the problems of safety and a convenient operating format. Many technologically successful projects that are described in the literature or stored in the files of research institutions never reached the health care practitioner because the innovators' enthusiasm outran their understanding of the market for their product.

#### NOTES

**1** The word *innovation*, as used here, refers to the creation of new devices or techniques, or the combination of old devices into new configurations or for new applications. There is, however, a more restricted definition that has come into use within the past decade.

> Economists define technological innovation as the initial commercial application of a new product or process. From the standpoint of the industrial firm, the activities leading to innovation involve a long-term investment decision process. This process incorporates the various stages of research, development, capital investment, and commercialization. A firm's investment in these activities is influenced by the same basic forces that govern outlays on other investment projects. Thus, investments for R&D and innovation will be determined by their perceived profits and risks relative to alternative investment opportunities as well as the cost and availability of funds for investment. (National Academy of Sciences, 1969)

Peter Hutt, former counsel of the Food and Drug Administration (FDA), illustrates the use of the term:

> In the pharmaceutical industry, innovation is thus best measured by the number of new chemical entity (NCE) drugs approved by the Food and Drug Administration (FDA) for marketing during any particular time. These NCE drugs represent, in the words of the National Academy, "the initial commercial application of a new product or process."
>
> During the period from 1950 to the present, pharmaceutical innovation in the United States has declined substantially. This reduction in pharmaceutical innovation is attributable to two interrelated factors.
>
> First, drug research is lagging behind the growth rate of the drug industry.
>
> Second, the cost of developing and obtaining approval of an NCE drug has also risen dramatically. (1982)

**2** There is an occasional exception. Some very large companies – International Business Machines, General Motors, Xerox, International Telephone and Telegraph – have developed biomedical devices for very small markets, perhaps on philanthropic impulse. Some have featured these contributions as part of their institutional advertising programs.

SELECTED BIBLIOGRAPHY

Abel, J. J., Rowndtree, L. G., and Turner, B. B. (1913–14). On the removal of diffuseable substances from the circulating blood of living animals by dialysis. *J. Pharmacol. Exp. Ther.* 5:275.
Allwall, N., Norvitt, L., and Steins, A. M. (1948). An artificial kidney: clinical experience of dialytic treatment of uremia. *Acta Med. Scand.* 132:587.
Cormack, A. M. (1963). Representation of a function by its line integrals with some radiological applications. *Appl. Phys 34*:2722.
Damadian, R. (1971). Tumor detection by NMR. *Science 171*:1151.
*The Economist*, October 9, 1982.
Eden, M., Green, J. E., and Sun, A. (1973). Feasibility of computer screening of blood film for the detection of malarial parasites. *Bull. World Health Org.* 48:211–18.
Geller, I. (1982). Business outlook: medical imaging. *High Technology 2*(6):82.
Golding, A. L., Nissenson, A. R., and Raible, D. (1979). Carbon transcutaneous access device (CTAD). *Proc. Dial. Transplant. Forum 9*:242–7.
Hounsfield, G., Ambrose, J., Perry, J., et al. (1973). Computerized transverse axial scanning. *Br. J. Radiol. 46*:1016.
Hutt, P. B. (1982). The importance of patent term restoration to pharmaceutical innovation. *Health Affairs 1* (2):6.
I.R. 100 awards for new products processes and materials (1982). *Industrial Research and Development* (October): 87–154.
Kolff, W. J., and Berk, H. I. J. (1944). Artificial kidney: dialyzer with great area. *Acta Med. Scand. 117*:121.
Lauterbur, P. (1973). Image formation by induced local interactions: examples employing nuclear magnetic resonance. *Nature 242*:190.
National Academy of Sciences (1979). *The Impact of Regulation on Industrial Innovation.* Washington, D.C.: National Academy Press, p. 8.

Office of Technology Assessment (In press). *Federal Policies and The Medical Devices Industry*. Washington, D.C.: U.S. Government Printing Office.

Patent news (1982). *Medical Devices Report 11*(37):8.

Quinton, W., Dillard, D., and Scribner, B. H. (1960). Cannulation of blood vessels for prolonged hemodialysis. *Trans. ASAIO 6*:104.

CHAPTER 5

# EMBRACING OR REJECTING INNOVATIONS: CLINICAL DIFFUSION OF HEALTH CARE TECHNOLOGY

H. DAVID BANTA

The process by which a technology (or procedure) enters and becomes part of the health care system is known as *diffusion* (Banta, Behney, and Willems 1981). This phase follows the stage of research and development, and may or may not follow careful clinical trials to demonstrate efficacy and safety.

Descriptive research has shown that the diffusion process for any technology usually follows an S-shaped or sigmoid curve that relates the percentage of potential to actual adopters (Rogers and Shoemaker 1971, pp. 129, 131–3) (Figure 1). Generally, there is an early phase of diffusion that is somewhat slower. This has been interpreted as indicating caution on the part of users (Rogers and Shoemaker 1971, p. 188), although it could also indicate problems in communicating information about the innovation (OTA 1976, p. 4). As experience or studies show that the technology has some benefit, acceptance increases. Finally, when most potential adopters have accepted the innovation, diffusion slows and the curve flattens.

This type of curve has been demonstrated to apply to a number of medical technologies, including intensive care units (Russell 1978, pp. 49–51), cardiac pacemakers (OTA 1976, p. 76), respiratory therapy (Russell 1978, pp. 74, 75), diagnostic radioisotope facilities (Rapoport 1978), gastric freezing (Fineberg 1979, pp. 173–200), and electroencephalographs (Russell 1978, pp. 84–5, 94–5). However, one should be cautious about expecting all medical technologies to follow this curve or to spread at a common rate. At least one medical technology has been shown to diffuse in a different pattern. When the diffusion is very rapid initially, the pattern has been called the *desperation–reaction model* (Warner 1975). In the case shown in Figure 2, chemotherapy for leukemia, the rapid diffusion seemed to occur because providers desired to help the patient and alleviate their mutual desperation. Faced with life-threatening illness and little available therapy, it may not be reasonable to expect physicians to be cautious. Later, as results of clinical tests and experience begin to influence

65

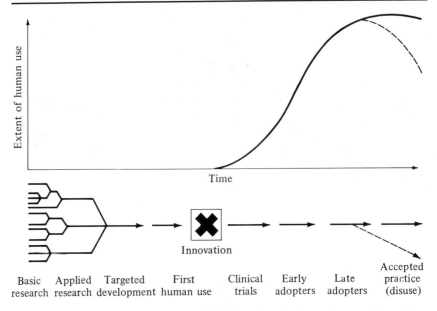

Figure 1. A scheme for development and diffusion of medical technologies. (From Office of Technology Assessment, U.S. Congress, *Development of Medical Technology: Opportunities for Assessment*. Washington, D.C.: U.S. Government Printing Office, 1976)

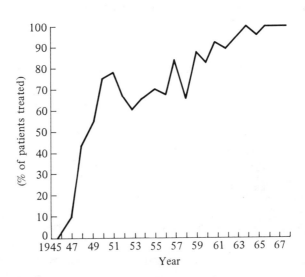

Figure 2. Diffusion of chemotherapy for leukemia. (From K. Warner, A 'desperation–reaction' model of medical diffusion. *Health Serv. Res. 10*:369, 1975)

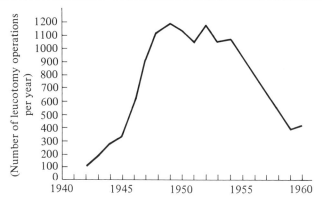

Figure 3. Leukotomy operations, England and Wales. (From G. Tooth and M. Newton, *Leucotomy in England and Wales 1942–54*, Reports on Public Health and Medical Subjects No. 104. London: Ministry of Health, Great Britain, 1961)

physicians' behavior, diffusion may slow. If results are positive, rapid diffusion may continue. If the evidence is not clear-cut or is negative, there may be slow diffusion or even abandonment.

As shown in Figure 1, some technologies are abandoned. The rate of tonsillectomy, for example, is presently declining (National Center for Health Statistics 1981, p. 250, Table 41). Such a decrease can result either from evidence of lack of benefit (unfavorable risk/benefit or cost/benefit ratio) or from the introduction of a more effective technology. The polio vaccine, for example, almost overnight entirely supplanted the costly "halfway technology" of rehabilitation centers (Thomas 1974, p. 36). Figure 3 shows the pattern of leukotomy in England and Wales. As evidence of side effects became available to temper earlier positive reports, leukotomy has become a rare procedure (Tooth and Newton 1961).

The importance of the diffusion curve of medical technology, what some have called the *life cycle* of a technology, is helpful in understanding these processes. In particular, from the standpoint of public policy, the goal is to ensure that beneficial technologies are rapidly disseminated and widely used, and that worthless technologies are not accepted at all. A subsidiary goal is to approach innovations cautiously and to discourage widespread use until evidence of benefit is available. Federal health policies have these aims, as well as others such as minimizing costs and protecting innovation. Later in the chapter, federal policies dealing with medical technologies will be discussed in more detail.

DEVELOPMENT OF THE COMPUTED TOMOGRAPHY (CT) SCANNER

Figure 4 presents schematically the development of the CT scanner. An important concept illustrated by the figure is that the development of technology can be very complex. In the case of the CT scanner, modern advances in the fields of x-ray instrumentation, computers, and mathematics were all necessary to produce

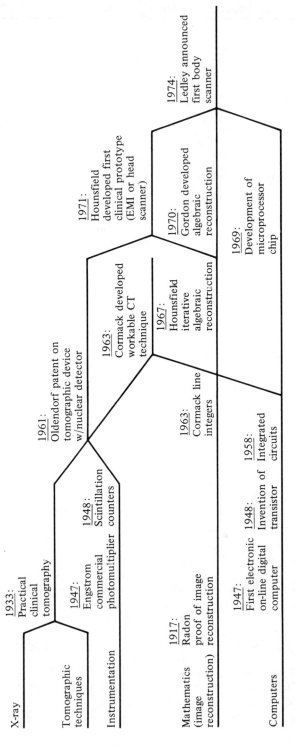

Figure 4. Development of the computed tomography (CT) scanner. (Modified from *Analysis of Selected Biomedical Research Programs*, vol. 2. Columbus, Ohio: Battelle Columbus Laboratories, 1976, p. K-9)

it (Battelle Columbus Laboratories 1976). In a broad sense, of course, the scanner's development depended on knowledge of human anatomy and physiology, physics, electronics, and so forth, which has developed over the centuries.

The CT scanner is a revolutionary diagnostic device that combines x-ray equipment with a computer and a cathode ray tube to produce images of cross sections of the human body (OTA 1978b, p. 3). The earliest x-ray films (and conventional x-ray films today) depended on the exposure of film to x-rays to measure the amount of radiation that passes through different parts of the body. Tomographic techniques, beginning with mechanical methods, overcame to some extent the two-dimensional nature of the x-ray and showed objects in a particular plane. William Oldendorf, a Los Angeles neurologist, first used a nuclear detector as part of a tomographic device (Henderson 1979). Simultaneously, instrumentation developed that made measurement of radiation easier. Mathematics made it possible to reconstruct images from large sets of data. In 1917, Radon showed that a two- or three-dimensional object can be uniquely reconstructed from the infinite set of all of its projections. However, producing the mathematical models capable of doing such reconstruction depended on the development of modern computers.

Cormack, a physicist, built the first workable CT instrument. However, his work received little attention from the medical community. Hounsfield, working in the Central Research Laboratory of EMI in London, developed a scanner that produced its first crude pictures in 1967. The British Department of Health and Social Security invested in the prototype instrument, which scanned only the head. The first one was used at Atkinson Morley Hospital in 1971. Results of the initial evaluations were reported in 1972, and the first commercial model was installed at the Mayo Clinic in the summer of 1973.

Shortly after the EMI scanner reached the market, Ledley at Georgetown University Medical Center announced the development of a CT body scanner, which was then marketed by Pfizer as the ACTA scanner. A number of companies scrambled to produce commercial CT scanners. In 1979, Cormack and Hounsfield were awarded the Nobel Prize in medicine for their work in developing the CT scanner.

## DESCRIPTION OF THE CT SCANNER

CT scanning builds on the principles of conventional x-ray films: Structures are differentiated by their ability to absorb energy from x-rays. The denser a structure is, the more energy it will absorb. Thus, less energy will reach the film or another receptor, and the image of that structure will be lighter. The CT scanner is similar, with a source of x-rays, a detector to determine how much energy passed through different parts of the body, a computer to collect, store, and process this data, and an imaging device to display the reconstruction of the part being scanned.

The first scanners took about 5 minutes to complete one scan. This is important because movement of patients or their internal organs can destroy the image. The earliest body scanners were hindered by this fact in attempting to depict the lungs and abdomen. However, most recent scanners produce an image in less than 5 seconds by using hundreds of contiguous detectors and a single x-ray fan beam. The CT scanner overcomes two shortcomings of conventional x-rays (Gordon, Herman, and Johnson 1975). First, in conventional x-rays, various organs overlap in the film and obscure each other. The CT scanner eliminates this problem. Second, conventional x-rays do not always differentiate between adjacent structures of similar density. CT scanning can make slight differences in density apparent. It is especially useful for visualizing soft, low-density tissues such as those in the brain. The most recent scanners can detect masses as small as 0.61 mm (OTA 1981, p. 60). They can thus locate tumors very early in their development.

The controversy stirred by the CT scanner has not concerned its technical merits. Clearly, it is a good technology. However, from the beginning, the rapidity of its diffusion and its expense made it a national policy issue in the United States.

## NUMBER OF CT SCANNERS

Figure 5 shows the diffusion of CT scanners in the United States from the first instrument installed in 1973 to May 1980, when 1,471 operational scanners existed in this country (OTA 1981, p. 60). At the end of 1974, only 45 scanners were in operation. At the end of 1976, the number had increased to 475. During 1977, about 40 scanners were installed per month. During 1978, however, the rate of installation fell by nearly half. In 1979 and the first 4 months of 1980, the rate fell a little more to about 17 scanners per month.

As of May 1980, all states had at least one scanner, although American Samoa, Guam, the Trust Territory of the Mariana Islands, and the Virgin Islands had none. The national average was about 6.7 scanners per million population. Washington, D.C., had the highest ratio, with 16.7 scanners per million population. States with high scanner/population ratios included Nevada (12.8), Florida (10.9), California (10.5), Missouri (9.4), North Dakota (9.1), Arizona (9.0), Nebraska (8.3), and New Mexico (8.0). States with the lowest scanner/population ratios included South Carolina (2.4), Rhode Island (3.3), Idaho (3.3), Delaware (3.4), Michigan (3.6), New Jersey (3.7), Kentucky (3.7), and Montana (3.8). Puerto Rico had only about 1.6 scanners per million population.

The number of scanners per million population is often used as a standard by which to compare scanner availability in the United States to that in other countries. Table 1 gives the number of CT scanners in the United States and in certain other industrialized countries early in 1979. These data reveal that the

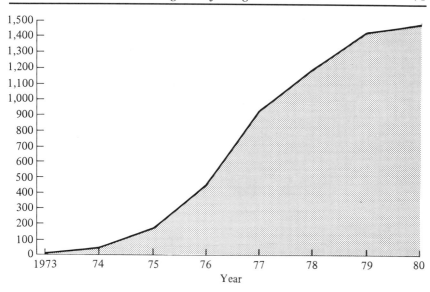

Figure 5. Cumulative number of CT scanners installed, 1973–80. (From Office of Technology Assessment, 1981)

Table 1. *Distribution of installed CT scanners, by country, 1979*

| Country[a] | Head | Body | Total | Scanners per million population |
|---|---|---|---|---|
| United States | 400 | 854 | 1,254 | 5.7 (Feb.) |
| Japan | 304 | 212 | 516 | 4.6 (Apr.) |
| West Germany | Unknown | Unknown | 160 | 2.6 (July) |
| Australia | 7 | 21 | 28 | 1.9 (Jan.) |
| Canada | 9 | 29 | 38 | 1.7 (May) |
| Sweden | 8 | 6 | 14 | 1.7 (Jan.) |
| Netherlands[b] | Unknown | Unknown | 20 | 1.4 (Jan.) |
| United Kingdom | 39 | 18 | 57 | 1.0 (Jan.) |
| France[c] | 20 | 10 | 30 | 0.6 (Jan.) |

[a]Ranked by scanners per million population in 1979.
[b]The Netherlands has planned to install 30 head scanners and 8 body scanners.
[c]In France, an additional 21 scanners were authorized in July 1979.
*Sources:* U.S. 1979 data: Office of Technology Assessment, U.S. Congress, *Policy Implications of the Computed Tomography (CT) Scanner: An Update,* GPO Stock No. 052-003-00793-2. Washington, D.C.: U.S. Government Printing Office, 1981. Canadian 1979 data: Health and Welfare Canada, unpublished data, 1979. Netherlands 1979 data: Ministry of Health and Environmental Protection, personal communication, 1980. Other 1979 data: H. D. Banta and K. B. Kemp, *The Management of Health Care Technology in Nine Countries.* New York: Springer, 1982, chaps. 2, 4–7, 9.

United States had the largest absolute number of CT scanners and the largest number per million population (Johnson 1978; OTA 1980). This information is not easy to interpret because the optimal number of scanners is not known. The United States also had the greatest number of other diagnostic technologies, such as conventional x-ray, and a larger number of surgeons per capita than countries such as Canada and the United Kingdom (Bunker 1970; Vayda 1973). In addition, by 1982 Japan had considerably more scanners per capita than the United States as a result of a large number of installations in 1980 and 1981.

In the United States, the crude scanner/population ratio is also misleading. Several of the states with high ratios are large, with a low population density. To assure reasonable access, these states must have a large number of scanners per population. Urban areas generally have more scanners, but one reason is that they generally contain large, specialized hospitals.

The United States is divided by the national health planning program into 203 Health Service Areas. By May 1980, only three of these areas had no CT scanner, and they were remote rural regions. Access throughout the country seems to be reasonably good. However, some areas, including the District of Columbia, have quite a large number of scanners per population.

In terms of institutional distribution, about 81 percent of scanners were in hospitals, and 18.9 percent were in private offices and clinics. The percentage of scanners in private offices has been relatively constant over time.

Of a total of 5,881 short-term general hospitals in the United States, 1,015, or 17.3 percent, had CT scanners in 1980. However, 48 percent of all hospitals had fewer than 100 beds, and another 24 percent had 100 to 199 beds. Of the 311 hospitals with more than 500 beds, 264, or 84.9 percent, had CT scanners. Seventy percent of the 243 hospitals with 400 to 499 beds had scanners, as did the almost 60 percent of those with 300 to 399 beds. Thus, coverage in the larger hospitals that tend to be more specialized and deal with sicker patients was fairly good. However, public hospitals tended not to have CT scanners. Of the 47 local government-supported hospitals with at least 500 beds, only 32 had CT scanners. Such large hospitals as Bellevue and Harlem Hospital in New York, D.C. General Hospital in Washington, D.C., and Cook County Hospital in Chicago did not have CT scanners.

Finally, it is interesting to consider the manufacturers of existing scanners. The CT scanner market has undergone dramatic changes since 1973, when EMI was the only company producing a commercial scanner. EMI dominated the U.S. and world markets through mid-1975 and made large profits on its head scanner. However, by May 1977, there were six other companies marketing CT scanners in the United States; by March 1978, 15 companies were selling them worldwide. Figure 6 shows the diffusion curve for CT scanners in the United States, including company names. One can readily see that by 1977, interest in the head scanner was falling, because buyers preferred the whole body scanner. Not only that, established x-ray equipment manufacturers such as General Electric had made significant inroads in the CT scanner market. The decline in scanner

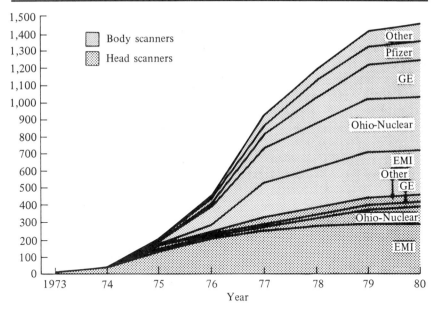

Figure 6. Cumulative number of CT scanners installed, by manufacturer. (From Office of Technology Assessment, 1981)

sales in 1977 and 1978 marked the end of the expansionary market, and companies paid the price for overestimating the size of the potential market. EMI had a $29.1 million profit in 1977, but lost almost $30 million in 1978 and 1979. EMI eventually was acquired by Thorn Electrical Industries, which divested itself of its EMI scanner business. Other companies that left the CT scanner field included Searle (ceased manufacture), Syntex (ceased manufacture), AS&E (sold out to Pfizer), Ohio-Nuclear (acquired by Johnson & Johnson), Neuroscan (ceased manufacture), Artronix (ceased manufacture), Varian (ceased manufacture), and Pfizer (ceased manufacture). A number of manufacturers had thus ample reason to regret ever having become involved in CT scanning. Since much of health technology development funding comes from private industry, this course of events may continue to have ripple effects for years to come.

### IMPLICATIONS OF THE DIFFUSION OF THE CT SCANNER

The diffusion of the CT scanner shown in Figure 6 has been more rapid than that of any modern medical technology that has been documented statistically. One comparison is provided by the spread of intensive care units in U.S. hospitals from 1960 to 1968. Their most rapid diffusion rate was slightly over 200 a year, or fewer than 20 per month, compared with an average of about 40 new scanners per month during 1977 (Russell 1978, pp. 49–51). The diffusion of nuclear medicine can also be compared with that of CT scanners. During the period

1952–69, it spread at a rate of fewer than 100 facilities per year, and at a rate of almost 200 facilities a year from 1969 to 1972 (Rapoport 1978).

The rapid dissemination of the CT scanner is particularly surprising considering its price. Early head scanners cost more than $300,000 and the latest body scanners up to $1 million. In 1978, the Office of Technology Assessment estimated that it would cost $276,000 to $468,000 a year to operate a CT scanner (OTA 1978b, p. 89, Table 20). Today that figure would have to be increased due to inflation. With more than 1,500 scanners, this country has made a capital investment in CT scanners on the order of $750 million, and spends around $1 billion a year on CT scanning.

Fees have generally been higher than the costs of CT scanning. Average fees in 1976 were between $240 and $260 for a head scan. A 1977 survey reported fees of $273 for a head scan and $286 for a body scan; fees of up to $476 for a head scan have been reported (Evens and Jost 1978; Johnson Associates 1976). Based on such figures, the Office of Technology Assessment estimated that average charges for CT examinations have exceeded estimated expenses by 39 to 229 percent (OTA 1978b, pp. 87–9). The estimated average profit in 1976 per scanner was between $51,000 and $292,000. These figures may be even higher today, although the volume of scans may have fallen, reducing revenues.

The rapidity of diffusion of the CT scanner was unfortunate because it prevented formal and detailed proof of its safety and efficacy (OTA 1978b, pp. 27–39). The available evidence did not come from well-designed, prospective clinical trials, but instead from analyses of clinical experiences. This evidence dealt almost entirely with diagnostic accuracy. Small attention was paid then, as now, to the effects of CT scanning on therapy planning or patient outcome (Abrams and McNeil 1978; OTA 1981, p. 28).

The CT scanner does have an important place in modern medicine. One study showed that the incidence of exploratory surgery in head injury was reduced sharply after the introduction of head scanning to Atkinson Morley Hospital in London (Ambrose and Gooding 1976). However, relatively few scans are done for head injury in this country. Most are performed for common conditions such as stroke, headaches, and cancer. One evaluation showed that CT scanning had little influence on either therapy or outcome for stroke patients (Larson, Omenn, and Loop 1978), but this fact has not lowered the rate of scanning by physicians of patients with stroke. Some reports indicate that as many as 20 percent of CT head scans are done for people with headache, but several well-designed studies show that virtually all patients with headache and a normal neurological examination have normal CT head scans.[1] The justifications for body scanning are even less thoroughly documented and harder to demonstrate. Many conditions affecting abdominal organs, additional organs to scan, and many alternative tests that might be as useful as CT scanning need to be compared. The most thoroughly documented use for CT body scans is radiation therapy for cancer, but apparently there has been no evaluation to show that it improves patient outcome.

Why did the CT scanner diffuse so rapidly? With its high cost, one would have expected some degree of caution. Although the early results were interesting, they did not seem to justify rapid spread for the purpose of saving lives or preventing the progress of disease. The reimbursement system amply rewarded those doing CT scans, so that profits for those who had the first scanners were considerable. The profit motive, however, does not seem to be an adequate explanation. Creditor and Garrett (1977) examined the scientific literature on CT scanning and compared it with the diffusion curve. They showed that rapid diffusion occurred well before the results of more than a few evaluations were available.

The remainder of this chapter deals with the research that has been done to explain the diffusion of medical technology, and thus shed light on questions such as those previously posed. Research results are not available in all cases to examine the factors related to CT scanner diffusion, but every relevant one will be stated. I will be speculative without trying to be overly cautious and scientific, and will use anecdotes where no scientific study is available. These speculations should be regarded as no more than that. The purpose of this chapter is to discuss diffusion, and not primarily the CT scanner. It will serve as a useful case in examining the rather theoretical sociological and economic literature on diffusion.

### COMMUNICATING INFORMATION ABOUT NEW MEDICAL TECHNOLOGY

Diffusion has two phases: the initial period, in which an individual or institution decides to *adopt* an innovation, and the subsequent period, encompassing the many decisions about how and how frequently to *use* it. Adoption has been studied far more thoroughly than use. Government attempts to channel technology have focused primarily on the adoption phase, as will become apparent later in this discussion. This is ironic, because the goal of public policy is to optimize the use of technology. However, it is much easier to control adoption than it is to influence use. Physicians are notoriously independent, and public and private policies have devised few effective mechanisms for changing their behavior.

One rarely used mechanism for changing both adoption and utilization is communication or education. Obviously, before adoption or rejection can occur, knowledge about a technology must be communicated to potential adopters. The literature on adoption describes it as occurring in stages (Rogers and Shoemaker 1971, p. 100; Kaluzny 1974):

1. Awareness, in which the potential adopter learns about the innovation and acquires some knowledge about it
2. Trial, in which the adopter is persuaded to think about or try out the innovation on a limited basis

3. Decision, in which the adopter decides to accept or reject the innovation in practice
4. Confirmation, in which the adopter seeks reinforcement for the decision

These stages have been called the *innovation–decision process* (Rogers and Shoemaker 1971, pp. 99–132). Research indicates that the factors influencing adoption of a new practice may be different at each stage. For example, Coleman, Katz, and Menzel (1966) found that commercial sources, such as direct mail and detail persons, were the sources of first knowledge about a drug, whereas professional sources, such as colleagues and medical journals, were dominant in the decision to try the drug. In practice, the critical distinction is between communications that inform adopters and those that persuade them to act.

The literature on drugs is fairly large,[2] and that on specific devices is growing.[3] In contrast, little is known about the communication or adoption of complex medical procedures that may not involve drugs or hardware. Likewise, little is known about how use is affected by communication. When an innovation is first adopted, many of its uses have not been demonstrated. The spread of information on these innovative uses has not been studied. This is a key factor for use of the technology.

Communication may be from multiple sources, including such broad channels as journal advertising and such narrow ones as face-to-face contact. Professional colleagues are potent influences on adoption, and professional face-to-face contact is the most effective influence on physician decisions to adopt.[4]

Little attention has been paid to the nature of the communication. Given the recent concern about medical technology, it would be useful to know if rejection of a technology is influenced in the same way as acceptance. The literature sheds little light on this question. Some reports suggest that new practices are adopted more rapidly than old ones are discarded.[5] Many articles report that the results of controlled clinical trials failed to influence practice.[6] It appears that a colleague's anecdote may often be a more important influence than professional literature.

The source of communication is also a key issue. Some physicians behave differently than others. This issue will be discussed later. The adoption process also differs if the adopting unit is an institution rather than an individual. This issue will also be discussed later.

Little direct attention has been paid to the CT scanner. Only 13 papers had been published on head scanning by June 1975, at which time almost 100 scanners had been installed (Creditor and Garrett 1977). This indicates how little influence the published literature may have. In the case of the scanner, initial evaluation results were reported in international meetings in Japan in 1972. Radiologists from the Mayo Clinic and the Massachusetts General Hospital, which acquired the first two scanners in the United States, attended the meeting and shortly afterward ordered scanners. This indicates that the published literature was probably of little importance in the scanner's early diffusion. There is a lag of at least a year in the publication of scientific articles. Although the scientific literature is the ultimate repository of scientific knowledge, it cannot be expected to have much influence in the early diffusion of an exciting innovation. In addition to the scientific papers presented at meetings, exhibits and face-to-face contact with colleagues provide opportunities for potential adopters to learn about innovations and begin to make adoption decisions (Gempel and Metzger 1977).

There is little literature concerning equipment sales representatives and their influence. However, all large companies making medical devices have many sales representatives who visit every good-sized hospital periodically. General Electric is the largest manufacturer of radiological equipment in the United States. Not surprisingly, when this company produced a scanner, it quickly became dominant in the market.

FACTORS INFLUENCING ADOPTION OF MEDICAL TECHNOLOGY

### Characteristics of the technology

Most of the literature on medical technology assumes that any adoption must be desirable and examines factors that hasten it. Such factors as advantage over previous methods, compatibility with the adopter's values, complexity of the technology, and observability or visibility of the results to others have been described (Tanon and Rogers 1975).

The CT scanner has many characteristics that would be expected to speed diffusion. Compared to its alternatives, such as pneumoencephalograms, CT scanning reduces the patient's discomfort and risk, as well as the physician's inconvenience. The scanner uses x-rays, a modality familiar to radiologists and technicians. (Ultrasound, which has some advantages over CT scanning, has been adopted much more slowly, apparently because of its unfamiliarity and difficulty of operation.) The results of CT scanning are striking and rather easy to interpret. Head scans, in particular, produce images of the brain that give information previously unobtainable without exploratory surgery.

### Characteristics of the adopter

Studies of individual adopters have focused on physicians and their acceptance of new drugs. Some studies have found that physicians who have a higher level of training and participate more actively in their medical community more readily adopted a new drug, whereas others have found little correlation (Tanon and Rogers 1975). These inconsistent results may be related to the appropriateness of the drugs studied. Researchers have paid little attention to this variable, but physicians, faced with a drug whose value they doubted, may have exercised prudence. The previously cited case of desperation also influences acceptance of a new drug.

Within organizations, adoption has generally been associated with practitioners and administrators with a higher level of training and a more cosmopolitan outlook (Kaluzny, Barhyte, and Reader 1975; Greer 1977). Decision making within organizations is spread among subgroups with differing interests.

All researchers agree that physicians are key decision makers. However, not all researchers agree on the role of physicians. Some have portrayed physicians as medically conservative, resistant to change, and skeptical of innovation (Coleman, Katz, and Menzel 1966, pp. 11, 12; Stross and Harlan 1979). Others have stressed physician dominance in the formulation of hospital policies as explaining their decision-making processes.[7] Harris (1977) stated that conflict among physicians is resolved not by strategic bargaining but by an agreement to expand the overall capacity and adopt innovations. Cromwell et al. (1975, pp. 197, 225, 227) hypothesized that administrators seek sophisticated equipment because it both raises the hospital's prestige and attracts physician specialists to the staff. They found adoption to be greater in states with more physicians per capita and more specialists per physician. Recent analyses have tended to assume that hospitals must cater to physicians' desire for new technology.[8]

These conflicting results and views are confusing. Greer's (1981) study of technology adoption in 25 voluntary hospitals in Milwaukee seems to shed light on this issue. She found that the assumption that all physicians are the same is false, and classified physicians as follows: (1) community physicians, concerned primarily with patients seen in private offices; (2) community specialists, who are largely office based, but who emphasize a specialty oriented to hospital services and technologies; (3) referral physicians, who restrict their practice to specialized procedures and are very dependent on the hospital; and (4) hospital-based physicians, who are entirely dependent on the hospital and typically have no private patients. Radiologists are members of the last group. Hospital-based physicians are very dependent on technology, readily accept new technology, and because of their proximity, and commitment to a particular hospital, greatly influence decision making in hospitals. After acquiring a new technology, they "sell" it to their practitioner colleagues. Greer's work conveys a sense of how the diffusion of new technology actually occurs, and may become the basis for new policy approaches to managing technology. Clearly, it is very applicable to CT scanners.

The role of the administrator in these decisions has also grown as hospitals have become larger and complex (Perrow 1972; Scott 1972). Greer (1981) confirmed the importance of the administrator. Administrators, like physicians, are a diverse group. Some are eager to acquire new technology, whereas others are more conservative. Clearly, the ability of administrators to influence hospital decisions increases as the organization and its environment become more complex. This finding is related to research on the structure of the institution.

Greater adoption of technology has been found in acute care hospitals (Kaluzny, Barhyte, and Reader 1975, pp. 29–43). Complexity, size, medical school affiliation, and diversity of tasks have all been found to be associated with greater adoption.[9] Because size is correlated with variables such as medical school affiliation and financial and personnel resources, the independent effect of each is unclear. These findings clearly are consistent with the data on CT scanners, which diffused first into larger hospitals.

With few exceptions, studies of organizational adoption of medical technologies have been confined to hospitals. Ambulatory care practices, whether solo physicians' offices or group practices, have received little attention. Health planning laws have generally excluded out-of-hospital settings from control. Yet technology is moving rapidly into physicians' offices, as indicated by the case of the gastrointestinal endoscope (Showstack and Schroeder 1981). As noted earlier, almost 19 percent of CT scanners are found in out-of-hospital settings

Group practices, particularly health maintenance organizations (HMOs) have stimulated national interest in recent years because of their potential ability to deliver medical care at lower cost (Fein 1967; Willems 1979). The purchase of a CT scanner by the Kaiser-Permanente health plan in northern California suggests that HMOs do acquire technology differently (Banta, Behney, and Willems 1981). In 1976, when Kaiser-Permanente decided to buy a scanner for its 1.3 million members, the state of California already had 60 scanners, with 2.8 per million population. Kaiser purchased its scanner only after its analysis indicated that performing its own scans would be less costly than doing them at an outside facility.

## Characteristics of the environment

Researchers who have studied technology adoption have stressed the importance of external factors such as financing methods, market conditions, and government programs.[10] An important part of the environment that has received little stress is patient need or demand (White 1974, 1975). Research has found little relationship between, for example, the incidence of disease and the adoption of relevant technology (Ginsberg 1972; Russell 1978, p. 127).

Economists have tended to attribute increases in medical technology and medical expenditures to the growth of third-party payment (Feldstein and Taylor 1977; Russell 1978, p. 127). Adoption of expensive technologies is fostered because third parties pay more than 90 percent of all hospital expenditures (National Center for Health Statistics 1978). The methods of payment, cost reimbursement to hospitals, and fee-for-service payments to physicians tend to foster acceptance of new technology. As indicated earlier in regard to the CT scanner, large profits are often built into reimbursement for new high-technology services. Research has confirmed that third-party payment stimulates technology adoption. Cromwell and his associates (1975, p. 229) found that the percentage of revenues from third-party payors was significantly and positively related to hospital adoption of expensive technology. Russell (1978, pp. 97, 128) found that the adoption of cobalt therapy and electroencephalography occurred more quickly in hospitals where the level of insurance coverage was higher and proceeded more rapidly as the level grew. As Medicare's contribution to a hospital's total costs rose, so did the adoption of cobalt therapy, intensive care beds, and diagnostic radioisotopes.

The nature of the market for hospital services may influence adoption. Russell (1978, p. 128) found that the concentration of market power in a few large hospitals did not appear to influence the adoption of a number of technologies, but that hospitals in more concentrated markets were less likely to adopt open heart surgery. Prior adoption of a technology in a locality was found to speed the adoption of intensive care units and electroencephalograms, but not other expensive technologies (Cromwell et al. 1975, p. 212; Russell 1978, p. 128). Although nothing definitive can be said about CT scanners, their concentration in large cities with several large hospitals is noteworthy. Competition among hospitals may be an important factor in the adoption of CT scanning.

With rising concerns about efficacy, safety, and costs, the federal government has created a number of programs designed to rationalize the development, evaluation, and adoption of expensive technologies such as the CT scanner. One is the Food and Drug Administration's Bureau of Medical Devices, established by law in 1976 to regulate the marketing of devices to assure efficacy and safety. The CT scanner is subject to performance standards under this legislation. The effects of this program on diffusion of technologies has not been studied, but it can be safely predicted that a regulatory program requiring prior evaluation of technology will slow diffusion (Schifrin and Tayan 1977).

The other major federal program regulates capital investment through health planning. Legislation passed in 1974 requires all states to have a certificate-of-need (CON) program that requires prior approval of institutional capital investment, including CT scanners. In an early study of CON laws, Salkever and Bice (1976, 1979) found reduced hospital expenditures on beds but unchanged overall hospital investment. Faced with greater control over beds, hospitals apparently channeled their investment to other technologies. Cromwell et al. (1975, pp. 188, 195) found that CON appeared to reduce adoption rates for expensive, widely adopted technologies, such as x-rays and cobalt and radium therapies, but did not affect other technologies examined. Planning legislation was not correlated with interstate differences in the adoption of CT scanners (Willems et al., 1979, pp. 116–43). In fact, impending legislation may have spurred adoption as providers rushed to place orders for scanners before laws came into effect. Such an effect may have occurred in California, for example, whose 1976 law exempted equipment already ordered (Banta 1980). In addition, it seems clear that CON, which generally excludes physicians' offices, fostered the purchase of scanners for that setting (OTA 1978b, p. 35). A particular problem faced by health planners in dealing with CT scanning, and a problem common to all new technology, was the lack of good data on efficacy and safety at the time that institutions wished to purchase scanners.

States have also attempted to control cost increases. A number of states have developed programs of prospective reimbursement or rate regulation, in which rates of payment are set in advance of the time period in which they will apply.

The theory is that if revenue is limited and choice among technologies is necessary, physicians and hospitals might reduce or forgo the use of technologies that have low marginal efficacy, that duplicate others, or that have less costly alternatives (Banta, Behney, and Willems 1981, p. 129). The effect on technology use of prospective reimbursement to hospitals has been conflicting (Applied Management Sciences 1978; Dowling et al. 1978), perhaps reflecting different forms of prospective reimbursement. Recent analyses, however, indicate that rate regulation has moderated cost increases in states with strong programs.[11]

A recent project has examined the general effects of regulation on hospital behavior (Urban and Bice 1981). The investigators developed an index of regulatory intensity because existing research papers on the subject examine single regulatory programs and ignore possible joint effects. The project found that price regulation, as conducted in a number of rate review programs, was the most powerful determinant of hospital behavior. The project looked specifically at the diffusion and distribution of CT scanners. The CON program was found to have essentially no effect on their diffusion and distribution. On the other hand, rate review did have a marked effect on the number and distribution of scanners.

A similar project examined the effects of different factors, including CON and rate review (Joskow 1981). Only rate regulation was found clearly to affect the diffusion of CT scanners. On average, the presence of rate regulation in a state was found to reduce the number of CT scanners by about 20 percent. There was little evidence of the effect of CON on the number of CT scanners. However, both rate review and CON apparently led to a substitution of office-based for hospital-based CT scanners.

### FACTORS INFLUENCING USE OF TECHNOLOGY

One reason for separating adoption and use is that no general relationship between them has been observed. Obviously, technology must be acquired to be used. However, adopted technologies are used at very different rates. It has been found that hospital beds tend to be filled regardless of health problems or the nature of an area (Roemer and Shain 1959). It appears that the ready availability of clinical laboratory tests has stimulated a rapid increase in the number done (OTA 1976, p. 11), and the large number of surgeons per capita in this country is associated with high rates of surgery (Bunker 1970; Vayda 1973). Although availability increases use, the amount of use generated is not clear. Cromwell and colleagues (1975, p. 225) found that Massachusetts hospitals used certain diagnostic equipment at only 50 to 60 percent of capacity. It seems clear that the use of operational CT scanners is considerably below capacity (OTA 1978b, p. 19). In addition, use varies remarkably. Wennberg and Gittelsohn (1973) found that the rates of common surgical procedures such as tonsillectomy, hysterectomy, and appendectomy in similar areas in New England vary by as much as 300 to 400 percent. Overall, as in the case of adoption, little relationship has been found between patient needs and the use of technology.

### The physician and use of technology

The physician has a high degree of autonomy. One of the attributes of any professional group is control over its technology (Smith and Kaluzny 1975). This makes it difficult to affect the group's use of technology.

Traditionally, the physician acts as the patient's agent. The physician's role is to defend the patient's interest against competing ones, such as cost containment (Mechanic 1977). The "social contract" binds physicians to provide the best possible care, apparently regardless of cost (Arrow 1963). The patient with full insurance coverage pays little for care, and the physician has little immediate reason to be concerned about the cost of technology.

The growth of specialties is strongly related to at least some technologies. Specialties such as radiology have developed because of technology. As mentioned earlier, radiologists have led the way in the adoption of CT scanning and have sold it to their clinical colleagues. The literature generally confirms a strong relationship between specialization and increasing use of technology (Banta, Behney, and Willems 1981, pp. 78–80). In part, this is because of the nature of training, with its emphasis on acute disease and specialized hospital care (Mechanic 1972).

Malpractice is frequently cited as a determinant of the use of technology (Committee on Technology and Health Care, Institute of Medicine 1979). Once the use of a technology has become part of accepted medical practice, physicians and hospitals often feel compelled to provide it routinely. Fear of malpractice seems to be associated particularly with the use of diagnostic technologies such as skull x-rays (Bell and Loop 1979) and clinical laboratory testing (Schroeder and Showstack 1979). Malpractice suits have been brought against Washington, D.C., and California hospitals without scanners.

Industry promotion, as mentioned previously, is a reason for the use of technology. Industry spends a great deal of money on both advertising and direct face-to-face contact with physicians and administrators (Silverman and Lee 1974; Banta, Behney, and Willems 1981, pp. 31–2). However, it is important to remember that information communicated by the industry appears to be more effective in developing awareness than it is in influencing adoption (and perhaps use).

A growing factor in the use of technology is the form of medical practice. Few reports specifically discuss the use of technology. Literature on the adoption of technology by hospitals and HMOs has already been reviewed. Most of the literature on use deals with HMOs. It has been demonstrated that HMOs have lower hospitalization rates than the population as a whole (Perrott 1971; Luft 1978). Surgery rates have also been found to be lower in some cases (Donabedian 1965; Luft 1982). The literature on diagnostic services is contradictory. For example, one study found radiological use to be lower in a hospital-based capitation group than in solo fee-for-service practices, but laboratory use to be higher (Diehr et al. 1976). Despite these contradictions, HMOs are seen as having great theoretical advantages in an era of limited resources. However, the physician's commitment to serving the best interests of the patient may conflict with the rationing and control of resources imposed by organizations. Care must be taken to ensure that the bureaucratization of medicine does not lead to a loss of many of the best features of health care.

Finally, as with adoption, the common methods of paying providers for services facilitate, if they do not encourage, the use of additional services because providers can increase the revenues by ordering more services. Payment methods also affect the distribution of services among different types of technologies. Fee scales reward the physician less generously for taking a patient's history, conducting a physical examination, or providing counsel than for using technology (Schroeder and Showstack 1978). Earlier in this chapter, data were presented to show the large profits associated with CT scanning, especially early in its diffusion and use.

A consensus exists that third-party coverage of care has increased the use of and expenditures on medical technology (Feldstein and Taylor 1977; Russell 1978). The spectacular rise in the use of ancillary services provided by hospital-based physicians, including radiologists and pathologists, is related to specialization, payment method, and third-party coverage. From 1968 to 1971, more intense use of nine such medical services accounted for about 40 percent of the increase in hospital operating costs (Redish 1974). Hospital-based physicians receive higher incomes from a greater volume of services, but their incomes are generally unrelated to the expense of providing them. Third-party payors readily pay for the services. And as indicated previously, hospital-based physicians appear to have extra leverage over hospital purchases of technology such as CT scanners.

This issue probably will be the focus of public attempts to control medical care expenditures. The payment system, which seems to contribute to the rapid diffusion of new technology, also appears to offer the main hope for control. The present system of care in the United States is composed largely of independent private parties, whereas the payment mechanism is largely collective, with a strong federal government role. Federal government attempts to reduce inflation in medical care costs have until now been largely regulatory, for example, the health planning program. These programs have failed to control costs. Regulating the reimbursement system or using it more actively to channel technology appears to offer more promise. One innovative effort just initiated was legislation, effective in October 1983, that changed the method of reimbursement to hospitals under the Medicare program. There is now in place a prospective payment system in which rates of payment for given illnesses are based on categories in which they fall called diagnostic related groups (DRG). Its explicit aim is to control costs and the use of technology.

Another public attempt to rationalize the use of technology is the Professional Standards Review Organization (PSRO) program. Established by a 1972 federal statute, PSROs are decentralized, physician-controlled organizations that review hospital-based care provided under the Medicare and Medicaid programs to assure its appropriateness. The program has focused on the use of beds and has affected their use (Congressional Budget Office 1979). Some PSROs have also reviewed the use of CT scanning services (OTA 1978b, pp. 37–8). This program, which has had little influence and may be phased out in the next several years, will not be discussed further.

### CAUSES OF THE RAPID DIFFUSION OF CT SCANNERS

Although little of the research cited deals explicitly with CT scanning, one can draw some tentative conclusions on why this technology diffused rapidly and in specific patterns. As noted, CT scanning was unquestionably an exciting technology that allowed physicians to do things that could not be done before. Radiologists were familiar with the interpretation of images, so that the technology fit in with existing practice and skills. As one would expect, the scanners went first to large, university-affiliated hospitals. Similarly, smaller hospitals that accepted the scanner early had staff or administrators who were interested in fostering new technology. Since the acquisition of CT scanning was promoted aggressively by influential hospital-based physicians, it had advantages over many other potential investments such as operating room technology. Fees for CT scanning were generous; indeed, large profits were obtained by the technologists involved. The only national program to constrain the use of CT scanners was the health planning program, which was politically weak, understaffed, and poorly financed. Fear of malpractice suits fostered the acquisition and use of scanners – increasingly as time went on. Industry was actively involved in the promotion of scanning and in arguing against government attempts to regulate it. In fact, the only restraint on the diffusion of scanners appears to be the state rate review programs. Which factors were predominant is impossible to say. Noteworthy, however, are the many factors facilitating diffusion.

### COMPETITORS OF THE CT SCANNER

When the CT scanner entered the market, it had no competitor capable of producing comparable images of the brain. This was not true of the body scanner. Multiple diagnostic tests were available for use in the abdomen, chest, and extremities. This has made the ultimate value of body scanning doubtful, even without the presence of direct competitors. Indeed, some new imaging techniques under development may ultimately displace the CT scanner entirely.

Widely used technologies in the imaging field include, in addition to CT scanning, conventional x-ray films, radionuclide scanning, and medical ultrasound. Emerging technologies include nuclear magnetic resonance (NMR) and

Table 2. *Overview of diagnostic imaging in the United States, 1977 and 1980*

| | Number of hospitals with capability | Number of procedures (millions) | | Costs (millions) | |
|---|---|---|---|---|---|
| | | 1977 | 1980 | 1977 | 1980 |
| Diagnostic x-ray | 7,000 | 158 | 171 | $5,300 | $7,600 |
| CT scanning | 1,000 | 1–1.4 | 3–4 | 300 | 875 |
| Nuclear medicine | 3,300 | 8.2 | 11.1 | 800 | 1,250 |
| Ultrasound | All | Approximately 4 | | NA | 360 |

*Note:* Estimates are approximate, for illustration only.
*Source:* Office of Technology Assessment, U.S. Congress: *Policy Implications of the Computed Tomography (CT) Scanner; An Update.* Washington, D.C.: U.S. Government Printing Office, 1981, p. 59.

positron emission transaxial tomography (PETT) scanning. Since all of these technologies produce images of the internal organs and body parts, it is difficult to determine when each is necessary; this problem will increase.

Radionuclide scanning involves the injection or ingestion of a radiopharmaceutical (a radioactive substance), the passage of time to allow the substance to disseminate widely or to concentrate in a particular organ or part of the body, and the detection of radioactivity by an external detector, usually a gamma scintillation camera. As shown in Table 2, radionuclide scanning is a rapidly developing field in medical diagnosis. It is finding new applications, for example, in scanning the heart and coronary arteries. An estimated 227,000 cardiac scans were performed in the United States in 1978, and a projected 1.5 million were performed in 1981 (Stason and Fortress 1982).

The use of ultrasound is growing even faster than that of radionuclide scanning. This technology involves the use of sound waves, which are thought to eliminate the risk of x-rays or radioactivity. Its major limitation is that it cannot penetrate bone or gas, and thus cannot be used to image the adult brain, the lungs, or structures surrounded by gas-filled bowel. However, ultrasound is finding many applications in areas of the body such as the abdomen, eye, breast, and coronary arteries. Ultrasound presents a particular problem because it is less expensive than other imaging technologies. This has helped lead to a possibly excessive proliferation in clinical settings such as obstetrics, ophthalmology, pediatrics, and neurology wards and practices. Other diagnostic imaging technologies are generally under the control of radiologists, and thus are to some extent in competition with each other.

It is difficult to argue against the search for a good diagnosis. It is also difficult to argue against the sequential use of a series of diagnostic tests without good research on the optimal path to a diagnosis. This problem will be compounded when the new technologies begin to diffuse rapidly. PETT scanning is an application of radionuclide scanning plus tomography techniques. It is a computer-controlled unit that maps the distribution of positron-emitting pharmaceuticals in order to construct detailed images of organ metabolism, physiology, and function. The present cost of a scanner and its associated equipment is as high as $2 million. There are presently more than 20 experimental units in the world, half of which are located in the United States (OTA 1978b, pp. 63–4).

NMR tomography uses a magnetic field and measures the resulting behavior of hydrogen nuclei in the body. A computer generates the images. This technology may provide metabolic information that is not now available. Presently, NMR tomography is an experimental technique with prototype machines being tested in a number of places in the United States and other countries. Many companies are interested in producing and marketing NMR scanners (OTA 1978b, pp. 64–6; OTA 1983).

## SUMMARY AND CONCLUSIONS

The case of the CT scanner is instructive in examining the diffusion of medical technology. This chapter in no way implies that the CT scanner should not have come rapidly into use. The fact that it was not carefully evaluated before being widely diffused is the norm for the United States. However, the CT scanner was actually evaluated more carefully than usual because of the attention it received.

The scanner illustrates very nicely many of the factors related to the diffusion of technology. In part because of strong financial incentives, technology tends to be adopted quickly in medical care, leading to rapid diffusion and insufficient time for evaluation. The result is that specific indications for the use of technology are seldom known. The problem is compounded by the small investment in technology evaluation made by the federal government (OTA 1978a). Although the CT scanner is not a typical medical technology, its visibility has made it useful for better understanding the factors that facilitate and impede the diffusion of medical technology. In addition, the possible policy approaches outlined in this chapter have been tested most specifically with the CT scanner. The approaches that so far appear to be successful are likely to dominate health care policy making in regard to medical technology in the years to come.

## NOTES

Readers should refer to the selected bibliography for complete references.

1 Alderson, Mikhael, Coleman, et al. 1976; Carerra, Gerson, Schnur et al. 1977; OTA 1978b.

2 Caplow and Raymond 1954; Worthen 1973; Christensen and Wertheimer 1979; Manning and Denson 1979.

3 Darrow and Bradford 1977; Bunker, Hinkley, and McDermott 1978; Fineberg, Gabel, and Sosman 1978; Russell 1978; Fineberg 1979; Manning and Denson 1979; Banta 1980.

4 Caplow and Raymond 1954; Menzel and Katz 1955–6; Coleman, Katz, and Menzel 1966; Worthen 1973; Inui, Yourtee, and Williamson 1976; Christensen and Wertheimer 1979.

**5** Chalmers 1974; Warner 1977; Fineberg and Hiatt 1979.

**6** Chalmers 1974; Bunker, Hinkley, and McDermott 1978; Banta and Thacker 1979; Fineberg and Hiatt 1979.

**7** Goss 1963; Perrow 1963; Freidson 1970; Gordon 1970; Smith 1979; Guest 1972.

**8** Lee 1971; Committee on Technology and Health Care 1979; Shroeder and Showstack 1979.

**9** Cromwell, Ginsberg, Hamilton, et al. 1975; Kaluzny, Barhyte, and Reader 1975; Russell 1976; Greer 1977; Rapoport 1978.

**10** Warner 1974; Gordon and Fisher 1975; Committee on Technology and Health Care 1979.

**11** Cromwell 1976; Biles, Schramm, and Atkinson 1980; General Accounting Office 1980; Melnick, Wheeler, and Felstein 1981.

SELECTED BIBLIOGRAPHY

Abrams, H., and McNeil, B. (1978). Medical implications of computed tomography ("CT scanning"). *N. Eng. J. Med.* 298:255–61, 310–18.
Alderson, P. L., Mikhael, M., Coleman, R.E., et al. (1976). Optimal utilization of computerized cranial tomography and radionuclide brain imaging. *Neurology 26*:803–15.
Ambrose, J., and Gooding, M. R. (1976). E.M.I. scan in the management of head injuries. *Lancet 1*:847–9.
Applied Management Sciences. (1975). *Analysis of Prospective Reimbursement Systems: Western Pennsylvania.* Prepared for the Office of Research and Statistics, Department of Health, Education, and Welfare, 1975. Quoted in J. Wagner: *Impact of Hospital Reimbursement Policy.* Project Proposal to the Health Care Financing Administration, Grant 18-P-97113/3-01, 1978.
Arrow, K. (1963). Uncertainty and the welfare economics of medical care. *Am. Economic Rev. 53*:941–73.
Banta, H. D. (1980). The diffusion of the computed tomography (CT) scanner in the United States. *Int. J. Health Serv. 10*:251–69.
Banta, H. D., Behney, C. J., and Willems, J. S. (1981). *Toward Rational Technology in Medicine.* New York: Springer, pp. 53–7.
Banta, H. D., and Thacker, S. (1979). Assessing the costs and benefits of electronic fetal monitoring. *Obstet. Gynecol. Survey 34*(suppl):627–42.
Battelle Columbus Laboratories. (1976). *Analysis of Selected Biomedical Research Programs. Volume II. Appendixes. Case Histories.* Columbus, Ohio, pp. K2–K6.
Bell, R., and Loop, J. (1971). The utility and futility of radiographic skull examination for trauma. *N. Engl. J. Med. 284*:236–9.
Biles, B., Schramm, C. J., and Atkinson, J. G. (1980). Hospital cost inflation under state rate setting. *N. Engl. J. Med. 303*:664–8.
Bunker, J. P. (1970). Surgical manpower. *N. Engl. J. Med. 282*:135–9.
Bunker, J. P., Hinkley, D., and McDermott, W. V. (1978). Surgical innovation and its evaluation. *Science 200*:937–41.
Caplow, T., and Raymond, J. J. (1954). Factors influencing the selection of pharmacy products. *J. Marketing 19*:18–23.
Carerra, G. F., Gerson, D. E., Schnur, J., et al. (1977). Computed tomography of the brain in patients with headache or temporal lobe epilepsy: findings and cost–effectiveness. *J. Comput. Assist. Tomogr. 1*:1–4.

Chalmers, T. C. (1974). The impact of controlled trials on the practice of medicine. *Mt. Sinai J. Med.* *41*:753–9.

Christensen, D. B., and Wertheimer, A. I. (1979). Source of information and influence on new drug prescribing among physicians in an HMO. *Social Sci. Med.* *13A*:313–22.

Coleman, J. S., Katz, E., and Menzel, H. (1966). *Medical Innovation: A Diffusion Study.* Indianapolis: Bobbs-Merrill, pp. 11–12, 59–60.

Committee on Technology and Health Care, Institute of Medicine. (1979). *Medical Technology and the Health Care System.* Washington, D.C.: National Academy of Sciences.

Congressional Budget Office. (1979). *The Effects of PSROs on Health Care Costs: Current Findings and Future Evaluations.* Washington, D.C.: U.S. Congress.

Creditor, M. C., and Garrett, J. B. (1977). The information base for diffusion of technology: computed tomography scanning. *N. Engl. J. Med.* *297*:49–52.

Cromwell, J. (1976). The impact of rate regulation on the diffusion of new technologies in hospitals. Discussion paper. Cambridge, Mass.: Abt Associates.

Cromwell, J., Ginsberg, P., Hamilton, D., et al. (1975). *Incentives and Decisions Underlying Hospitals' Adoption of Major Capital Equipment.* Cambridge, Mass.: ABT Associates, pp. 197, 225, 227.

Darrow, W. W., and Bradford, W. R. (1977). Adoption of Thayer-Martin culture medium by physicians in office-based practice. *Sexually Trans. Dis.* *4*:144–9.

Diehr, P., Richardson, W. C., Drucker, W. L., et al. (1976). Utilization: ambulatory and hospital. In *The Seattle Prepaid Health Care Project: Comparison of Health Services Delivery.* Seattle: University of Washington. Quoted in H. Luft, Why do HMO's seem to provide more health maintenance services? *MMFQ/Health Soc.* *56*:140, 1978.

Donabedian, A. (1965). *A Review of Some Experiences with Prepaid Group Practice.* Research Series No. 12. Ann Arbor: School of Public Health, University of Michigan.

Dowling, W., House, P., Lehman, J. M., et al. (1976). Prospective reimbursement in downstate New York and its impact in hospitals—a summary. Seattle: University of Washington. Quoted in J. Wagner: *Impact of Hospital Reimbursement Policy.* Project Proposal to the Health Care Financing Administration, Grant 18-P-97113/3-01, 1978.

Evans, R. G., and Jost, R. G. (1978). Economic analysis of body computed tomography units including data on utilization. *Radiology* *127*:151–5.

Fein, R. (1967). *The Doctor Shortage: An Economic Diagnosis.* Washington, D.C.: Brookings Institution.

Feldstein, M., and Taylor, A. (1977). *The Rapid Rise of Hospital Costs.* Washington, D.C.: President's Council on Wage and Price Stability.

Ferber, R., and Wales, H. G. (1958). *The Effectiveness of Pharmaceutical Promotion.* Urbana, Ill.: University of Illinois.

Fineberg, H. V. (1979). Gastric freezing—a study of diffusion of a medical innovation. In Committee on Technology and Health Care, *Medical Technology and the Health Care System.* Washington, D.C.: National Academy of Sciences, pp. 173-200.

Fineberg, H. V., Gabel, R. A., and Sosman, M. B. (1978). Acquisition and application of new medical knowledge by anesthesiologists: three recent examples. *Anesthesiology* *48*:430–6.

Fineberg, H. V., and Hiatt, H. H. (1979). Evaluation of medical practices: the case for technology assessment. *N. Engl. J. Med.* *301*:1086–91.

Freidson, E. (1970). *Professional Dominance: The Social Structure of Medical Care.* Chicago: Aldine.

Gempel, P. A., and Metzger, J. B. (1977). *Body Computerized Tomography (CT), Review of Clinical Experience.* Cambridge, Mass.: Arthur D. Little.

General Accounting Office. (1980). *Rising Hospital Costs Can Be Restrained by Regulating Payments and Improving Management.* Washington, D.C.: U.S. Government Printing Office, Sept. 19.

Ginsberg, P. (1972). Resource allocation in the hospital industry: the role of capital financing. *Social Security Bul. 35*:20–30.

Gordon, G., and Fisher, G. L. (1975). *The Diffusion of Medical Technology.* Cambridge, Mass.: Ballinger.

Gordon, P. J. (1970). The top management triangle in voluntary hospitals, I and II. *J. Acad. Management 4*:205–14; *5*:65–75.

Gordon, R., Herman, G. T., and Johnson, S. A. (1975). Image reconstruction from projections. *Sci. Am. 233*:56–68.

Goss, M. E. W. (1963). Patterns of bureaucracy among hospital staff physicians. In *The Hospital in Modern Society*, E. Freidson, ed. New York: Free Press, pp. 170–94.

Greer, A. L. (1977). Advances in the study of diffusion and innovations in health care organizations. *MMFQ/Health Soc. 55*:505–32.

Greer, A. L. (1981). Deus ex machina: physicians in the adoption of hospital medical technology (manuscript). Milwaukee: Urban Research Center, The University of Wisconsin–Milwaukee.

Guest, R. H. (1972). The role of the doctor in institutional management. In *Organization Research on Health Institutions*, B. S. Georgopoulos, ed. Ann Arbor, Mich.: Institute for Social Research.

Harris, J. (1977). The internal organization of hospitals: some economic implications. *Bell J. Economics 8*:467–82.

Henderson, H. (1979). A sideways look at scanners. *New Scientist 84*:782–5.

Inui, T. L., Yourtee, E. L., and Williamson, J. W. (1976). Improved outcomes in hypertension after physician tutorials: a controlled trial. *Ann. Intern. Med. 84*:646–51.

J. Lloyd Johnson Associates. (1976). *The Demand for Computed Tomography and Impact on Diagnostic Imaging Market.* Northfield, Ill., p. 43.

Jonsson, E. (1978). Letter. *N. Engl. J. Med. 229*:655.

Joskow, P. L. (1981). *Controlling Hospitals Costs: The Role of Government Regulation.* Cambridge, Mass.: MIT Press, pp. 162–8.

Kaluzny, A. D. (1974). Innovation in health services: theoretical framework and review of research. *Health Serv. Res. 9*:101–20.

Kaluzny, A. D., Barhyte, D. Y., and Reader, G. G. (1975). Health systems. In *The Diffusion of Medical Technology* G. Gordon and L. Fisher, eds. Cambridge, Mass: Ballinger, pp. 29–43.

Larson, E. B., Omenn, G. S., and Loop, J. W. (1978). Computed tomography of the brain in patients with cerebrovascular disease: impact of a new technology on patient care. *Am. J. Roentgenol. 131*:35–40.

Lee, M. L. (1971). A conspicuous productions theory of hospital behavior. *South. Econ. J. 38*:48–58.

Luft, H. (1978). HMO's and medical costs: the rhetoric and the evidence. *N. Engl. J. Med. 298*:1336–43.

Luft, H. S. (1982). Health Maintenance Organizations and the Rationing of Medical Care. *Milbank Memorial Fund Quarterly 60*:268–305.

Manning, P. R., and Denson, T. A. (1979). How cardiologists learn about echocardiography: a reminder for medical educators and legislators. *Ann. Intern. Med. 91*:469–71.

Mechanic, D. (1972). *Public Expectations and Health Care.* New York: Wiley-Interscience, pp. 30–3.

Mechanic, D. (1977). The growth of medical technology and bureaucracy: implications for medical care. *MMFQ/Health Soc. 55*:61–78.

Melnick, G. A., Wheeler, J., and Feldstein, P. J. (1981). Effects of rate regulation on selected components of hospital expenses. *Inquiry 18*:240–46.

Menzel, H., and Katz, E. (1955–6). Social relations and innovations in the medical profession: the epidemiology of a new drug. *Public Opinion Q. 19*:337–52.

National Center for Health Statistics, National Center for Health Services Research. (1980). *Health United States. 1978*. DHEW Publication No. (PHS) 78-1232. Hyattsville, Md.: Department of Health Education, and Welfare, p. 402, Table 162.

National Center for Health Statistics, National Center for Health Services Research. (1981). *Health United States. 1980*. DHHS Publication No. (PHS) 81-1232. Hyattsville, Md.: Department of Health and Human Services, p. 250, Table 41.

Office of Technology Assessment (OTA). (1976). *Development of Medical Technology Opportunities for Assessment*. Publication No. OTA-H-34. Washington, D.C.: U.S. Government Printing Office, p. 74.

OTA. (1978a). *Assessing the Efficacy and Safety of Medical Technologies*. Publication No. OTA-H-75. Washington, D.C., U.S. Government Printing Office.

OTA (1978b). *Policy Implications of the Computed Tomography (CT) Scanner*. Publication No. OTA-H-56. Washington, D.C.: U.S. Government Printing Office, p. 3.

OTA. (1980). *The Implications of Cost-Effectiveness Analysis of Medical Technology. Background Paper 4: The Management of Health Care Technology in Ten Countries*. Publication No. OTA-BP-H-7. Washington, D.C.: U.S. Government Printing Office, p. 207, Table 3.

OTA. (1981). *Policy Implications of the Computed Tomography (CT) Scanner: An Update*. Publication No. OTA-BP-H-8. Washington, D.C.: U.S. Government Printing Office, p. 60.

OTA. (1983). *The Emergence of NMR Imaging Technology: A Clinical, Industrial, and Policy Analysis*. Washington, D.C.: U.S. Government Printing Office (draft).

Perrow, C. (1963). Goals and power structure: a historical care study. In *The Hospital in Modern Society*, E. Freidson, ed. New York: Free Press, pp. 112–46.

Perrow, C. (1972). *Complex Organizations: A Critical Essay*. Glenview, Ill.: Scott, Foresmen.

Perrott, G. (1971). *The Federal Employees Health Benefits Program*. Washington, D.C.: Department of Health, Education and Welfare.

Rapoport, J. (1978). Diffusion of technological innovation among nonprofit firms: a case study of radioisotopes in U.S. hospitals. *J. Econ. Bus. 30*:108–18.

Redisch, M. (1974). Hospital inflationary mechanisms. Presented at the meeting of the Western Economic Association, Las Vegas, Nevada, June 10–12.

Roemer, M., and Shain, M. (1959). *Hospital Utilization Under Insurance*. Chicago: American Hospital Association.

Rogers, E. M., and Shoemaker, F. F. (1971). *Communication of Innovations: A Cross-Cultural Approach*. New York: Free Press, pp. 99–133.

Russell, L. (1976). The diffusion of new hospital technologies in the United States. *Int. J. Health Serv. 6*:557–80.

Russell, L. B. (1978). *Technology in Hospitals, Medical Advances and Their Diffusion*. Washington, D.C.: Brookings Institution, pp. 49–51.

Salkever, D., and Bice, T. (1976). The impact of certificate-of-need controls on hospital investment. *MMFQ/Health Soc. 54*:185–214.

Salkever, D., and Bice, T. (1979). *Hospital Certificate-of-Need Controls: Impact on Investment, Costs and Use*. Washington, D.C.: American Enterprise Institute of Public Policy Research.

Schifrin, L., and Tayan, J. (1977). The drug lag: an interpretive review of the literature. *Int. J. Health Services 7*:359–74.

Schroeder, S., and Showstack, J. (1978). Financial incentives to perform medical procedures and laboratory tests: illustrative models of office practice. *Med. Care 16*:289–98.

Schroeder, S., and Showstack, J. (1979). The dynamics of medical technology use: analysis and policy options. In *Medical Technology: The Culprit Behind Health Care Costs?* (S. Altman and R. Blendon, eds.). DHEW Publication No. (PHS) 79:3216. Hyattsville, Md.: U.S. Department of Health, Education, and Welfare, pp. 178–212.

Scott, W. R. (1972). Professionals in hospitals: technology and the organization of work. In *Organization Research on Health Institutions*, B. S. Georgopoulos, ed., Ann Arbor, Mich.: Institute for Social Research, pp. 139–202.

Showstack, J., and Schroeder, S. (1981). Evaluating the costs and benefits of a diagnostic technology. The case of upper gastrointestinal endoscopy. *Med. Care 19*:498–509.

Silverman, M., and Lee, P. (1974). *Pills, Profits, and Politics*. Berkeley: University of California Press, p. 55.

Smith, A. (1979). Professional dominance and health care decisions. Sixth International Conference on Social Science and Medicine. Amsterdam: Leuwenhorst Congress Center, August 5–10.

Smith, D., and Kaluzny, A. (1975). *The White Labyrinth*. Berkeley: McCutchan.

Stason, W. B., and Fortress, E. (1982). Cardiac radionuclide imaging and cost effectiveness, in Office of Technology Assessment: *The Implications of Cost Effectiveness Analysis of Medical Technology*, Case Study 13. Publication No. OTA-BP-H-9. Washington, D.C.: U.S. Government Printing Office.

Stross, J. K., and Harlan, W. R. (1979). The dissemination of new medical information. *J.A.M.A. 241*:2622–4.

Tanon, C., and Rogers, E. (1975). Diffusion research methodology: focus on health care organizations. In *The Diffusion of Medical Technology*, G. Gordon and L. Fisher, eds. Cambridge, Mass.: Ballinger, pp. 51–77.

Thomas, L. (1974). *The Lives of A Cell: Notes of a Biology Watcher*. New York: Viking Press, p. 36.

Tooth, G., and Newton, M. (1961). *Leucotomy in England and Wales 1942–54*, Reports on Public Health and Medical Subjects No. 104. London: Ministry of Health, Great Britain.

Urban, N., and Bice, T. W. (1981). Measuring regulation and its effects on hospital behavior (manuscript). Seattle: University of Washington.

Vayda, E. (1973). A comparison of surgical rates in Canada and in England and Wales. *N. Engl. J. Med. 289*:1224–9.

Warner, K. (1974). The need for some innovative concepts of innovation: an examination of research on the diffusion of innovations. *Policy Sci. 5*:433–51.

Warner, K. E. (1975). A 'desperation–reaction' model of medical diffusion. *Health Services Res. 10*:369–79.

Warner, K. E. (1977). Treatment decision making in catastrophic illness. *Med. Care 15*:19–33.

Wennberg, J., and Gittelsohn, A. (1973). Small area variations in health care delivery. *Science 182*:1102–8.

White, K. (1974). Contemporary epidemiology. *Int. J. Epidemiol. 3*:295–303.

White, K. (1975). Opportunities and needs for epidemiology and health statistics in the United States. Presented at the Invitational Conference on Epidemiology as the Fundamental Basis for Planning, Administration and Evaluation of Health Services, Baltimore, March 2–4, 1975.

Willems, J. (1979). The relationship between the diffusion of medical technology and the organization and economics of health care delivery. In *Medical Technology*, J. Wagner, ed. DHEW Publication No. (PHS) 79-3254. Hyattsville, Md.: National Center for Health Services Research, pp. 92–104.

Willems, J., Banta, D., Lukas, T., et al. (1979). The computed tomography scanner. In *Medical Technology: The Culprit Behind Health Care Costs?* S. Altman and R. Blendon, eds. Publication No. (PHS) 79:3216. Hyattsville, Md.: U.S. Department of Health, Education and Welfare, pp. 116–143.

Worthen, D. B. (1973). Prescribing influences: an overview. *Br. J. Med. Ed.* 7:109–17.

Zaltman, G., Duncan, R., and Holbek, J. (1973). *Innovations and Organizations.* New York: Wiley.

# PART IV

# ORGANIZING TECHNOLOGY IN CLINICAL SETTINGS

# TECHNOLOGY'S FRONT LINE:
# THE INTENSIVE CARE UNIT

JAMES J. HASSETT

Ever since Sanctorius of Padua produced the first systematic measurements of pulse rate and body temperature in the seventeenth century, the practice of measurement in medicine has progressed. Recently, dramatic advances in clinical measurement have been made in concert with technological advances in electronics, nuclear science, and data processing. The basic advance has been the application of technological principles developed for nonmedical purposes to patient care.

Technology-oriented clinical units have been organized around a variety of unifying principles. The organ system involved, the technology employed, or the responsible medical specialty offered organizing criteria that resulted in the development of administratively distinct clinical units commonly called *intensive care units (ICU)*.

The original ICUs were organized to handle acute illnesses that involved significant morbidity and mortality. These units responded to the special needs of seriously ill patients either as extended recovery room areas (ICU) or high technology monitoring areas (cardiac care unit, or CCU). The subsequent development of the initial areas has paralleled that of the burgeoning medical technology field. The original ICU has been subdivided into a medical unit (MICU), a respiratory unit (RICU), and a pediatric unit (PICU) or neonatal unit. The surgical units (SICU) are subdivided into neurosurgical units, trauma or burn units, and cardiac postoperative units. The dialysis units have developed independently, but reflect this trend. Theoretically, there could be a special unit for each acute illness or system. Recently, in an effort to reflect the differing levels of intervention and technology, "step-down" ICUs with a partial monitoring capability have been designed. Although there is much technological overlap among all of these units, many have developed specialized techniques, protocols, and strategies of intervention. The administrative organization of an ICU mainly reflects mandated special requirements, as in the neonatal or dialysis units, the managerial roles of the specially trained physicians, or the unique technology involved, as in the hyperbaric chamber. The CCU has responded to a different set of needs because it deals with a unique organ system and limited pathology.

Elaborate technological systems have spawned the development of additional technology. To cope with this, physicians have had to improve their technological background or delegate responsibility to technological specialists. This is similar to the situation that produced the radiological specialist 60 years ago. As the organization of an efficient data base increased, data management and retrieval became important. As data input overwhelmed the traditional physician, he abandoned his decision-making role to interested specialists who later sought computer assistance in pattern recognition and analysis, and developed diagnostic and therapeutic routines for the highly repetitive problems.

The ICU was originally designed to provide a high level of assessment and control in order to allow effective intervention in acute life-threatening illnesses. Technological advances became the mainstay of this effort. Consequently, the purposes of technology in this setting are to permit the continuous evaluation of critical physiological function and feedback control of therapeutic interventions; to quantify subtle changes in delicate clinical conditions; to anticipate presumed or possible pathophysiology before it is clinically obvious; and to provide therapeutic support for vital organ systems.

The original advances in technology responded to these needs of the developing ICU. Because the principal problem is to acquire, organize, and frequently assess physiological parameters that change rapidly in acutely ill patients and have a strong relationship to morbidity and mortality, all units have developed technology for the automated direct and indirect measurement of blood pressure, heart rate, and heart rhythm; to enhance cardiac pump physiology; to allow mechanical support and control of ventilation; and to provide laboratory evaluation of basic systemic physiology. The technology applied to acute medical illness is usually electrically powered and performs the basic functions of continuous organ system monitoring, advanced life support, and organ system support and evaluation.

It should also be emphasized that the special care unit is not divorced from other technological advances in diagnosis and therapy, such as diagnostic imaging, which are located elsewhere in the hospital. ICU technology has to be relatively portable so that the monitors and life support systems may be continued when the patient is temporarily moved to other areas in the hospital (e.g., operating room, x-ray radiology room, or radiation therapy unit). Certain ICU technologies, including hyperbaric chambers and membrane oxygenators, are still searching for adequate clinical applications. They were developed and applied to specific medical problems, but have such specialized and isolated indications that they are rarely used.

PURPOSES OF TECHNOLOGY APPLICATION

*Continuous organ system monitoring*

The parameter usually monitored is pressure or electrophysiological function. The open system water manometer has been replaced by electrically controlled pressure transducers, which may monitor any fluid phase in a closed or semiclosed system (blood pressure, cerebrospinal fluid pressure, etc.). Continuous electrocardiographic monitoring is the single most common parameter followed. When linked to an adequate alarm mechanism, these monitored functions provide an effective surveillance system.

The general characteristics of such a system are that the physiological functions to be monitored have to be predictable; the signals generated should be reproducible within a limited reference range; limited recall of previously entered data and adequate display of current data must be present; an adequate sentry or alert mechanism with a low incidence of false-positive or false-negative alarms must be available; the equipment should be reliable and have interchangeable units with low down time; and the system as a whole should have a low risk/benefit ratio.

These systems are highly reliable and precise, with an error rate of less than 2 percent. The benefit of the monitoring system is measured in terms of the information gained. However, the system is not a substitute for decision making, and may provide too much information to allow proper analysis. It cannot assign significance to an abnormal signal or establish a high probability of disorder, both of which are necessary to direct effective action. Monitoring systems become much more important when they have the following features: data storage for posttherapy review and assessment; no hard wire connections and thus considerable mobility; minimal invasiveness and tissue destruction associated with data acquisition; increased protection against infective invasion; and a reliable portable power supply.

*Advanced life support*

This function has had the greatest recent development. External cardiac defibrillation and cardiac pacemakers have been joined by the intraaortic balloon pump. The pressure-cycled mechanical ventilator has been replaced by the electrically driven, volume-cycled respirator with high-frequency positive pressure ventilation (HFPPV), positive end-expiratory pressure (PEEP), and intermittent mandatory ventilation (IMV) – three options significantly altering the goals, strategies, and protocols of the ventilator with beneficial results. These varied technological developments have been matched only by the increasingly technological pharmacological support of inotropic and antiarrhythmic agents, antacids, antibiotics, and antifungal agents.

### Organ system support and evaluation

Indicator dilution cardiac output determination, enteral and parenteral alimentation systems, fluid and electrolyte support, hemodialysis, and mechanical ventilation, are among the many techniques used to support threatened life. They require sterile procedures and adequate calibration with precise instrumentation. The latter depends on technological advances in laboratory evaluation.

### LEVELS OF TECHNOLOGY APPLICATION

ICU patients can be classified by the level of technology applied, the degree of bodily invasion required, the amount of intervention, and the reliance on the technology needed for survival. The basis of this classification is a progressive use of the monitoring system, which provides a rationale to intervene in the pathophysiology being monitored, and thus achieve a more optimal result. There are three levels of technology:

1. Minimally invasive (watchful expectance). This level is characterized by intermittent venous sampling of standard chemical and hematologic variables, frequent monitoring of basic vital signs and simple body functions, continuous monitoring of cardiac rhythm, and basic nutritional and respiratory support.
2. Moderately invasive (active intervention). This level is characterized by the following (in addition to those for level 1): continuous indwelling monitors, initial support of a single organ failure, and pharmacologic support of monitored function.
3. Maximally invasive (full court press). This level is characterized by the following (in addition to those for levels 1 and 2): progressive monitor and technological support of individual organs in multiple system organ failure, and pharmacological intervention in advanced disease or in the iatrogenic misadventures of prior technology.

### SELECTION OF TECHNOLOGY AND ITS LIMITATIONS

Technology is applied in the ICU according to the following principles: (1) the technology used depends on perceived, possible, or actual patient risk; (2) use of technology is initiated or discontinued in response to appropriate clinical cues; (3) acquired data are assimilated into the decison-making process; (4) the level and extent of the technology are matched to the pace and natural history of the disease process.

The principles of selection of the type and level of technology are based on the characteristics of the physician, the patient, and the technology itself. The *physician*-based principles include (1) prior experience and prejudice and (2) hospital protocol imposed by a physician group or ancillary support. The selection based on the *patient's* status includes (1) the patient's actual or presumed fate without intervention, (2) the natural history of the disease or its outcome, (3) the relative ease of intervention, (4) known or possible effects of preexisting concurrent disease, and (5) patient triage factors including available technology and patient competition for space. The selection of technology based on *technology* includes (1) technology to monitor the technology, (2) continuance of technological intervention initiated outside the unit, and (3) possible side effects of previously applied or anticipated technological intervention.

Patients are selected for the level of technology by prearranged strategies that may be limited by space or technology availability, previously designed protocols, or professional preference and convenience. This may result in a suboptimal application of technology.

For example, some units will place intraarterial cannulas to facilitate phlebotomy during mechanical ventilation when multiple blood analyses are being performed. As a secondary gain to this method of angio-access, continuous blood pressure monitoring is usually performed simultaneously; this may not be essential to patient management. ICUs which deal with large volumes of critically ill patients with similar problems have achieved uniformity of response by establishing protocols. In these units, the level of technology is prearranged and applied indiscriminately. The postoperative cardiac surgical unit dealing with many aortocoronary bypass patients is the best example. Swan-Ganz catheterization for pulmonary capillary wedge pressure measurement and thermodilution cardiac output determination are, however, frequently limited by monitor availability.

When the significance of the data cannot be assessed and decisions cannot be made with confidence, the physician normally initially chooses a level of technology that is higher than necessary. Generally, the level is then readjusted according to the clinical requirements. Underestimation of the level of technology required usually results in higher morbidity. Blind application of protocols may result in technological overkill but is a useful strategy in high-volume teaching units.

Patients move easily from one level of technology to another by the progressive addition or deletion of more involved systems. The technological escalation or deescalation is usually determined by the physician's examination but is sometimes controlled by the protocol. Technologies tend to be applied in closely related groups. Therapeutic technologies stimulate the use of monitoring or evaluating technologies, which are included in response to the clinical conditions. The initial support systems of level 1 are relatively uncomplicated and are applied to patients whose clinical condition requires a high level of nursing support or close monitoring. Level 2 results from a more critical illness at the point of admission, progression of the admitting condition, or failure or complications of therapy. Most commonly, an indwelling monitor is used to measure arterial or venous pressure. The organ most commonly supported is the respiratory system. Inotropic support of cardiac function is the most common form of pharmacology applied.

Level 3 includes hemodialysis and the use of an intraarterial balloon pump, with pharmacological support of sepsis, its complications, and multiple system organ failure. Level 3 is rarely the initial level of technology used; most patients commonly enter at level 2 and are advanced to level 3.

Because there are few established and accepted criteria for initiation or maintenance of technology or technological support, in the absence of protocols of patient selection, the level of technology applied and the duration of application are individually determined by the responsible physician. When bed availability is not a crucial factor, there is a tendency to maintain the monitoring technology longer than is absolutely necessary to avoid the risk of placing a marginal patient in an unmonitored bed. The use of bed availability as a triage criterion for patient selection or disposition sometimes results in premature or inappropriate decisions on either the level or continuance of technological support, and may lead to therapeutic tragedies or to longer intervals of required intervention.

Since the ICU functions well in therapeutic modes but poorly in diagnostic modes, acutely ill patients in whom the etiology of the illness is not obvious tend to be assigned to an inappropriate level of technology. As the degree of inappropriate assignment increases, so does the risk of iatrogenic disease. With increasing data, the physician experiences sensory overload and can no longer discriminate or organize information effectively, further increasing the iatrogenic problem. The degree of acute illness and the potential side effects of therapy make these problems crucial to patient outcome. If adequate diagnosis requires transport away from the technology, life support must be portable or the risk of evaluation or diagnosis must be weighed against the gain in information. When appropriate diagnosis may result in reduction of the risks of iatrogenic problems, the risk of patient transport is justified.

The patient is attached to or supported by a technology that is accessible by a tube. The "theory of tubes" has become a shorthand comment on the relationship of the acuteness of the illness, the level of technology, and the dependence of the patient on the technology for survival. This theory relates the seriousness of the illness and the probability of a negative outcome to the ratio of natural orifices to the tubes placed in the patient. Although this is a sarcastic comment, its predictability seems obvious.

## TYPES OF ICU PATIENTS

There are three types of ICU patients. The first type has an acute surgical illness and is admitted for postoperative care. When the ICU is utilized in this situation, the majority of patients will require level 1 or level 2 technology and achieve a reasonable success rate. The second type of ICU patient has acute illness without surgical therapy. Utilization of the ICU for these patients also usually requires level 1 or level 2 technology and results in a reasonable success rate. The third type of patient is usually a therapeutic failure of the first two types or has such severe illness that the outcome must be guarded. These patients classically require level 3 technology initially or enter at a lower level and rapidly progress to level 3.

The increasing levels of technological intervention are generally accompanied by escalating cost (personnel, money, time, machinery), a progressively decreasing probability of success, a progressively increasing morbidity and mortality, an increasing sophistication of technological surveillance, and a progressive multiple system failure.

Escalating the level of technology to the level of illness implies that the increased activity will result in a finite increase in beneficial outcome, or at least a more acceptable outcome than would be expected without the added technology. This is correct only in some cases. In other situations, an increased level of intervention results in the creation of a group of patients who depend completely on the technology for their survival.

Patients at levels 1 and 2 have predictable and acceptable morbidity and mortality. Progression to level 3 may result in increased survival, but is usually accompanied by a progressive increase in morbidity and mortality.

At a certain point, the probability of success is inversely proportional to the level or duration of the technology applied. All of these patients demonstrate progressive multiple system organ failure. Application of technology also creates a group of patients who are considered to be survivors, that is, who demonstrate a beneficial outcome, but who are so disabled by their illness that they are no longer productive and require a high level of continued medical support.

PROBLEMS AND EFFECTS OF THE TECHNOLOGICAL ADVANCES IN THE ICU

*Accelerated progress of technology*

New technological advances raise new questions and result in the development of new technological systems to deal with them. The classic example is the progressive development of technology to evaluate and support the respiratory system. The pressure-cycled ventilator of 1970 was controlled by rudimentary evaluation of blood oxygen and $CO_2$ levels and by chest x-rays. This system was replaced by volume-cycled, electrically controlled mechanical ventilators capable of producing positive end-expiratory pressure (PEEP) and intermittent mandatory ventilation (IMV) controlled by modern blood gas analyzers or transcutaneous oxygen monitors. These ventilators are now challenged by high-frequency ventilation and lung water computers.

*Social and ethical conflicts*

*Ethical* problems include patient selection and triage criteria, initiation or withdrawal of support, and assessment of the benefit as measured by the quality or duration of life. *Social* pressure to utilize available technology without selection or professional discretion results in the uncontrolled use of technology, which severely limits resource allocation.

Both social and ethical conflicts arise from the limited resources and the professional obligation to select patients for therapy or discontinuation of therapy. The basic social pressure is to apply the technology indiscriminately and to continue its application regardless of the result or cost. The technology now exists to support the functions of specific organs long after the possibility of life independent of the support system has ceased. However, we have neither the social mandate to discontinue support nor the resources to continue it without denying its use to subsequent patients.

### Emotional and psychological effects

Increasing therapeutic futility and frustration are created by the establishment of a technological buffer between the patient and the health care team. The abundance of data creates indecision, with a variety of conflicting signals regarding patient outcome and the ability to predict manipulated future lifestyles of patients. The human–machine interface jeopardizes the human component of health care, requiring the health care team to take as much of an interest in the technology as they do in the patients or their illness. The use of technology and monitoring systems does not reduce personnel, but it does allow more efficient utilization of the staff. Preoccupation with technical details results in seeming indifference to patients, and their families. Moreover, a society of patients dependent on technology for survival is created.

The patient who is perceived by the staff to exhibit less human qualities may become transformed into an extension of the technologies applied. This may sound like science fiction, but it is a reality. As the patient becomes more unresponsive, the stress of attempting to maintain the technology jeopardizes the emotional commitment required for the patient's care.

### Physician-related problems

Preoccupation with data acquisition and organization does not allow one to determine the significance of the technology applied, its implications and consequences, or the appropriateness of the data to the clinical condition. Unfortunately, the belief that more accurate diagnosis would result in a better prognosis may cause an inappropriate application of technology in cases where the data acquired have no significant impact on the decisions to be made. Appropriate application of the available technology must be included in the basic construction of all special care units, including the development of protocols and algorithms to help the new or minimally experienced physician to deal with increasingly sophisticated data packages. The amount of the data available sometimes overwhelms the decision-making process, rendering discrimination and organization difficult. Attempts to organize data into recognizable patterns in order to render decision making more efficient are usually computer based and suffer from a higher cost and a new set of inherent problems. Diagnosis and daily patient management are still based on the physical examination. The frequent discrepancy between the monitored or computer processed data and the information based on the physical examination may result in physician indecision, and eventually is resolved only by direct examination of the patient using clinical expertise and attention to detail. Following such an experience, it is not surprising that many physicians distrust the monitoring systems, thus missing potentially useful information. Alternatively, overwhelmed by the data generated, they often relinquish responsibility to more technically skillful physicians, losing control of their patient's care.

### Patient effects and hazards

All special care units involve a substantial amount of electrical equipment, which presents a significant hazard to the patient. The patient must be protected against the dangers inherent in the use of these technologies.

The worst potential hazard is the threat of sepsis, which directly results from the invasive nature of technological life support. However, many patients who now lead productive lives owe their survival to the special care unit, its personnel, and its technology.

#### FUTURE PERSPECTIVES

Technology-oriented clinical units offer the physician the same inherent promises that technology has offered society as a whole. Unfortunately, the implication of relative immortality or the avoidance of the consequences of remediable illness with the ease and convenience of highly technological support (Buck Rogers mentality) is not uniformly possible. Poor patient selection and misuse of technology result in decreased effectiveness, an increased wait for service, and a higher demand than was originally intended or is possible to meet. Improvements will not overcome the limitations of current technology even if the new is much more reliable, efficient, and inexpensive than the old. Unfortunately, as the use of technology in medicine increases, it creates the development of additional new technologies to monitor, regulate, and control current technologies. The problems we are facing are not technological, but sociological and psychological. Technology has saved many lives but has also produced much stress. This requires a reassessment of our goals to achieve more realistic application of medical technology.

Future developments should occur in a much more effectively computerized organization for assessment and evaluation of diagnostic data, miniaturization of equipment, and reduction of both invasiveness and dependency on traditional hospital units for routine, reliable control. The ICU should remain in the forefront of technology utilization for the benefit of patients who cannot be treated elsewhere.

## SUMMARY

Technology-oriented clinical units exist to monitor, support, and assist basic organ function. The specific technologies utilized depend on the mission and intent of the special care unit involved. Technology creates a series of problems, not all of which are correctable. Nevertheless, it appears obvious that the overall benefit from these units far outweighs the risks.

### SELECTED BIBLIOGRAPHY

Chernow, B., and Lake, C. R. (1983). *The Pharmacologic Approach to the Critically Ill Patient*. Baltimore: Williams & Wilkins.

Shoemaker, W. C. (ed.). (1980–3). *Critical Care Medicine*, vols. 1–4. Baltimore: Williams & Wilkins.

Shoemaker, W. C., Thompson, W. L., and Holbrook, P. R. (1984). *Textbook of Critical Care*. Baltimore: Williams & Wilkins.

CHAPTER 7

# ACTION WITH DISPATCH: TECHNOLOGY IN THE EMERGENCY DEPARTMENT

MICHAEL ELIASTAM

Although the potential for technology application in the emergency department (ED) is extensive, the use of modern technology capable of improving its function has not been adequate. However, the new specialty of emergency medicine is likely to increase the rate of technological application rapidly in the next decade. This chapter provides a brief history of the emergency medical service system, a description of its functions, particularly where modern technology is applied, a discussion of the major issues affecting its use and misuse, and finally, a speculative look at the ED of the year 2001.

Use of technology in the ED exemplifies the interaction of health care providers, technology, and patients. The interaction starts in the prehospital care setting, continues in the ED, and affects patients after they have been discharged from the ED or transferred to a hospital ward. The ED is a community resource, not only as a locus of direct care but also as a provider of information and education. To understand its current place in the health care delivery system, one must understand the development of the emergency medical service system.

## RECENT HISTORY OF EMERGENCY MEDICAL CARE DEVELOPMENT

ED patient visits increased fourfold in the decade after World War II, and the rising rate of utilization persisted nearly to the present. Only recently has ED utilization decreased (by about 10 percent), apparently due to deterioration in the nation's economic status, which affects the patient's use of health care dollars.

The factors responsible for increased utilization include patients' difficulty in finding physicians at night, on weekends, and during holidays; recognition by the public that hospitals are open at all times; increased motor vehicle accidents and firearm incidents; physicians' use of the ED for treatments formerly performed in their offices; third-party payment for ED care; the ready availability

105

of x-ray and laboratory services that, when utilized, make third-party reimbursement more likely; population growth; and the development by patients of a perspective of health care as a right rather than a privilege.

This increase in visits to the ED initially imposed great hardship on existing facilities and staff. Inadequate departments manned by well-intentioned but poorly trained staff, hampered by inadequate equipment, were forced to deal with burgeoning numbers of people needing and or demanding attention.

Care by ambulance crews was often inadequate and occasionally made the patient's condition worse. An estimated 10 percent of spinal cord injuries occurred after accidents as a result of careless handling of patients. Ambulance-to-hospital communication was primitive, and hospitals rarely knew in advance of the impending arrival of seriously ill or injured people. The ambulance siren was often the first notification to the ED staff of imminent patient arrival.

In 1966 the National Academy of Sciences (NAS) issued a scathing report, "Accidental Death and Disability: The Neglected Disease of Modern Society." Reflecting on the prevalence of trauma morbidity and mortality in young adults, it stated that highway death rates in this group far exceeded those of the Vietnam War. The Vietnam War and the preceding Korean conflict had produced efficient systems for evacuation and transportation of battle casualties to well-equipped military hospitals, making it possible for well-trained medical teams using modern medical technology to reduce the mortality and morbidity significantly. The NAS report emphasized the tremendous loss to the nation's productivity that resulted from death and disability in its young adults. That same year, the U.S. Congress passed the National Highway Safety Act, which authorized the Department of Transportation to fund ambulance services, physician-to-paramedic communication systems, training programs, and statewide planning. The first civilian trauma unit was established at Cook County Hospital in Chicago in 1966.

The 5 years beginning in 1971 produced much activity. California passed a law establishing a pilot paramedic program based on the mobile coronary care unit developed by Pantride in Belfast, Northern Ireland. Reports by Yale University Medical School and the NAS prompted a coordinated national effort to deal with the crisis of injury and illness. The federal government set up Emergency Medical Services (EMS) demonstration projects in several states, allocating $16 million for systems development. The White House urged cities to develop centralized communication networks with a simplified access telephone number, 911. The Congress passed Public Law 93-154, the Emergency Medical Services System Act of 1973, authorizing the expenditure of $185 million over 3 years for regionalized life support emergency services. The Federal Communications Commission identified radio frequencies for exclusive EMS use. The American Medical Association urged its members to improve trauma care, and recommended that emergency medicine be considered a new specialty.

In 1976, Congress not only renewed the Emergency Medical Services Act but also authorized $260 million for emergency system development, research, and training. Emergency medicine was recognized as a specialty in 1979, and the first board examination was administered in 1980.

This financial and political support produced major changes in emergency care. Most of these changes have benefited patients by increasing their access to services and improving the quality and quantity of care delivered. Unfortunately, some of the results have been negative. The ready availability of ambulances and EDs stimulated inappropriate use and resulted in excessive costs, which were passed on to patients in the form of higher health insurance premiums and hospital charges. Overall, however, the benefits appear to exceed the costs by far, with significant reductions in mortality and morbidity in specific conditions such as heart attacks, poisoning, and trauma. Much remains to be done to ensure that emergency care is delivered to those who need it in the most efficient way possible. The intelligent use of technology is and will remain one of the most important ways to achieve this goal.

## THE EMERGENCY DEPARTMENT

Conceptually, the ED should be considered an arena in which a number of different actors with appropriate training and equipment play a role. The initial evaluation and care are given by a team consisting of physicians, nurses, and/ or technicians, backed up by laboratory and clerical personnel. They are provided usually by the emergency physician, the patient's primary care physician, or both. Consultant physicians are utilized in two ways. First, for critically ill or injured patients, policies are established mandating that specialty physicians be consulted to ensure efficient, safe, definitive care. The best example of this is trauma care, in which trauma teams are organized to provide surgeons, anesthesiologists, and other professionals on an immediate-response basis to join with the emergency physician in the resuscitation of seriously injured people. Cardiac arrest teams are another example. Second, for noncritically ill or injured patients, specialty consultants are often requested to provide more intensive evaluation and treatment, either in the ED or on the hospital ward to which the patient is admitted. For example, an orthopedic surgeon might be requested to reduce and cast a major fracture in the ED, and the patient would go home with instructions to return to the orthopedist's office for follow-up care. Patients with diseases such as pneumonia or myocardial infarction, which are serious enough to require admission to the hospital, need a specialist internist to assume responsibility for the hospital care and postdischarge follow-up care.

Many classifications of types of patients using the emergency department exist. One useful system is: (1) critically ill or injured patients, (2) those with urgent complaints, and (3) those with nonurgent complaints. This classification reflects the major problem that occurs with any effort to categorize ED patients. The judgment that a condition is ''urgent'' or ''nonurgent'' often differs when made by a physician and a nurse, compared to that made by the patient or family. The number of true emergencies and urgent complaints is far smaller than the number of apparent emergencies and urgent complaints identified by patients or families.

Almost every ED has at least one registered nurse present in the department at all times. Depending on the volume of patient visits, the remainder of the staff comprises additional registered nurses, licensed vocational or practical nurses, laboratory, electrocardiographic, and x-ray technicians, social workers, and administrative and clerical personnel. In very busy EDS with over 100,000 visits per year, these personnel may be permanently located in the department. In moderate-sized facilities (25,000 to 75,000 annual visits), some of these personnel may be responsible for providing their services such as electrocardiography (ECG) or x-rays to several areas of the hospital, including but not limited to the ED.

The care provided to the patient by the ED team usually begins with triage (a French word meaning "to sort,") performed by a nurse who decides which patients should be treated first and which ones can safely wait until the more urgent cases have been given care. Accurate, safe triage is quite difficult because it requires that a decision be made with limited information and without undue delay. Many EDs have triage policies including specific criteria to be used to decide who can wait and who cannot. For example, any patient with one of the following symptoms is considered to need prompt evaluation: pulse above 120 per minute, systolic blood pressure below 90, pediatric patients with a temperature above 104°F, evidence of altered mental status, and chest pain.

Triage criteria vary in each ED because they are based on the resources available within the ED and on alternatives available in the community. For example, some EDs do not send any patient to an alternative source of care, whereas other treat only patients with emergency and urgent complaints, referring all others to clinics elsewhere in the institution or in the community.

Patient registration follows triage. An ED record is created, including relevant demographic and financial information. Evaluation is the next step. This includes history-taking, physical examination, performance of x-ray studies and laboratory tests, and the use of consultants when necessary. Treatment is then instituted. Definitive care may be initiated immediately, or deferred to allow a period of observation, which may result in improved understanding of the patient's disease. Often the condition is self-limiting, and by the end of the observation period the patient may not require definitive treatment.

Disposition of the patients is then decided. For those to be admitted to the hospital, disposition means deciding into which ward to admit the patient. Options include coronary care units (CCU), intensive care units (ICU), and regular wards, which may be designated as special care areas such as orthopedics or internal medicine. For those patients not admitted to the hospital, disposition is often a complex problem. Every patient discharged from the ED must have a full understanding of the diagnosis made, the care given in the department, the take-home medication and medical care instructions, and the follow-up evaluation arrangements that have been made by the physician. Often it is necessary to involve social workers or public health nurses in the follow-up care, which may include visits to the home by these professionals or the acquisition of additional drugs or equipment from sources outside the hospital.

Information transmittal concludes the sequence of events. Every patient's ED record has multiple copies that are distributed to the hospital's medical records department, the follow-up physician's office or clinic, the billing office, and the ED's record file.

## USE OF TECHNOLOGY IN THE EMERGENCY DEPARTMENT

There is a range of technology utilization across the many different kinds of hospital departments, and often the amount of technology being used depends more on the interest and preference of the department administrators than it does on patient needs or departmental structure. Two major types of technology exist in most departments: (1) patient registration and billing, and (2) prehospital care information transmitted from the field to the hospital.

The use of technology for medical emergencies generally begins with the telephone. Patients call for emergency help by dialing a regional emergency number, increasingly the simple three-digit number 911, which goes directly to a central communication location for transfer to the fire department and/or ambulance center nearest the patient. A recent innovation, still experimental, is the installation of automatic pressure-activated devices on handicapped and disabled people in their homes. If the person collapses and falls on the device, which is strapped to the body, it activates an alarm attached to the telephone, which automatically signals the local communication center. The device can also be set to signal the communication center automatically if it is not deactivated by the individual at a specific time each day. Fire departments often use computer-aided dispatch systems to identify the fire station nearest to the patient and, based on the information given by the caller, to select and dispatch any additional vehicles carrying special equipment that may be needed. This is especially important in motor vehicle accidents in which extrication and fire suppression are needed, or when contamination by hazardous material is possible.

At the scene of the emergency, a combination of medical and communication technology provides lifesaving care. Paramedics acting under the supervision of physicians and nurses at a base station hospital resuscitate and stabilize critically ill or injured patients. Medical equipment includes complex items such as cardiac monitors and defibrillators, as well as relatively simple items such as pneumatic antishock trousers and esophageal obturator airways. In addition to voice communication, some emergency systems use telemetry to send ECG signals to the base station hospital for physician confirmation of the paramedic's assessment. Radio communication also allows the base station hospital's physician to distribute multiple victims to more than one receiving hospital in order to avoid overloading an individual hospital.

Electronic recording devices tape all communications between the patient and the communication center, between the units speeding to the scene and the communication center, and between the paramedics and the hospital.

Most EDs use a computerized billing system that either requires patient information to be manually entered after registration or receives this information directly from the data system into which the patient is first registered. Insurance information on patients who have used the hospital on a prior occasion is already in the system, and the patient's financial record is updated. Charges for use of the ED, supplies and equipment, and any special care are manually entered by the nurses or clerk for eventual submission of a bill for hospital services. The physician's fees for professional services are entered in a similar way by the physician providing the care, and bills for such services can be either combined with the hospital bill or processed separately. The computer is used extensively for these procedures, as well as for the provision of billing-related information to state (Medicaid) and federal (Medicare) reimbursement agencies.

Communication systems between the ED and the hospital medical records department transmit the patient's identifying information. The patient's prior medical records can thus be retrieved and brought to the ED for use by the physician. This helps prevent the ordering of unnecessary diagnostic tests and improves diagnostic accuracy by providing relevant prior medical and social historical information.

Digital technology is currently being applied to traditional equipment to improve ease of reading, accuracy, recording capability, and interpretation of serial data. An example is the use of a regular blood pressure cuff applied to the arm and connected to a digital recorder, which displays the blood pressure and pulse on a minute-by-minute basis and uses a printer to provide a permanent record. This noninvasive system is very accurate for most patients and often eliminates the need for invasive techniques such as arterial cannulation.

Another example is the ECG. Computers have been programmed to interpret ECGs taken remotely elsewhere in the hospital or in another hospital. The preliminary interpretation is done by the computer and confirmed by the cardiologist, who also scrutinizes unusual ECGs identified by the computer.

An interesting development in emergency medicine is the linkage of the ED to the laboratory. The patient's blood sample is taken to the laboratory, where computerized automated blood analyzers transmit results to terminals in the ED so that physicians can obtain the results immediately. Similar systems exist for x-rays; the radiologist's interpretation can be transmitted simultaneously when the dictated radiology report is transcribed.

Given the nature of emergency medicine, up-to-date medical information for diagnosis and treatment is essential. A recent innovation is the use of microfiche to provide rapidly accessible, regularly updated information for management of poisoning and toxic substance exposure. The system has a comprehensive index of all known toxic substances and drugs listed by their generic names, proprietary names, and, for abuse-prone drugs, their "street" names. Each drug or substance has a cross-indexed section on pharmacology and clinical management. A system similar to this one has recently been developed for all emergency medicine clinical information, and is currently being tested.

An everyday piece of technology, the standard telephone, has recently been incorporated into a new way of treating poisoning cases. To reduce unnecessary hospital visits, poison control centers have developed programs in which trained nurses and pharmacists handle patients who call in because of recent ingestion of toxic substances. After the toxic potential of the substance has been evaluated using the microfiche system described above, regular monitoring by telephone is done while a family member administers an emetic and reports the patient's response. When necessary, a nurse visits the home to monitor directly the patient's condition. Patients who should be evaluated in the ED are directed to the nearest appropriate facility immediately.

The field of interaction between physicians and computers for diagnostic assistance has not developed extensively in emergency medicine. However, one system has been used quite widely. Acid–base balance and electrolyte dysfunction interaction programs, developed in the early 1970s, are used by some emergency physicians through a telephone link to a computer in an academic medical center. The patient's laboratory values are entered by the inquiring physician, and the computer displays the likely diagnoses, suggests further tests needed, and outlines recommended therapy.

### PROBLEMS WITH TECHNOLOGY

The excessive use of technology in medicine has resulted in unacceptably high costs for health care. The ED is no exception. Under ideal circumstances, new technology should make medical practice cost effective and valuable for the patient. Unfortunately, this is not always true.

Overuse and inappropriate use, not underuse, are the major problems. Two major reasons, fear of malpractice and an academic orientation to avoid "missing something," are crucial factors causing excessive use of technology.

Panels of tests and multiple x-rays are ordered, producing a plethora of data, much of which is not very useful and often expensive. The indiscriminate use of batteries of tests can generate misleading or inaccurate information upon which further actions, such as the ordering of more tests, are based. Often no treatment is available or even indicated for certain abnormal test results, and the information only serves to confuse the physician and create anxiety in the patient.

A good example is the blood uric acid level. Although the normal concentration is 6 mg%, there is no scientific evidence regarding the impact of a level above 6 mg% but less than 10 mg%. Some evidence exists to support a clinical decision to treat patients with values greater than 10 mg% with drugs to reduce this level. However, physicians often feel obliged to investigate further a blood uric level above normal, that is, above 6 mg%, to evaluate patients for evidence of kidney stones, to look for rare metabolic disorders associated with elevated uric acid levels, and to "treat" these levels. In most cases, both the physician and the patient would have benefited by being ignorant of the existence of "elevated" uric acid levels.

It is important to recognize that inaccurate diagnostic results are not due to machine error alone. They may result from the inexperience of the technician performing the test and from transcription errors when results are transmitted from the diagnostic department to the emergency physician.

Physicians are not well educated about the interpretation of a single laboratory result. In addition to the danger of false positives and false negatives, few physicians appreciate how the prevalence of a particular disease in the population from which the patient is drawn influences the predictive value of the particular test result. A poor understanding of these principles often results in unnecessary additional diagnostic studies (see Chapter 12).

The policy of deferring certain diagnostic studies to the follow-up visit pending reevaluation of the patient after observation or preliminary treatment is sound if the patient can be depended upon to return if symptoms worsen. However, if the patient is not reliable, emergency physicians are often motivated to order more tests and studies. Many patients with mild to moderate ankle sprains or twists do not have associated ankle fractures. Under ideal conditions, the patient should not be x-rayed, but instead instructed to rest, elevate the limb, and return if symptoms persist or worsen after 3 to 5 days. The latter group, a much smaller one, should then be x-rayed to rule out fracture. Failure to diagnose the fracture on the initial evaluation, rather than 3 to 5 days later, has no effect on the final outcome of these patients. Unfortunately, physicians who fear charges of malpractice for not diagnosing a fracture promptly, or delayed return of patients despite worsening symptoms beyond the 3-to-5 days limit, with consequent morbidity to the ankle, are reluctant to eliminate x-ray examination of these patients on the initial evaluation.

Finally, in many cases the time required for tests seldom allows the results to be available to the physician without detaining the patient for unnecessarily long periods in the ED. Transmitting this test information to the follow-up site often requires elaborate and costly systems, a sometimes wasteful situation because the information may be of little value.

Treatment is often unnecessarily aggressive, and therefore costly and occasionally harmful. Trauma teams may be guilty of the last when they use aggressive resuscitation on less than seriously injured patients. This may include doing venous cut-downs and performing peritoneal lavage on patients whose injuries require only a peripheral intravenous line and careful observation. This situation can arise from a desire to avoid undertreating a patient whose serious injury is not readily apparent, and/or a desire to perfect resuscitation techniques to ensure their proficiency for the truly needy patient.

## THE EMERGENCY DEPARTMENT IN THE YEAR 2001

Based on current knowledge of applications of computer-based technology for emergency medicine, I will attempt here to make a best guess of what will probably develop in the next two decades. Predictions of this kind are hazardous, since unforeseen innovations can radically alter the rate of development of computer applications.

In addition to far more reliable radio communications, the year 2001 will see the use of a movie camera transmitting via satellite live pictures of the patient in the field. This will result in more accurate decision making and treatment.

- The automated alarms for high-risk citizens in the community, mentioned above, will be improved, and the reduction in false alarms will facilitate the devices' widespread acceptance and use. Also, systems for the visually and hearing diabled will be integrated into community emergency responses.

Micro- and minicomputers will be used to enter patients' demographic and financial information into a hospital data bank, allowing patients' names, pertinent social and medical information, and clinical evaluation status to be displayed on terminals throughout the ED. Physician and nursing personnel will be able easily to identify and track patients during their stay. The screen will identify the location of patients, those awaiting laboratory results, and those who appear to have been in the ED for an inordinate amount of time. The system will interface with the laboratory and x-ray departments so that laboratory results and x-ray interpretations can be transmitted electronically to the ED for physician use. More sophisticated systems will generate labeled laboratory and radiology requisitions, and allow the entry of free text by the physician to describe the patient's historical and examination data, as well as serial clinical and diagnostic information.

Hand-held computers will provide summary lists of differential diagnoses, formulas for various biomedical calculations, and the dosages of commonly used drugs. Microcomputers will provide diagnostic programs covering the major clinical conditions. In addition, traditional textbooks will be stored in easily accessible programs and frequently updated to provide the most current medical information. The more important medical journal articles will be integrated into this medical knowledge system. A universal index will replace the existing manual system, which is laborious and cost ineffective.

Existing diagnostic technology will be linked electronically to experts in remote sites, who will interpret the findings and transmit their diagnoses back to the ED. The most likely technology for this development is imaging, especially ultrasound, a noninvasive, safe diagnostic tool. Ultrasound machines are able to simplify the diagnosis of many conditions such as pericardial effusion, gallbladder disease, abdominal masses, and renal stones. A hand-held ultrasound probe operated by a trained person will transmit signals to a diagnostic center, where physician ultrasound experts will correlate the signals with pertinent clinical information and interpret the clinical situation.

This type of system will have multiple uses, including utilization within a hospital to avoid the necessity of transporting patients from the ED to the ultrasound department, which can be unsafe and result in inefficient use of space and personnel in the ultrasound facility. Keeping the patient in the ED is safer because clinical surveillance is continuous and the time needed for the ED patient's ultrasound examination is significantly reduced. Only a brief period is required for the physician expert's interpretation of the transmitted clinical information and ultrasound signals. The system will also facilitate more accurate diagnosis in rural hospitals, from which ultrasound signals and clinical information will be transmitted to regional medical centers, or possibly to the homes of physican experts for interpretation.

Miniaturization and simplification of use will result in the development of blood and urine auto-analyzers suited to ED use by appropriately trained personnel. Common blood and urine tests will be performed accurately, inexpensively, and quickly in the ED to speed up patient evaluation and treatment.

## QUALITY ASSURANCE PROGRAM

If the systems described thus far do develop as predicted, preliminary evaluation of the quality of patient care will be largely done using the computer. The system will identify patients with specific conditions to allow in-depth review of the medical records. Utilization data such as evaluation and treatment times, number of laboratory and x-ray tests, patient/personnel ratios, and referral information will be easily accessible, and thus more useful for quality-of-care evaluation. The system will be used to store apparently random deviations in quality of care and to facilitate aggregation of these deviations so that trends can be identified and corrective action taken when necessary. The system will not only perform relatively crude screening functions, but will reduce greatly the need for costly manual screening of medical records to identify cases for in-depth review.

For example, patients with chest pain falling into selected age categories could be identified by the system, and divided into those admitted and those discharged. The appropriateness of tests used to evaluate these patients could be analyzed, as could their clinical status at a specified time period after the ED visit. Variations in practice should be identified by comparing the specific actions taken for a particular patient by an individual physician against standards and criteria developed by peer physicians and other clinical experts. Thus, physicians who appear to perform less or more than the standard number of tests and examinations, or who appear to admit or discharge their chest pain patients inappropriately, can be identified and given an opportunity to justify their practices. Often these apparent deviations from standard practice are in fact indicative of excellent medical care, because of the difference in the characteristics of the particular patients when compared to those of the data base from which the standards and criteria are derived.

## CONCLUSION

Technology, which appears to be ideally suited for the ED, has only recently made an impact on emergency care. Although its benefits have exceeded its costs, new technology has made ED care expensive, often unjustifiably. Its income-generating potential for both the physician and the hospital, and its relative availability, have contributed to cost-ineffective health practices. It is likely that incorporation of technology into ED care will proceed at an increasing rate, and its use will depend heavily on the characteristics of the hospital. Rural hospital EDs will utilize technologies to provide services that are not immediately available elsewhere, whereas urban hospital EDs will adapt and apply the more sophisticated technologies already in use elsewhere in the hospital. The future of cost-effective ED technology probably lies with increasing miniaturization and the availability of communication satellites. New solutions create new problems. The misuse of technology will diminish as technical improvements and better-educated providers and consumers develop side by side.

SELECTED BIBLIOGRAPHY

Brown, K., Shoos, K., and Clarke, C. Jr. (1961). The changing emergency ward. *Am. J. Surg. 101*:336–42.

Gavaler, J., and Van Thiel, D. (1980). The non-emergency in the emergency room. *J. National Med. Assoc. 72* (1): 33–6.

Karas, S. (1980). Cost containment in emergency medicine. *J.A.M.A. 243*: 1356–59.

King, E. T. (1965). The emergency services and the changing pattern of general practice. *Med. J. Aust.* (July suppl) 8:8–9.

Noble, J. Jr., Wechsler, H., La Montagne, M., et al., eds. (1973). *Emergency Medical Services: Behavioral and Planning Perspectives.* New York: Behavioral Publications.

*Regional Emergency Medical Communications Systems* (1978). National Academy of Sciences Final Report of the Committee on Regional Emergency Medical Communications Systems. Washington, D.C.: Assembly of Life Sciences, National Academy of Sciences.

Sadler, A., Sadler, B., and Webb, S. (1977). *Emergency Medical Care: The Neglected Public Service, The Connecticut Experience.* Cambridge, Mass.: Ballinger.

U.S. Statutes at Large, 93d Congress, first session vol. 87. (1973). PL 93-154 Title XII – Emergency Medical Services Systems, Nov. 16, 1973, p. 594.

# PART V

# APPLYING TECHNOLOGY IN CLINICAL PRACTICE

CHAPTER 8

# THE UNWANTED SUITOR:
# LAW AND THE USE OF
# HEALTH CARE TECHNOLOGY

WILLIAM J. CURRAN

## THE LEGAL CLIMATE

One of the most serious occupational hazards for medical practice in the United States in the 1980s is the steady increase in malpractice suits. Twenty-five years ago, fewer than 2 in 100 physicians had suits brought against them annually. Currently, in some states, the number of suits is alleged to be 1 in 4 or 5 physicians each year. The vulnerability of hospitals over the last quarter century is even more dramatic. Up to the mid-1950s, most hospitals, which were charitably organized or publicly operated, were not sued at all; they were generally immune from patient injury lawsuits. Today, immunity of both charity and public institutions has been removed in most states. The federal government, formerly immune, is also subject to suit for malpractice in Veterans Administration and other federal hospitals.

The national crisis in medical malpractice dates, however, only from 1975 (An Overview of Medical Malpractice 1975). Prior to that time, the private insurance industry managed to cope with the increasing rate of suits and the inflation in financial awards per suit. In the mid-1970s, however, the private casualty insurance system for medical patient injuries virtually collapsed. Many companies went bankrupt or stopped writing policies in the medical and hospital fields. The remaining companies raised their premiums dramatically, from 3 to 10 times their previous levels. In testimony before the U.S. Senate in December 1975, Dr. Roger Egeberg, special assistant to the Secretary of Health, Education and Welfare, estimated that the total cost of malpractice insurance to physicians and hospitals in 1975 was about $500 million (Continuing Medical Malpractice Insurance Crisis 1975). He estimated that it would rise to $1 billion in 1976 and to $2 billion within a few years. The reaction of the state legislatures was to pass statutes to make insurance coverage more widely available to physicians

119

and hospitals and to reform the court system to aid the medical care industry in coping with unjustified claims. The situation has since eased somewhat, but the general inflation in the economy has caused malpractice premiums to continue to rise in most parts of the country.

## THE BASIS OF LEGAL LIABILITY

The law of medical professional liability has been reformed, but the basic foundation for a lawsuit against a physician or hospital remains the same: The basis of liability is *negligence*, or the failure to maintain an accepted standard of medical care (Louisell and Williams 1960; Holder 1978). This theory of vulnerability is also known as a *fault test*, as distinguished from a contractual guarantee or warranty of a successful outcome for all patient care. By contrast, the manufacturing industry carries a warranty standard for products sold on the open market unless the contracts of sale specifically reduce the degree of liability.

When a lawsuit is brought against a physician, four elements are required for a patient to recover damage:

1. Proof of the existence of a particular accepted and required standard of care for the procedure or practice involved
2. Proof that this accepted standard was violated, that is, that a *lower standard* was applied, or that the proper practice was applied erroneously or carelessly
3. Proof of a causal relationship between this violation and the patient's eventual injury
4. Damage to the patient, that is, physical and/or mental injury, usually with consequent financial loss in terms of medical bills and the loss of a job or income, plus the pain, discomfort, and disability due to the injury itself

## ACCEPTED STANDARDS OF MEDICAL PRACTICE

The key element in the legal requirements set out above is the first. No lawsuit against a physician or hospital can be maintained without proof that there was an accepted standard of care within the profession that was violated. Accepted standards may vary with the type of practice involved and, to some degree, with the location of the practice.

The legal concept of a professionally accepted practice is rather conservative. It has often been said that under this formulation, a physician "cannot be too far behind or too far out in front" of the majority of his or her colleagues in general practice or in the particular specialty in question. The physician who is found to lag behind other doctors rarely has an adequate excuse for such conduct. There is a professional obligation to keep up with the state of the art in one's field and to abandon practices that may be harmful to patients. In former years, there was a law that tended to protect physicians practicing in rural, isolated communities from lawsuits for negligence in not following improved practices and not abandoning outmoded, ineffective, potentially damaging ones. This was called the *locality rule*. It demanded that the courts apply the accepted practices of the physician's local community or other like communities (Nations and Surgent 1973). It was felt that small-town doctors could not be expected to adopt quickly the advances of their urban colleagues who had access to more modern facilities and teaching hospitals. This protective rule is fast disappearing from malpractice law throughout the United States. It has been replaced by a more general requirement of a regional or national standard of care for most common procedures. One of the strong supports for the movement toward this national standard was the success in the 1970s of the Regional Medical Programs installed during the Johnson administration. The purpose of these programs, which were conducted with large federal appropriations, was to bring currently accepted medical advances in practice and technology within the reach of all physicians.

### LEGAL ATTITUDES TOWARD CLINICAL EXPERIMENTATION IN TECHNOLOGICAL RESEARCH

As indicated above, U.S. courts frown upon physicians' practices that are unproved or uncommon. Litigated cases have often involved procedures or technology developed and utilized only by the defendant doctors, without acceptance by their colleagues and generally without adequate proof that they were more successful than the traditional methods applied. When patients have been harmed by these practices, the doctors have been found financially liable for improper care. In a popular textbook on medical malpractice, Louis Regan warned his medical readers: "In the treatment of the patient, there must be no experimentation" (Regan 1956).

In an important and influential court case, *Brown v. Hughes* (1934), the use of nonproven, experimental techniques was equated with rash action and virtual recklessness on the part of the doctor. Up to this point, the few court decisions that existed could have been interpreted to treat experimentation as an outlawed area of medical practice if it deviated significantly from accepted standards. To a large extent, experimentation carried with it *strict liability* without proved fault for any injury to the patient. If the patient were to suffer as a result of the use of advanced techniques, the physician, not the patient, assumed responsibility for injury if a mishap occurred during the procedure.

It is probable that writers such as Louis Regan, with their overcautious approach to advising readers, misread the legal precedents. The courts in these early years did not review and decide cases involving responsible efforts at clinical innovation at major teaching centers. The few cases brought to court were extreme examples of admittedly disreputable physicians, often in solo practice, who preyed upon desperate patients with worthless medications, dangerous surgical procedures, or strange science fiction devices. The literature concerning malpractice nevertheless tended to interpret these limited precedents as discouraging not only clearly irresponsible actions but also the application of any new technological advances, at least in their early stages of clinical development, at the "peril" of their users.

## TECHNOLOGICAL EXPERIMENTATION AND INFORMED CONSENT

A more rational legal approach to clinical innovation and the use of advanced technology began to appear in the legal literature after World World II. The new approach drew its support from *judicial dicta* (commentary by judges in cases decided on other issues) and from law journal papers by respected writers (Cady 1952; Ladimer 1955). This commentary stressed the fact that the litigated cases did not involve responsible leaders in academic medicine seeking new knowledge and utilizing accepted medical standards for such work. Also, it was pointed out that the exploiters and medical quacks found guilty of malpractice nearly always used fraudulent methods to deceive their patients into accepting the worthless remedies. In order to function properly, therefore, responsible clinical innovators would need to avoid these errors (Beecher 1966). A legally supportable methodology would include:

1. Following a well-designed research plan or experimental protocol of high scientific quality with reasonable potential for yielding valuable new knowledge
2. Utilizing clinical investigators of experience and superior scientific reputation
3. Seeking and receiving the informed consent of the patient who was subject to the innovative procedure

As a model for accepted practices in clinical research the commentators seized upon the *Nuremberg code*, a set of principles for accepted experimental practices formulated for legal purposes at the trials of Nazi war criminals after World War II (*U.S. v. Brandt et al.* 1947). This code put particular stress on enlightened, informed consent and on the avoidance of dangerous medical procedures.

In the past 20 years, there have been very few medical malpractice cases involving responsible clinical investigation. In fact, the total number of appellate court cases in the United States and Canada is no more than five. These few cases have uniformly endorsed the more rational approach outlined above. However, the important law in this field has not been developed under the common law and in malpractice litigation. Rather, it has been formulated almost entirely under federal statutes and regulations concerned with governmental financial support for medical research and federal control of the testing and marketing of therapeutic drugs and technological devices (Curran 1969). Research centers and teaching hospitals have been required to establish committees to review and approve all experimentation on human subjects and subject patients prior to the beginning of any such work by clinical investigators. Where such regulatory committees have been used, the courts have found the experimental activities to be proper and responsible (*Bailey v. Lally* 1979).

## THE LEGAL OBLIGATION TO USE ACCEPTED MEDICAL TECHNOLOGY

Despite the cautions noted above in regard to unproved, unaccepted technologies, U.S. courts have never hesitated to require physicians and hospitals to apply medical technologies once they were generally accepted. In fact, where the technology does not involve excessive danger to the patient, is readily available, and is reasonably reliable for its purposes, the courts have demanded its use. The most outstanding example of this judicial tendency has been in the application of diagnostic radiology. U.S. courts accepted x-ray evidence very quickly after the technology was introduced. X-ray pictures became common in support of medical testimony in personal injury trauma cases to provide objective proof of bone fractures suffered in railway, automobile, and other accidents. By the 1930s, it was no longer necessary to offer evidence in court of the reliability of x-rays and their acceptance in medical practice. This fact was taken for granted, and the x-ray results were readily presented. When medical malpractice cases were filed when physicians had failed to x-ray and the patient was later discovered to have fractures that went untreated, the courts had little patience with the defendants. In many cases, the courts have ruled that it is common knowledge that x-rays should be taken when bone fracture was or should have been suspected. The courts have also described the failure to utilize diagnostic x-rays as so clearly negligent as to constitute *res ipsa loquitur*, or the action "speaks for itself," an obvious failure to follow accepted medical practice.

In later years, this type of common knowledge or *res ipsa loquitur* description was applied to other medical technologies. For example, in *Corn v. French* (1955), the Nevada Supreme Court ruled that it was common knowledge that a tissue biopsy should be performed before surgery for a radical mastectomy. The postoperative study revealed no malignancy in the breast removed.

In an effort to avoid charges of malpractice for failure to use accepted technologies, many physicians have been alleged to overutilize x-ray diagnosis and other medical tests. This overutilization has been a part of *defensive medicine*, the use of unnecessary procedures and technology merely as a means of presenting a good record of practice should the patient encounter problems that might later be alleged to have been caused by malpractice.

### FURTHER DEVELOPMENTS IN COURT-ESTABLISHED RULES

The majority of case law on malpractice involving a failure to utilize accepted medical technology has allowed the defendant doctor to present evidence in rebuttal of the charge that the technology should have been applied. Usually, the plaintiff relies solely on a common knowledge or *res ipsa loquitur* rule to force the physician to explain the failure. The plaintiff often does not, or cannot, present an expert medical witness to support the case against the doctor. The defendant doctor generally testifies personally and/or calls other experts to support his or her decision not to use the technology. The physician may have relied on a general physical examination and clinical signs and symptoms, plus clinical judgment, in making the diagnosis or the decision to treat in a particular way. Also, the physician may have used other forms of technology believed to be superior to the one not utilized. It should also be realized that the physician is *never* guilty of malpractice in failing to use accepted technological aids, even if he or she was clearly violating common practice, unless the patient is *harmed* as a result. If the patient does not have pathology that could have been revealed by the test, then there is no legal liability. For example, in the radical mastectomy surgery case noted above, *Corn v. French*, there would have been no malpractice suit if the postoperative study of the tissue had indicated malignancy.

However, in certain cases, U.S. courts have required the defendant to apply available technology that would have prevented the plaintiff's injury or loss. In these cases, the court rejected the defense that the accepted practice was *against* the use of the technology, and found that the entire group or industry was clearly negligent in not adopting the technological advances available. This line of cases originated in a famous decision by Justice Learned Hand in the Second Circuit Federal Court of Appeals in 1932. In the case of T. J. Hooper, Justice Hand dealt with a case involving a tugboat collision in New York harbor in a dense fog. Evidence indicated that use of radio might have given the tugs warning of the fog and aided in the emergency. The defendant's tugboat had no radio. In rebutting the charge that the boat should have been equipped with a radio, the defendant pointed out that no tugboat in that busy harbor had as yet installed radios. Justice Hand rejected this offer of proof and held that "reasonable prudence" required that such easily installed equipment, with proved reliability and utility, should have been adopted years before. He wrote that the courts would *require* such precautions be taken even in the event that "a whole calling may have unduly lagged in the adoption of new and available devices." He concluded that the use of some devices or technology may be "so *imperative* that even their *universal disregard* will not excuse their omission."

This rule of reasonable prudence has been enforced only infrequently against an entire industry's accepted standards, but it has not been ignored. Has it an application to the medical field?

The entire medical care industry was shocked when the Hooper rule was applied in 1974, in the supreme court of Washington state, to the field of ophthalmology. In the case of *Helling v. Carey and Laughlin*, the plaintiff had gone to the defendants, partners in ophthalmology, with complaints about her contact lenses and with frequent complaints of irritation and pain. She was seen over the period 1963 to 1968. Her problems were generally attributed to troubles with her contact lenses. Only in late 1968, when the plaintiff was 32 years of age, did the defendants, after the plaintiff's further complaints about blurred vision, conduct extensive tests of her field of vision and her eye pressure because of the possibility of glaucoma. On that occasion, the plaintiff was found to have advanced glaucoma and to have already lost considerable vision. At the time of the trial, the plaintiff's condition had worsened and was irreversible.

The defendant doctors countered the charge of negligence in not applying the pressure test for glaucoma with undisputed evidence that ophthalmologists across the country did not routinely test patients under 40 years of age for glaucoma. It was admitted, however, that such tests were done at earlier ages when the patient's complaints and examination caused suspicion of this disease. Dr. Carey testified that glaucoma was found in patients under 40 in only about 1 case in 25,000.

The supreme court of Washington rejected the defendant's evidence. It was found that the entire specialty field was failing to use reasonable prudence in not routinely conducting pressure tests, at least on all patients of this patient's age and with her complaints. The court described five reasons for imposing the requirement:

1. The technology in question was highly accurate.
2. The test procedure was not dangerous to the patient.
3. The test procedure was painless to the patient.
4. The entire procedure was relatively inexpensive.
5. The disease that the technology was designed to detect was extremely grave, in this case involving blindness.

The reaction of the medical and insurance communities to the case and its rule of reasonable prudence was highly critical. The case has generally been credited with contributing considerably to the "insurance crisis" of the next year, 1975.

No other courts have followed the Helling decision directly. Furthermore, the legislature in Washington was expected to reform the law in order to avoid the future application of such a rule by the state's courts. A statute designed to accomplish the change was enacted in 1976, but the state's supreme court justices did not find that it had succeeded (*Gates v. Jensen* 1979). The statute required the court to find, for malpractice, that the defendant doctors "failed to exercise that degree of skill, care, and learning possessed by other persons in the profession." The court found the key word to be *possessed*. They discovered that the legislature had rejected an earlier version of the law, in which the word was *practiced*. On this basis, the court concluded that the physicians possessed the skills and technologies, but had refused to apply them to patients under age 40. This refusal was still found to be a violation of the rule of reasonable prudence on the part of physicians in Washington. Up to the time of this writing, the Washington legislature has not acted further on this issue.

### THE PATIENT'S ROLE IN TECHNOLOGY APPLICATIONS

The application of technology to medical practice does not concern the clinical investigator or attending physician alone. The patient also has a role in the choice of procedures, practices, medications, and therapeutic technologies. The intelligent patient may request that the doctor consider the use of certain new approaches, including recently developed technologies. The attending physician need not accept the suggestions, but should consider them seriously. One requirement of a fully informed consent is the presentation to the patient of reasonable alternatives to the course of treatment that the attending doctor advises. These alternatives should include technologies that the particular physician does not use and perhaps does not fully accept or understand. For example, the alternatives for an advanced heart disease patient might reasonably include referral to a distant medical center where open heart surgery and/or heart transplantation may be practiced.

Probably the most well-known lawsuit in this area was the malpractice action against Dr. Denton Cooley in Houston for his first attempt to use an artificial left ventricle cardiac replacement in his patient, Mr. Haskell Karp. Dr. Cooley explained the new technology carefully to his patient, an intelligent man who had suffered severe cardiac problems for many years. Mr. Karp came to Houston to be cared for by Dr. Cooley. The patient wished to try a cadaver heart transplant, but none was available at the time. His condition worsened, and he became increasingly impatient for an organ transplant. Dr. Cooley then offered to use an artificial heart implant that would suffice until a cadaver heart became available. The patient requested the artificial instrument. Dr. Cooley and other physicians discussed the matter with the patient. The patient also consulted a rabbi who had counseled him since he was first admitted to the hospital. The rabbi testified that Mr. Karp was aware of the risk involved and knew that this was the first human application of the cardiac pump. The rabbi said that Mr. Karp had told him that the chances were at least 80 to 20 against his survival, but that he was glad of the possibility of a normal life. He said that he was proud to be the first recipient of an artificial heart.

Dr. Cooley decided to go ahead. He first attempted a surgical operation called a *wedge procedure*, but it was unsuccessful. He then inserted the mechanical device. The patient was sustained for over 30 hours on the pump. A cadaver organ was then implanted, and sustained the patient for about another 30 hours, until he died.

Suit for wrongful death was brought against the surgeon by the wife of the patient, who charged that neither Mr. Karp nor she was fully informed of the risks of the innovative procedure. After a nine-day trial, the judge dismissed the case against Dr. Cooley. He ruled that no malpractice was proved and that the patient had given his informed consent to the innovative technology being used in his case. On appeal to the Fifth Circuit Federal Court of Appeals, the judge's decision was upheld. The prestigious Fifth Circuit Court reviewed the conversations with the patient and the written informed consent that he had signed. The judges were clearly impressed with the thoroughness of the hospital and the surgeons in informing the patient of the risks he was running and the remoteness of his chances for a complete recovery or survival. The wife had testified at the trial that she thought that the artificial instrument was little more than a "newer model" of a heart-lung machine and that Mr. Karp was really going to have a cadaver transplant. The Fifth Circuit Court ruled that the wife's understanding was not required in the matter. The key involvement was that of the intelligent, rational patient himself, and the court had no doubt that Mr. Karp understood the situation fully.

The Cooley decision is of primary significance legally to the field of medical technology. It indicates important judicial support for careful consent practices, including the use of written consent forms, to involve patients adequately in decisions to apply innovative medical procedures.

There is another issue concerning patient consent, or even patient urging, in the use of clinical technology, either long accepted or innovative. This issue is the patient's *refusal* of the procedure. What is the physician's obligation when the patient refuses what seems to be an obviously beneficial procedure?

If the patient is rational, the refusal must be respected, even if it seems unwise or even foolhardy to the doctor. This rule of law is quite well settled, although it is offered largely as *judicial dictum* in cases where the patient either did not refuse, or the refusal was found to have sound logical support (*Lane v. Candura* 1978).

A recent case in California presented a novel application of the right of patient refusal. In this case, *Truman v. Thomas* (1980), the woman patient refused on more than one occasion to submit to a pap smear designed to detect cervical cancer. The physician was a general practitioner who had cared for the patient over a 6-year period including delivery of one of her two children. He testified that he had frequently said to the patient, "You should have a pap smear." She had declined the test. On at least two occasions, Dr. Thomas had performed pelvic examinations on the patient, asking her at this time if she wanted a pap smear. She had refused, saying that she didn't think she could afford the cost. Dr. Thomas testified that he had offered to defer any payment, but Mrs. Truman still refused. She had always paid cash for medical services at the time they were rendered, either to her or to her children.

Mrs. Truman visited a urologist in April 1969 because of a urinary tract infection. While examining her, the urologist discovered that her cervix was extremely rough and that she was having heavy vaginal discharges. He advised her to see a gynecologist as soon as possible. Mrs. Truman did not follow his advice, but he telephoned her several months later and made an appointment on her behalf with a gynecologist. It was now 6 months since she had seen the urologist and at least 7 months since she had last seen the defendant, Dr. Thomas. The gynecologist, in his first examination of Mrs. Truman, found a large mass in the cervix too advanced for surgery. It proved to be malignant. The tumor was not successfully treated, and she died some 8 months later.

Mrs. Truman's two minor children sued Dr. Thomas in a wrongful death action for not preventing her death. They argued that he should have made greater efforts to persuade her to have periodic pap smear examinations during the years he was seeing her.

Surprising as it seemed to many, the supreme court of California, one of the most liberal high courts in the country in supporting financial awards for personal injury plaintiffs, agreed with this argument and found that the defendant could be liable for malpractice.

The basis for this unusual finding against Dr. Thomas was that he breached his duty to his patient in not warning her more forcefully of the consequences of allowing a grave disease, cervical cancer, to develop undetected over a period of time. Dr. Thomas, admittedly, had only *suggested* that she needed the test. On her refusal, he had respected her decision. At the trial, he indicated that he believed Mrs. Truman and all of his female patients were well aware of the purpose of a pap smear: to detect cervical cancer. After her refusal on at least one or two occasions, Mrs. Truman had responded, "I just don't feel like it." On the occasion of the pelvic examinations, when performance of the test would have been quite easy and convenient, she added that she could not afford the cost. Dr. Thomas, as indicated earlier, had offered to delay payment and urged her to have the test. She still refused, and he took no further action. On no occasion did he counsel her further or warn her of the danger of cancer.

The supreme court of California nevertheless sent the matter back for trial (or settlement) on the basis that there were still some issues of fact to be determined by the jury. For a verdict in favor of the plaintiffs, the jury would need to find that, had Mrs. Truman been warned properly of the potential danger in refusing, she would have consented to the tests periodically over the years and her cancer could have been prevented. For a verdict in favor of Dr. Thomas, the jury would need to find that Mrs. Truman, even if properly warned or already aware of the danger, would still have refused the tests. The California supreme court gave its own rather pointed interpretation of the latter alternative. The court observed that the jury could find on behalf of the doctor (no malpractice) only if they decided that the patient would have "*unreasonably refused* a pap smear in the face of adequate disclosure."

It should also be noted that the procedure involved in the Truman case met all the criteria that so impressed the much more conservative court of Washington state in the Helling decision examined earlier. It was a simple, painless diagnostic test; it was accurate; it was inexpensive; and it was designed to detect a disease or a process that could lead to grave consequences for the patient.

The California decision remains unique among the group of cases involving allegations of failure to warn patients. In all of the other suits, the patient had consented to the treatment and had suffered some ill effect from the application of the technology. In some of the cases, the possible dangers were very remote and the benefits were direct and substantial. Nevertheless, liability has been found because of the failure to warn and thus to give the patient an opportunity to refuse. In only one case of which I am aware did a high court refuse to demand such an outcome. The Oklahoma supreme court found that a failure to warn patients of an extremely remote (1 in 5 to 8 million) risk of paralysis from poliomyelitis immunization could not be grounds for a successful suit even when the patient was paralyzed (*Cunningham v. Charles Pfizer and Co.* 1974). The court found that rational patients (and parents of minor children) would not refuse the immunizations and the clear benefits received from them even if warned of these extremely remote dangers.

It should be clear from the preceding discussions that U.S. courts place a very high value on patient participation in decisions to apply either accepted or new treatments and technologies. Investigators and attending physicians should warn patients of *any level* of danger, especially if related to grave consequences of severe disability, pain, or death. Physicians should also make patients aware of reasonable alternatives to the treatment suggested, including new technology of clear value to the patient.

### LIFE-SUPPORT SYSTEMS AND BRAIN DEATH

This last section is concerned with certain other, more indirect legal consequences of the application of technological advances in medical clinical practice.

One of the most striking consequences in terms of increased court litigation in recent years has been the development of complex, highly effective life-support systems, particularly heart-lung machines. More and more patients can be resuscitated and kept alive with life-support equipment. The application of these technologies is not inexpensive. In fact, it is very high in terms of equipment, equipment maintenance, hospital space, and personnel. The courts are now being called upon to intervene in what were very private, personal decisions to begin, continue, or terminate such treatment in patients with no real prospect of total recovery.

The first and still the most successful of the legal changes in this area has been the widespread adoption of a new definition of death using the concept of *brain death*. Adoption of this new criterion of death has enabled medical facilities to discontinue life support systems for patients who have hopelessly lost all brain function and consciousness. Both legislatures and courts rapidly accepted the concept after its development by the Harvard University Ad Hoc Committee on Brain Death, of which the writer was privileged to be the legal member (1968). The committee, chaired by Dr. Henry K. Beecher, set forth medical, ethical, and legal criteria for determining brain death and turning off clinical instrumentality that was prolonging decisions on ending treatment. In 1978, the National Conference of Commissioners on Uniform State Laws adopted a brief enabling statute that was recommended to all states as a basis for legalizing the new concept of brain death. Modifications were made in the draft language in 1980. None of the statutes adopted in the 27 states that have enacted laws have made the mistake of including actual medical criteria for determining death. The 1980 draft of the national commissioners, for example, directs that the determination of irreversible cessation of all functions of the brain be made "in accordance with accepted medical standards." It should be noted that the concept of accepted standards drawn from common law is thereby incorporated into the statute.

The brain death concept covers only a small percentage of the patients, particularly elderly patients, who are sustained or resuscitated, or who have been kept alive by various applications of medical technology. More and more of these difficult cases are finding their way into court because doctors and patients are unsure of what to do. The relevance of these dilemmas to our discussion in this chapter comes from the fact that so many physicians and hospitals consider themselves to be seriously vulnerable to a malpractice suit if they do not continue to offer treatment. Many physicians believe that the standard of accepted practice requires them and the hospital or nursing home to "opt for life" when any means is available to sustain it.

It is arguable that neither medical ethics nor malpractice law has ever required an unwavering, universal devotion in medical care to continuing life support under all circumstances. Ever since the general recognition of the papal commentary of 1958, it has been considered ethically proper to utilize only ordinary care, not extraordinary measures, to prolong life in the dying patient who is in pain and unable to function with dignity. The definition of extraordinary measures that need not be utilized has never been very clear, at least not as clear as some rather literal-minded medical practitioners and hospital administrators would like. However, they have seemed to be closely identified with high technology and the utilization of resources that could be considered scarce and expensive.

The court decisions in this field are all quite recent. They tend to fall into two groups: (1) those that have demanded close court supervision of such decision making when patients could not decide for themselves, and (2) those that have placed more trust in the medical community, aided perhaps by hospital-based ethics committees, in making such decisions in the patient's best interests. The courts have also resorted to appointing special guardians for patients; these persons substitute for the patient and decide what care is to be given. Regardless of the judicial approach taken, nearly all decisions have allowed *removal* of life support systems. None of them has stated that all measures to sustain life must be continued. Only one high court case that I have reviewed has required treatment to continue in a contested matter: an order to continue blood transfusions in a 53-year-old man who was severely retarded (with a mental age of about 18 months). The patient had cancer of the bladder and was receiving chemotherapy. He was in pain that was generally relieved by medications. The highest court of New York State refused to allow discontinuance of treatment, which, it found, would "allow an incompetent patient to bleed to death" because his mother thought it "*best* for one with an incurable disease" (emphasis added) (In the Matter of John Storar 1981). Nevertheless, the same high court, in the same combined opinion, allowed removal of a mechanical respirator that was being used on an 83-year old retired Catholic priest. The patient had sustained severe brain damage in a hernia operation and was not expected to recover consciousness. He was not brain dead, however. The New York court ordered treatment discontinued on the basis of "clear and convincing evidence" that the patient had earlier given his rational and well-thought-out opinion that he did not wish treatment to be continued if such circumstances occurred. In a few states, statutes have been enacted to allow persons to adopt and sign "living wills" containing instructions to discontinue, or not to begin, treatment in such events. The statutes often describe the treatment that should not be given as "extraordinary means of sustaining life."

### LEGAL COUNTERMEASURES: COST CONTAINMENT AND CONTROLS ON OVERUSE OF MEDICAL TECHNOLOGY

No one active in the medical care field today can be unaware of the change in attitude in recent years regarding high technology in medical practice and hospital care. For many years, the thrust of public policy was always expected to support improved clinical procedures and technologies. Medical research has been supported strongly in the U.S. Congress for decades through the National Institutes of Health. Other countries had looked especially to the United States for the development of new medical breakthroughs. Nevertheless, there have been signs of weakening of public support. The pharmaceutical industry for years has been pointing to a new drug development lag in the United States due to increasingly tight regulatory controls on the pharmaceutical industry by the federal Food and Drug Administration. Conservative administrations beginning with that of Richard Nixon have been slowly but surely reducing federal commitments to medical research and the training of medical clinical investigators as well as basic medical scientists.

The most widespread change in national public policy, however, has come within the past 5 years or so with the development of legally installed medical and hospital cost control programs (Havighurst 1977). Once begun, these programs have commonly been strengthened and expanded to cover further areas of medical costs. One of the main targets of the cost control regulations in every state has been expensive medical technology such as computerized tomographic scanners discussed in Chapter 5 (Curran 1981).

The cost containment programs have not been concentrating merely on controlling capital investment in high-technology, high-cost medical equipment. They have sought to reduce substantially the number and kind of technological aids used by physicians and hospitals that may prove to be unnecessary. For example, the regulators may seek to reduce the habit of repeating diagnostic tests when the results are positive, and to eliminate those tests that seem to have little or no significance in the actual treatment decisions of physicians. Also, administrators of health insurance plans are requiring more second opinions of other physicians before approving serious and expensive procedures.

It has been observed that the courts, in dealing with medical malpractice and applying accepted standards of care, have not yet caught up with this emphasis on cost containment. This clash of philosophies has not yet been aired in the courts. We would expect that the courts, in reviewing malpractice cases wherein patients have been severely harmed, will not be totally sympathetic to vigorous cost containment at the expense of coldly calculated patient risk. Nevertheless, the courts can be expected to listen to medically supported arguments concerning reasonable decisions about the utilization of scarce medical resources on a cost effectiveness basis. The most important courtroom battles over the application of medical technology to patient care may well occur in the remaining years of the 1980s.

## SELECTED BIBLIOGRAPHY

An overview of medical malpractice. (1975). Committee Report, U.S. House of Representatives, Committee on Interstate and Foreign Commerce. Washington, D.C.: U.S. Government Printing Office.

*Bailey v. Lally*, 581 F. Supp. 203, 1979. (The case involved the use of prisoners in medical research. The U.S. Court of Appeals held the practices to be proper under the approval of a university-based ethical review committee.)

Beecher, H. K. (1966). Ethics and clinical research. *N. Engl. J. Med. 274*:1354–60.

*Brown v. Hughes*, 94 Colo. 295, 30 P. 259 (1934).

Cady, E. J. (1952). Medical malpractice: what about experimentation? *Ann. W. Med. Surg. 6*:164–70.

Continuing medical malpractice insurance crisis, 1975. (1975). Hearings Before the Subcommittee on Health, U.S. Senate. Washington, D.C.: U.S. Government Printing Office.

*Corn v. French*, 71 Nev. 280, 289 P.2d 173, 1955.

*Cunningham v. Charles Pfizer and Co.*, 532 P.2d 1377, 1974.

Curran, W. J. (1969). Governmental regulation of the use of human subjects in medical research: the approach of two federal agencies. *Daedalus 98*:542–95.

Curran, W. J. (1981). The health planners and computerized tomography: high technology, cost control, and judicial review. *N. Engl. J. Med. 303*:626–7.

Defining death, report on medical, legal and ethical issues in the determination of death. (1981). President's Commission for the Study of Ethical Problems in Medicine and Biomedical and Behavioral Research. Washington, D.C.: U.S. Government Printing Office, p. 73.

*Gates v. Jensen*, 92 Wash. 2d 246, 595 P.2d 919, 1979.

Havighurst, C. (1977). Health care cost-containment regulation: prospects and an alternative. *Am. J. Law Med. 3*:309–26.

*Helling v. Carey and Laughlin*, 83 Wash. 2d 514, 519 P. 2d 981, 1974.

Holder, A. R. (1978). *Medical Malpractice Law*, 2d ed. New York: Wiley.

*T. J. Hooper* 60 F. 2d 732, 1932.

In the Matter of John Storar. (1981). New York Court of Appeals. Reprinted in a collection of cases in Curran, W. J., and Shapiro, E. D., *Law, Medicine and Forensic Science*, 3rd ed. Boston: Little, Brown, 1982, p. 868.

Ladimer, I. (1955). Ethical and legal aspects of medical research on human beings. *J. Pub. Law 3*:35–80.

*Lane v. Candura*, 376 N.E. 2d 1232, 1978.

Louisell, D., and Williams, J. (1960). *Medical Malpractice*. New York: Matthew Bender (supplemented regularly).

Nations, W. H., and Surgent, H. (1973). Medical malpractice and the locality rule. *Texas L. J. 14*:129–49.

Pope Pius XII (1958). The prolongation of life, in Reiser, S. J., Dyck, A. J., and Curran, W. J., (eds.) (1977), *Ethics in Medicine: Historical Perspectives and Contemporary Concerns*. Cambridge: MIT Press, pp. 501–4.

Regan, L. J. (1956). *Doctor and Patient and the Law*, 3rd ed. St. Louis: C. V. Mosby, p. 370.

Report of Harvard Medical School Ad Hoc Committee to examine the definition of brain death: a definition of irreversible coma. (1968). *J.A.M.A. 205*:337–41.

*Truman v. Thomas*, 27 Cal. 3d 285, 1980.

*U.S. v. Brandt et al.* (1947). *Trials of War Criminals, The Medical Case*, Washington, D.C.: U.S. Government Printing Office. vol. 2, pp. 181–3. The code is reprinted in Reiser, S. J., Dyck, A. J., and Curran, W. J., (eds.) (1977), *Ethics in Medicine: Historical Perspectives and Contemporary Concerns*. Cambridge, Mass.: MIT Press, 1977, p. 272.

# CHAPTER 9

# THE MACHINE AND THE MARKETPLACE: ECONOMIC CONSIDERATIONS IN APPLYING HEALTH CARE TECHNOLOGY

WARREN BUTT and DUNCAN NEUHAUSER

Physicians are expected to treat patients as thoroughly as possible. As the 1949 ethical code of the World Medical Association states: "A doctor owes a patient . . . all the resources of his science." However, the economic realities of resource scarcity make this ethical aspiration impossible. The problem is to determine which expenditures are most beneficial. The following story of a Swedish heart transplant patient illustrates this point.

A nearly complete National Health Service paid for through taxes is the cornerstone of the welfare system of Sweden, a country with a per capita income slightly higher than that of the United States. Eight million Swedes are basically well satisfied with their "free" health service run by the government.

In December 1980, local experts decided that a 26-year-old man in Stockholm would benefit from a heart transplant. In the absence of this surgery, his life expectancy was estimated to be 6 months. This operation was not done in Sweden at the time, and the surgeon with the most experience was Dr. Norman Shumway at Stanford University. The physicians involved appealed to the senior administrators and politicians responsible for medical care in Stockholm County. Without mentioning the patient's name, the doctors asked the county to pay to have this man operated on in California, where the average life expectancy for patients with heart transplants was 2.6 years.

While the senior officials hesitated, the newspapers discovered this event and even found out the name of the patient, who was promptly interviewed. As a result, it was decided that the county should pay for his California heart transplant. They did so. The total cost was $80,000, and the patient lived for 26 days. The Swedish government is wondering what it should do to prepare for the next such request.

When Swedish doctors, administrators, and politicians decided to send this patient to Stanford University for a heart transplant, they indicated that the operation was not only helpful but among the best of the limited number of beneficial purchases society could afford.

Because of their method of evaluation, no one will ever know whether their decision was correct. It is unclear how this decision was made. Although doctors, politicians, administrators, and presumably public opinion all influenced it, who was ultimately responsible? Was the decision made to benefit the patient, to satisfy the doctors' intellectual curiosity, to maintain political-occupational security for politicians and administrators, or for some combination of these reasons? Finally, how did these people decide between this and other potential expenditures such as new schools or road improvements?

Proper analysis of such a case requires a comparison of the benefits and disadvantages of the available options. This chapter will explore two very different approaches to this problem: competition in a free marketplace and cost benefit/cost effectiveness analysis.

## THE THEORETICAL COMPETITIVE MARKET

Every time we make a decision, we do not systematically quantify our desires (or utility values, in economic terms). If we did, deciding when to get up in the morning, when to leave for the office, what to eat, and the myriad decisions made before going to work would take forever. Instead, we use judgment to weigh intuitively our sometimes conflicting desires.

Analysis becomes even more difficult when decisions must be made cooperatively, as in a doctor–patient relationship. In these situations, many economists also prefer to avoid quantifying utility values. Instead, they use the model of the marketplace under conditions of pure competition. Here, producers and consumers (doctors and patients) use their judgment independently, as in the previous example, to sell and buy freely so as to gain maximum utility (satisfaction). The key: Both parties measure and judge their desires internally in deciding whether to buy or sell.

The market system, to function perfectly, requires many independent profit-maximizing buyers and sellers of the same product of constant quality, all of whom are fully informed about prices, the product, its quality, and their own preferences. Furthermore, the buyers and sellers must be able to interact freely.

## THE MEDICAL CARE MARKET

Health economics is largely concerned with how the market for medical care departs from pure competition and what misallocations develop. This departure occurs when assumptions in the theoretical model fail owing to poor distribution, external problems, scarcity, or inadequate information.

*Poor initial distribution of resources.* The competitive model ignores the desirability of any initial distribution of resources. It does not guarantee minimum standards of care. For example, a poor person cannot buy adequate health care in the marketplace. That is why there are Social Security, city hospitals, and government health payments for the poor (Medicaid).

*External problems.* The marketplace does not consider, via costs and profits, the effects upon parties not directly involved in a transaction. These effects may be positive or negative. Vaccines have a *positive external* effect, for they stop disease spread not only to the recipient but also to those he or she contacts. These third parties receive benefits without paying for them. Vaccines will be underallocated unless some agency (government) intervenes offering, for example, government grants for lower prices.

*Scarcity.* Although there is always an inability to purchase all of the desired items for society at large, through insurance or prepaid plans an individual may pay little or none of the cost of treatment. Others with the same policy pay for his or her treatment. Although insurance reduces the patient's risk of not being able to afford treatment in cases of health catastrophe, it frequently leads to overallocation.

*Inadequate information.* Unlike theoretical consumers, patients rarely understand the quality or cost of treatment alternatives. Our medical care system makes attainment of this information too difficult, time-consuming, or expensive. Without proper understanding, patients cannot be expected to make reasonable choices.

The competitive market, like Darwinian evolution, assumes the survival of the fittest and an individual's possession of the skills to take care of himself. Opponents of the market approach usually reject this as inappropriate for the sick and injured.

Many of the competitive market assumptions may fail, and the consequences of this failure are disturbing. Advocates of the competitive market attempt to correct inadequacies in the free market allocation system rather than abandoning it for nonmarket techniques. A sampling of their recommendations is outlined in Table 1. A checklist of questions (Table 2) is included to help readers focus on problem areas in the competitive market approach.

### ECONOMIC EVALUATION OUTSIDE THE MARKETPLACE

Rather than modeling health care upon a competitive market in which patients and doctors buy and sell medical services, some observers choose a different model: that of the paternalistic expert. Patients unable to guide themselves through illness call on a doctor, from whom they expect altruism, empathy, and sound scientific knowledge. They also want the doctor to listen to them and respect their individual needs. Unfortunately, not all doctors act on their patients' behalf.

Table 1. *Proposals to make the medical market function competitively*

| Proposal | Source |
|---|---|
| Eliminate all licensing of health workers. Licensing creates a monopoly. | Friedman (1962) |
| Require a very large deductible for health insurance (10 percent of a family's yearly income). | Feldstein (1981) |
| Allow employees to choose from among several competing health insurance plans and health maintenance organizations. If they choose a lower-cost plan, they keep the savings. | Enthoven (1980) |
| Give people eligible for Medicare and Medicaid vouchers that they can use to buy the private health insurance or health maintenance plan of their choice. | |
| Provide more information to patients so that they can make more informed choices. | |
| Vastly reduce the role of the U.S. Food and Drug Administration in approving drugs. | Peltzman (1974) |
| Promote the sale of human blood. | Johnson (1976); Titmus (1971) |

Table 2. *Checklist market approach*

1. Do patients have options for health care? Do these options provide alternative services at different prices?

2. Are patients clearly capable of making necessary decisions? If not, is there a way to restructure health services so that patients can become capable?

3. Are patients well enough informed to make decisions? Is the necessary information available?

4. Do patients feel comfortable shopping for health care? Can they freely question doctors and nurses? What social dynamics prevent this?

5. Does society protect itself when the interests of the individual and the community conflict?

6. If health care is a right, do all patients have enough money to obtain minimal care?

7. Do cost incentives encourage patients and doctors to conserve (leading to proper resource allocation)?

8. Can patients reasonably bear the cost of health care in all circumstances? (Are insurance plans available to protect patients from catastrophies?)

9. Do laws (such as malpractice laws) protect patients and doctors? Do these laws motivate protective behavior in conflict with wise allocation?

For example, fee-for-service delivery encourages doctors to perform procedures that are not always consistent with patients' best interests. Also, not all doctors are worthy of trust; some are incompetent. Some of them do not listen to patients' desires. Informal decision making provides few guarantees against these and other dangers. It is hard to scrutinize intuitive decision making.

Formal methods of quantifying patients' utility payoffs address these needs. They explicitly define to all (patients, other doctors, juries) what criteria are used. Through such techniques, knowledgeable patients can verify whether this analysis reflects their concerns. These methods, by their very design, clarify who benefits by the procedure. Finally, cost analysis provides a guide to help physicians analyze the logic of a decision rule.

### Formal cost analysis

Although our focus is on the benefits and costs of potential outcomes, these techniques would be of very limited value if they were separated from techniques of decision analysis. To decide on an appropriate action, both the importance of an outcome and its frequency must be considered. For example, penicillin allergy leading to death is unquestionably a terrible outcome; fortunately, its low frequency tempers concern. To place cost analysis in perspective, a very brief outline of its relation to decision analysis is presented. (For an in-depth consideration, see Weinstein and Stason 1977.)

### Decision analysis

Decision analysis assumes a decision maker who desires to achieve as much benefit as possible and has limited resources available for this purpose. The decision maker reconstructs conditions as they would occur in the marketplace, but brings knowledge and rationality to the process.

There are six principal steps in every analysis: (1) development of a decision tree; (2) measurement of the probability of reaching each outcome; (3) measurement of the cost and benefits of each possible outcome (payoff value); (4) multiplication of the payoff values by the probabilities to give the expected utilities of each event; (5) summation of all of the expected utilities associated with each decision option; and (6) the choice of the option with the greatest utility.

Steps 1 and 2 determine the probable occurrence of each possible event. Step 3 is our focus: the measurement of the value of each outcome. Steps 4, 5, and 6 involve only computation. (The reader who feels uncomfortable with probabilities or decision trees is referred to Chapter 10 or to Weinstein and Stason 1977.)

Decision analysis has traditionally been divided into two parts – cost benefit and cost effectiveness – based on the method of measurement. The difference between cost–effectiveness and cost–benefit analysis is that cost effectiveness measures the output (effect) in nonmonetary terms. For example, years of life saved or cases found are cost effectiveness measures. By contrast, in cost–benefit analysis, benefits are measured in financial terms. Thus, years of life saved or cases found must be given a dollar value. This is a problematic process.

Cost benefit and cost effectiveness may both be subdivided into two types, one-outcome and multifactorial outcome measurements. One-outcome studies measure only one value of interest. For instance, a one-output cost–effectiveness study of the effects of cimetidine, a new drug to prevent gastrointestinal bleeding, might measure only the years of life saved per cost of cimetidine treatment. Other important factors, such as reduced pain and gain of work time, are ignored.

Multifactorial outcome measurements attempt to measure more and sometimes all effects of treatment. These cost–effectiveness studies measure benefits on a utility scale per cost of treatment. This utility scale is generated by asking a patient about his preferences in given medical predicaments. This information is then used to generate an independent scale that indicates how the patient intuitively measures all of the outputs (effects) of treatment. In contrast, multifactorial cost–benefit analysis measures the total benefit *in dollars* to both the individual and society per cost of treatment.

### CRITERIA FOR CHOICE

#### Cost–effectiveness versus cost–benefit analysis

A cost–effectiveness measure by itself does not provide an adequate basis for making a choice; a cost–benefit measure does. In *cost–benefit* analysis, both costs and benefits are measured by a common variable – usually dollars – in such a way that they are easily compared. When benefits exceed costs, the option is wise. By contrast, cost–effectiveness measures do not share a common denominator. For example, a cost–effectiveness study of cimetidine shows that it saves X days of life per dosage regimen. Before deciding whether to administer it, the value of these days must be compared to the cost of the regimen. Some analysts bypass this issue by choosing options with the highest effectiveness/cost ratio until their money runs out. This approach is useful if one has a fixed expenditure budget.

#### Multifactorial versus unifactorial measurement

In theory, multifactorial outcome measurement applied to all effects is ideal. Single-outcome studies assume that only the one effect measured is significant. For example, a single-outcome study of cimetidine's effect on the years of life saved disregards the importance of its side effects – nausea and vomiting. However, unifactorial measurement is simpler and often satisfactory (Table 3).

### VALUING OUTCOMES

What is the value of a life saved? Cost–effectiveness analysis allows us to set

Table 3. *Correlation of study types with measurement indexes*

| | Cost effectiveness (Cost of treatment/unit of outcome) | Cost benefit (Cost of treatment/dollar value of outcome) |
|---|---|---|
| Single-outcome measurements | Cost of treatment per year of life saved | Cost of treatment per dollar value of life saved |
| Multifactorial outcome measurements | Cost of treatment per effect on utility scale | Costs of treatment per dollar value of treatment effects |

this question aside. Cost–benefit analysis, however, attempts to consider all parameters of medical care, including quality of life after treatment, ability to return to work, and so on. To do this, a common denominator, such as dollars, is used. Any unit can be used, however, as long as it measures both costs and benefits. To demonstrate the wide range of methods used to weigh outcome, let us consider the question posed earlier: "What is the value of life?"

Because, fortunately, we do not buy and sell human beings, we must choose other estimates. Here are three ways this value is calculated.

1. Determine lost earnings discounted to present value. This assumes that a human being's value to society is measured by his or her contribution to the gross national product, and is measured by an earning stream discounted to present value.
2. Ask people to choose among possible alternative states of existence. By asking people to choose between options such as full health but a reduced life span and a longer life span with disability, one can quantify their relative preferences for medically related outcomes. This process is called *utility analysis*.
3. Observe decisions actually made that influence survival in populations. This approach assumes that a decision not to install a safety device such as air bags in automobiles implies, among other things, that the cost per life saved was too high. A decision to do so implies that the cost per life saved is worthwhile. Economists have undertaken such studies and have observed great variations in the imputed value of a life from a few hundred to tens of millions of dollars. The following is an example of such a decision.

This is the first hospital visit for this 88-year-old man, who entered the emergency room of a large urban hospital Friday night at 9 P.M. He requests admission now while his normal support, his daughter and son-in-law, are on vacation. His other near relatives are 2,000 miles away. On cursory examination, he shows no signs of physical or emotional distress. He has 2+ lower body muscle strength, which restricts him to a wheelchair. He says that he has been in a chair "ever since I fell and busted my hip a long time ago." The patient has reduced remote memory; he is unable to remember his birth date, his birthplace, or his children's names. Due to poor ambulation and diminished mental acuity, he appears to be incapable of performing independently the activities of daily life. His unused Medicare and third-party insurance fully cover his hospitalization costs, which would be approximately $400 a day for 5 days, at least until his daughter returns.

1. Should the physician on duty admit this patient? What techniques can we use to approach this problem?
2. What are the alternatives to hospital admission?
3. Currently, there frequently is no alternative. Why not?
4. Analyze this decision with respect to the costs and benefits for the patient, the doctor, the third-party insurer, and society as a whole.
5. How many of the assumptions of pure competition are violated here?
6. Design a more competitive market system that would correct these problems.

### ETHICAL QUANDARIES

Cost–effectiveness and cost–benefit analysis force us to confront several ethical issues directly. Here are two examples:

1. Although no one is particularly satisfied with any approach to measuring the value of life, some consider the entire practice unethical. Thomas Shelling suggests that the ethical quandary occurs when a person A tries to decide what person B's life is worth. He says that in making such evaluations, one should think of the value of one's own life: The life you save may be your own. Others argue that virtually any medical decision implicitly establishes a value of life. Is it any more ethical to do so informally without quantification?
2. Is the decision maker responsible to society or to the patient? Occasionally, there may be a conflict of interests. For example, a Medicaid patient may pay only a fraction of his or her bill. In evaluating the cost/benefit ratio, should the cost to the patient or the cost to society (the full cost of the service) be considered?

### EXAMPLE: PHARYNGITIS

Perhaps the easiest way to understand cost–benefit analysis is to apply it to a medical problem. The treatment of sore throat is analyzed here because the original study by Tompkins and associates is available for scrutiny in the *Annals of Internal Medicine*. The cases on upper respiratory infections that follow and options to increase the life span allow the reader to review the preparation of decision trees as discussed in Chapter 10 and to investigate different methods of weighing outcomes. They also show the reader how to use information from the Tompkins cost–benefit analysis to develop a simpler single-outcome cost–

effectiveness model for the pharyngitis problem. Table 5, which follows the two cases, points out problem areas for this and other cost analyses.

## UPPER RESPIRATORY INFECTIONS: THE USE OF DECISION TREES

Upper respiratory infections (URI), including pharyngitis, are the most prevalent cause of acute illness in the United States. Fortunately, pharyngitis is usually self-limiting. The prime preventable complication is acute rheumatic fever, (ARF), after β-hemolytic group A streptococcal infection. Standard prophylaxis is treatment with penicillin (PCN).

Three approaches to such patients have been used:

1. Culture all throats; if the cultures are positive, administer PCN.
2. Immediately administer PCN to all patients.
3. Do not treat. This decision has been made because of the declining risk of acute rheumatic fever, the risk of an allergic reaction to PCN, and the cost of throat cultures.

Draw a decision tree for this decision (see Fig. 1). Some needed facts and simplifying assumptions are presented. The facts are not sufficient to develop a complete tree and the expected values. Consider what other information is needed.

1. Assume that the patient does not have nonrheumatogenic complications, such as an abscess.
2. Assume that clinicians cannot meaningfully predict, through physical examination, the likelihood of β-hemolytic group A streptococcal infections. Whether this is true is debatable.
3. Seventeen percent of the population are carriers of β-hemolytic group A streptococci in their normal throat flora. They are not at risk for developing acute rheumatic fever.
4. Approximately 10 percent of throat cultures give false-negative results.
5. To simplify this analysis, assume that allergic reactions to PCN are defined as (a) mild, (b) severe, or (c) causing death.
6. To simplify, do not try to separate out the different outcomes in acute rheumatic fever.
7. Do not attempt to determine the probability of each outcome.

## COST–BENEFIT ANALYSIS

Tompkins et al. developed one of the first multifactorial cost–benefit analyses, which was published in 1978. It was important because it questioned and provoked controversy over long-accepted dogma. It included the costs of medical care, the value of the patient's lost time, and the costs to the patient in lost productivity. It ignored the patient's pain and suffering and asked readers to decide whether the outcomes seemed reasonable.

The following section (including Table 4) demonstrates how Tompkins et al.

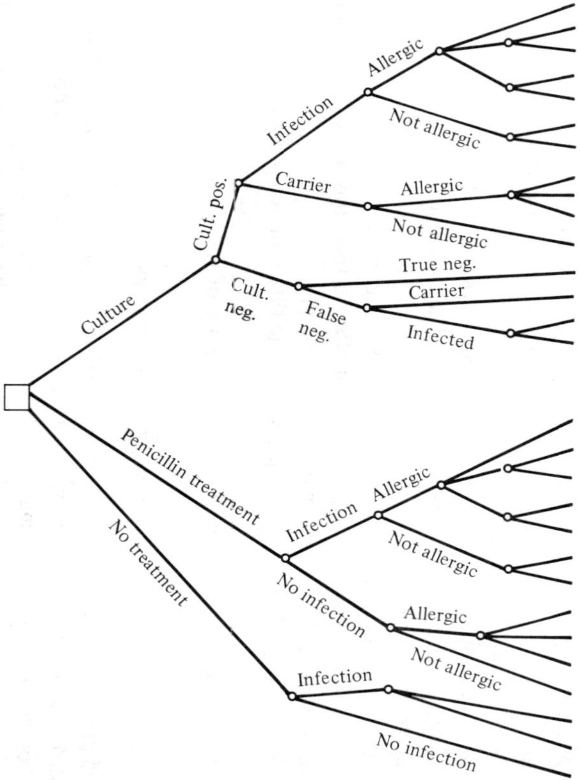

| Outcome | Tompkins est. ($) 1977 | ($) derived from col. 1 | Third World est. ($) |
|---|---|---|---|
| Death | 72,019.50 | 1 + 2 + 3 + 4 | 2401.75 |
| Serious allergy and ARF | 11,405.50 | 1 + 2 + 3 + 5 + 7 | 128.31 |
| Serious allergy | 845.50 | 1 + 2 + 3 + 5 | 11.75 |
| Mild allergy and ARF | 10,594.50 | 1 + 2 + 3 + 6 + 7 | 118.31 |
| Mild allergy | 34.50 | 1 + 2 + 3 + 6 | 1.75 |
| ARF | 10,579.50 | 1 + 2 + 3 + 7 | 118.31 |
| Well | 19.50 | 1 + 2 + 3 | 1.75 |
| Death | 72,019.50 | 1 + 2 + 3 + 4 | 2401.75 |
| Serious allergy | 845.50 | 1 + 2 + 3 + 5 | 11.75 |
| Mild allergy | 34.50 | 1 + 2 + 3 + 6 | 1.75 |
| Well | 19.50 | 1 + 2 + 3 | 1.75 |
| Well | 16.50 | 1 + 2 | 1.40 |
| Well | 16.50 | 1 + 2 | 1.40 |
| ARF | 10,576.50 | 1 + 2 + 7 | 117.96 |
| Well | 16.50 | 1 + 2 | 1.40 |
| Death | 72,017.50 | 1 + 3 + 4 | 2401.35 |
| Serious allergy and ARF | 11,403.50 | 1 + 3 + 5 + 7 | 127.91 |
| Serious allergy | 843.50 | 1 + 3 + 5 | 11.35 |
| Mild allergy and ARF | 10,592.50 | 1 + 3 + 6 + 7 | 117.91 |
| Mild allergy | 32.50 | 1 + 3 + 6 | 1.35 |
| ARF | 10,577.50 | 1 + 3 + 7 | 117.91 |
| Well | 17.50 | 1 + 3 | 1.35 |
| Death | 72,017.50 | 1 + 3 + 4 | 2401.35 |
| Serious allergy | 843.50 | 1 + 3 + 5 | 11.35 |
| Mild allergy | 32.50 | 1 + 3 + 6 | 1.35 |
| Well | 17.50 | 1 + 3 | 1.35 |
| ARF | 10,574.50 | 1 + 7 | 117.56 |
| Well | 14.50 | 1 | 1.00 |
| Well | 14.50 | 1 | 1.00 |

Figure 1. Pharyngitis decision tree. See note on p. 149. (From R. K. Tompkins, D. C. Burns, and W. E. Cable 1977).

Table 4.

| | | Unit costs (1977) | |
|---|---|---|---|
| A. | Throat culture | $2.00 | Based on costs of a prepaid group clinic in New Hampshire |
| B. | Penicillin | 3.00 | |
| C. | Cost of a patient's time per visit | 4.50 | 60 minutes travel time plus 30 minutes in the doctor's office at $3 per hour, the value of the patient's time |
| D. | Diagnostic office visit | 10.00 | |
| E. | Therapy-only visit | 4.00 | Relevant for return visit under the first decision if intramuscular penicillin injection is used |
| F. | Daily cost of hospitalization | 94.00 | Includes hospital and medication costs and physician's fees |

| | Medical care strategy costs | | |
|---|---|---|---|
| | Decision: Culture first | | |
| G. | Culture negative: A + C + D | = | $16.50 |
| H. | Culture positive: A + B + C + D | = | 19.50[a] |
| | Decision: Treat everyone | | |
| I. | B + C + D | = | 17.50 |
| | Decision: No treatment | | |
| J. | C + D | = | 14.50 |

[a]For oral penicillin. For intramuscular penicillin, two visits are required for a positive culture. (A + B + C + D) + (B +C + E) = $28.
*Source:* Adapted from R. K. Tompkins et al.

(p. 483) formulated payoff values. We will quote from the Tompkins paper to describe how the other adverse outcome costs were calculated.

### Adverse medical outcome costs

Tompkins et al. use $72,000 as the value of a life and therefore the cost associated with death.

### Cost of acute rheumatic fever

The estimated cost of the initial acute rheumatic fever attack ($10,560) is the sum of the following factors:

Table 5. *Cost analysis checklist*

1. Most decision analyses ignore factors important to patients. One-output studies always ignore factors such as lost work time, plus pain endured. Multifactorial output studies often omit difficult-to-measure factors such as the pain suffered by the patient and the anxiety endured by the patient's friends and family. How do these omissions affect the analysis?

2. Are individual payoff values appropriate? If not, use sensitivity analysis to determine whether changing the payoff value affects the decision.

3. Did the study discount the payoff values? The benefit achieved today is valued more highly than the same benefit achieved tomorrow. Ask children whether they would like to have candy now or tomorrow. Children typically want it now. Patients may be more concerned with immediate relief of pain and anxiety than with taking hypertension medications or using dental floss in order to avoid future medical problems. Discounting is the technique by which future costs and benefits are reduced relative to a present value.

4. Do values reflect individual patients' concerns? Decision analysis should reflect patient desires amalgamated with professional wisdom. Payoff values, then, should be modified to reflect each patient's unique condition.

1. The cost of hospitalization for acute rheumatic fever for an estimated 11 days ($1,034) plus 90 days of total disability ($2,160), giving a cost of $3,194 for a single episode of acute rheumatic fever.

2. The cost of maintaining penicillin prophylaxis (benzathine penicillin every 4 weeks) for those patients who survive until age 35. The average duration of prophylaxis will be 25 years for 96.1 percent of the patients. Approximate yearly cost of prophylaxis is $150 ($11.50 × 13 office visits per year) [for a total of $3,604 rounded with no discounting].

3. The cost of recurrent acute rheumatic fever attacks despite adequate prophylaxis; rate of recurrence per patient year 0.004 × 25 patient years × $3,194 per case of acute rheumatic fever = $319.

4. The cost of allergic reactions during penicillin prophylaxis. The data from Miller, Stancer, and Massell indicate that there will be an average of 1.041 mild allergic reactions per patient during the 25 years of prophylaxis: 1.041 × $15 = $15.

5. The calculation of the cost due to class IV rheumatic heart disease assumes that: patients with severe rheumatic heart disease will require at least four visits per year to a physician (at $25 per visit); that they will be hospitalized for 14 days on two occasions each year; that they will survive an average of 6.2 years, but will be totally incapacitated until their deaths. These assumptions imply that the cost of class IV rheumatic heart disease includes both the cost of premature death ($72,000) and the cost of medical care for 6.2 years ($16,938) for a total of $88,938 per case of rheumatic heart disease. Each patient who has an acute rheumatic fever attack has a 14/771 probability of developing class IV rheumatic heart disease as calculated

below. Therefore, the potential cost of this complication of the initial acute rheumatic fever attack is $14/771 \times \$88,938 = \$3,428$.

### Cost of allergic reactions

Data are unavailable to ascertain accurately the cost of the potential allergic reactions to penicillin. The estimate is based on the following assumptions.

1. Individuals with serious allergy (anaphylaxis and serum sickness) may require hospitalization for approximately 7 days ($658) and will have an equivalent disability period ($168). These assumptions yield an estimated cost of $826.

2. Mild allergies (predominantly urticaria) will not require hospitalization nor generate any disability; but will necessitate a diagnostic office visit, symptomatic treatment (eight 25-mg capsules Benadryl at $0.07 per capsule), and will cost 90 min. of patient time. Total estimated cost, $15.

To summarize, ARF cost $10,560, serious allergy $826, and mild allergy $15.

Tompkins et al. found that the correct treatment depended on the prevalence as follows:

| Prevalence | Preferred treatment plan |
|------------|--------------------------|
| 0–5% | No treatment |
| 5–20% | Culture |
| 20% or greater | Penicillin treatment first |

A good exercise is to critique these figures, make corrections, and reanalyze the decision to determine its importance. This kind of analysis, in which probabilities and payoffs are changed to examine their impact on the decision, is called *sensitivity analysis*.

### UPPER RESPIRATORY INFECTION: THE USE OF A COST–EFFECTIVENESS MODEL

A. Develop a cost–effectiveness model to decide which option (culture, treatment, or no treatment) will increase patient's life span.

1. Assume that death from PCN allergy occurs immediately. Assume that the treatment and reaction occur at the time of pharyngitis infection.

2. Death from acute rheumatic fever occurs in 1.8 percent of patients. They live, on average, 6.2 years after developing the initial pharyngitis infection.

3. Assume that other patients live 50 more years on average. Try to reason through the results before calculating them.

B.  If the chance of death due to PCN allergy in an allergic individual is 10,000 times the normal level, how will the decision rule be affected?

A.  This analysis may be performed by altering only the payoff values. Our goal is to measure the expected life span of each endpoint. On average, all people with serious or mild allergies and well persons live for 50 years. Patients who die due to allergy have the same life span. Survival of acute rheumatic fever involves two types of patients: the 1.81 percent of those who live 6.2 years on average before succumbing to congestive heart failure, and the other 98.2 percent who live the full 50 years. The expected life span for any acute rheumatic fever patient equals the weighted average of these two groups.

$$\frac{98.19\% \times 50 \text{ years} + 1.81\% \times 6.2 \text{ years}}{100\%} = 49.2 \text{ years}$$

This discussion can be summarized as follows:

| Input | Weighted value (years) |
|---|---|
| Death due to allergy | 0 |
| Serious allergy | 50 |
| Mild allergy | 50 |
| Acute rheumatic fever | 49.2 |
| Well | 50 |

Inserting these payoff values into the Tompkins et al. decision tree, we obtain the following result:

| Prevalence | Treatment |
|---|---|
| Less than 5% | No treatment |
| More than 5% | PCN treatment |

B.  Increasing the chance of death due to PCN allergies to 10,000 times the original level discourages the use of PCN, either directly or following culture. Hence, no treatment is the best treatment in all prevalence groups. This can be verified by inserting the numbers as before, changing only this one probability value.

## CONCLUSION

The basic ideas behind cost effectiveness are rather simple. They are sometimes made more complicated to achieve greater accuracy. Sometimes difficulty reflects ethical dilemmas. As long as physicians know that their time is not the only scarce resource, and as long as they consider what the benefits of medical treatment are, then it is likely that they will achieve more cost effective medical care. The formal mathematical techniques of analysis are a way of checking to see if costs and benefits have been determined. It potentially allows other physicians, patients, administrators, and lawyers insight into the decision-making process. The peculiarities of the payment system for medical care distort the use of medical treatments. These distortions also suggest the need for this kind of reasoning in the absence of market alternatives.

In his 1984 commencement address before the Case Western Reserve Medical School Frederick Robbins, the president of the Institute of Medicine, underscored the new emphasis on cost effectiveness. He likened misallocation to malpractice and proposed that the Hippocratic oath be modified to require cost-effective care. Decision analysis is both a language and a technique to help health care providers reach this goal.

### NOTE

Column two in Figure 1 shows how the dollar values in column one were derived. (1) The value of the patient's time and the cost of an office visit, $14.50, see (J) in Table 4; (2) the cost of a throat culture, $2.00, see (A) in Table 4; (3) the cost of penicillin, $3.00, see (B) in Table 4; (4) the value of life saved or the cost of a death, $72,000; (5) the cost of a serious allergy, $826; (6) the cost of a mild allergy, $15.00; (7) the cost of acute rheumatic fever attack, $10,560. The Third World values in column three can be decomposed in the same way. The Third World estimates are hypothetical costs. They are shown to demonstrate the large possible differences in outcome values and to highlight the ethical and moral issues raised by placing a dollar value on life. The reader is urged to choose other values that may more closely adhere to their personal values and to recalculate the results. Because the calculations involved in this decision tree are laborious, this decision has been programmed for an Apple II microcomputer and is available for purchase for $10 from Biomatrix c/o Kathy Smyth-Staruch, Ph.D., 2401 Queenston Road, Cleveland Heights, Ohio 44118.

### SELECTED BIBLIOGRAPHY

Bunker, J., Barnes, B., and Mosteller, F. (1977). *Costs, Risks and Benefits of Surgery*. New York: Oxford University Press. (Decision analysis and cost effectiveness analysis applied to common surgical procedures.)

Cullis, J., and West, P. (1979). *The Economics of Health: An Introduction*. New York: New York University Press. (Chapter 8 deals with cost–benefit techniques and Chapter 9 with valuing human life.)

Culyer, A. J., Wiseman, J., and Walker, A. (1977). *An Annotated Bibliography of Health Economics* (English Language Sources). New York: St. Martin's Press.

Drummond, M. F. (1980). *Principles of Economic Appraisal in Health Care*. Oxford: Oxford Medical Publications, Oxford University Press. (An introduction to cost–benefit and cost–effectiveness analysis in medical care with several examples. Paperback.)

Eastaugh, S. (1981). *Medical Economics and Health Finance*. Boston: Auburn House.

(Chapter 3 deals with cost–effectiveness and cost–benefit analysis, Chapter 4 with technology assessment. There is a glossary of terms and extensive references.)

Enthoven, A. (1980). *Health Plan*. Reading, Mass.: Addison-Wesley.

Feldstein, M. (1981). *Hospital Costs and Health Insurance*. Cambridge, Mass.: Harvard University Press.

Feldstein, P. J. (1979). *Health Care Economics*. New York: Wiley.

Friedman, M. (1962). *Capitalism and Freedom*. Chicago: University of Chicago Press. (Chapter 9 deals with medical licensure. Paperback.)

Fuchs, V. (1974). *Who Shall Live? Health Economics and Social Choice*. New York: Basic Books. (A popular nontechnical view.)

Griffiths, D. A. T., Rigoni, R., Tacier, P., et al. (1980). *An Annotated Bibliography of Health Economics* (West European Sources). New York: St. Martin's Press.

Jacobs, P. (1980). *The Economics of Health and Medical Care: An Introduction*. Baltimore: University Park Press. (Chapter 14 deals with cost–benefit analysis. Paperback.)

Johnson, D. B., ed. (1976). *Blood Policy: Issues and Alternatives*. Washington, D.C.: American Enterprise Institute for Public Policy Research. (Paperback.)

Miller, J. M., Stancer, S. L., and Massell, B. F. (1958). A controlled study of beta-hemolytic streptococcal infection in rheumatic families. II. Penicillin prophylaxis among rheumatic fever subjects, comparing different regimens. *Am. J. Med.* 25:845–56.

Miqué, J.-L. and Bélanger, G. (1974). *The Price of Health*. Toronto: Macmillan. (Chapter 7 deals with cost–benefit analysis. Paperback.)

Mooney, G. (1977). *The Valuation of Human Life*. London: Macmillan. (An introduction to cost–benefit analysis in medical care.)

Neuhauser, D. (1980). Cost effective clinical decision making and the medical care manager. *Hosp. Health Service Admin.* 25:55–61. (Implications for managing health services.)

Newhouse, J. (1978). *The Economics of Medical Care*. Reading, Mass.: Addison-Wesley. (An introduction to health economics. Paperback.)

Office of Technology Assessment. Washington, D.C.: Congress of the United States, Series of papers on technology assessment.

*The Implication of Cost-Effectiveness Analysis of Medical Technology*. August 1980.

Background paper 1. *Methodological Issues and Literature Review*. September 1980.

Background paper 2. *Case Studies*, 1981. (This consists of 16 separately bound short case studies of different medical technologies.)

Background paper 3. *The Efficacy and Cost Effectiveness of Psychotherapy*. October 1980.

Background paper 4. *The Management of Health Care Technology in Ten Countries*. October 1980.

Peltzman, S. (1974). *Regulation of Pharmaceutical Innovation*. Washington, D.C.: American Enterprise Institute for Public Policy Research.

Shelling, T. (1967). The life you save may be your own. In *Problems in Public Expenditure Analysis*, S. Chase, ed., Washington, D.C.: Brookings Institution, pp. 127–61.

Titmus, R. (1971). *The Gift Relationship: From Human Blood to Social Policy*. New York: Random House.

Tompkins, R. K., Burnes, D. C., and Cable, W. E. (1977). Analysis of the cost-effectiveness of pharyngitis management and acute rheumatic fever prevention. *Ann. Intern. Med.* 86:481–92.

Van Eimeren, W., and Köpke, W. (1979). *Bestandsaufnahme Gesundheits system-for-schung* (State-of-the-art report, *Health Systems Research*). Munich: Institute for Medical Information Processing, Statistics, and Biomathematics. (An extraordinary computerized, cross-referenced, multilanguage health services research bibliography.)

Ward, R. (1975). *The Economics of Health Resources*. Reading, Mass.: Addison-Wesley. (An introduction to health economics. Chapter 8 is on cost–benefit analysis.)

Weinstein, M., Fineberg, H., Elstein, A., et al. (1980). *Clinical Decision Analysis*. Philadelphia: W.B. Saunders. (Decision analysis applied to medicine. Chapter 8 deals with the costs of care. A bibliography is included.)

Weinstein, M., and Stason, W. (1977). Foundations of cost effectiveness analysis for health and medical practices. *N. Engl. J. Med. 296*:716–21.

# CHAPTER 10

# THE TECHNOLOGICAL STRATEGIST: EMPLOYING TECHNIQUES OF CLINICAL DECISION MAKING

MARK J. YOUNG, SANKEY V. WILLIAMS, and
JOHN M. EISENBERG

During the past 10 years, there has been increasing interest in understanding how clinicians make decisions, as well as in helping them to analyze the difficult clinical decisions they face every day. In response, the new field of medical decison making has emerged as an amalgam of health economics, cognitive psychology, operations research, and clinical epidemiology. The last decade has also witnessed growing concern about the use of medical technology. The number of diagnostic tests has increased, and new types of clinicians have joined physicians in making decisions about diagnosis and treatment. Accordingly, there has been an increasing awareness of the need to develop aids for the use of the new technology, as well as clinical guidelines for the new health professionals, such as nurse practitioners and physician's assistants. The greater availability of computers and the growing comfort of professionals in using computers in their practices have made possible advanced decision-making systems that would not have been available a decade ago. This chapter reviews the use of several of the new ways of deciding on diagnostic and therapeutic strategies, particularly with the use of medical technology. These new methods include simultaneous multivariate equations, decision analysis, patient data banks, artificial intelligence, and clinical algorithms.

## MULTIVARIATE ANALYSIS

Many medical decisions, such as making a diagnosis or estimating a prognosis, require the simultaneous consideration of multiple factors, each with a different degree of importance for the decision. For example, in deciding whether a patient with chest pain has myocardial infarction, there are many factors that will influence the decision, such as age, sex, past history, and location of the pain. Similarly, in predicting the prognosis of a patient with an acute myocardial infarction, it is necessary to consider the age of the patient, the presence or

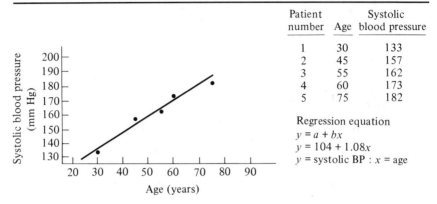

| Patient number | Age | Systolic blood pressure |
|---|---|---|
| 1 | 30 | 133 |
| 2 | 45 | 157 |
| 3 | 55 | 162 |
| 4 | 60 | 173 |
| 5 | 75 | 182 |

Regression equation
$y = a + bx$
$y = 104 + 1.08x$
$y$ = systolic BP : $x$ = age

Figure 1. Linear regression of systolic blood pressure on age.

absence of heart failure, the location of the infarct, and the previous state of health. Multivariate analysis is a technique that identifies important variables and assigns them weights that are based on their relative importance. This information can be used to develop a mathematical model for making a diagnosis or prognosis. Complex mathematics and computer calculations are required to design the models, but often the models can be applied by practicing physicians without reference to these resources. Therefore, multivariate analysis has the potential to help the clinician decide when to use diagnostic and therapeutic technology.

We will discuss multiple regression, which is the central technique in multivariate analysis, explain its relationship to other multivariate techniques, and show how multivariate analysis might be used in clinical medicine.

### Principles of multiple regression

Multiple regression is an expansion of simple linear regression. In simple linear regression, an equation is developed to describe the relationship between a single independent variable and a single dependent variable. For instance, if we determine the age and blood pressure of a group of patients, we can develop an equation that specifies a straight line that relates age to blood pressure. The equation has the general form $y = a + bx$ where $y$ is the dependent variable, blood pressure, and $x$ is the independent variable, age. The intercept on the $y$ axis is $a$ and the slope of the line is $b$. Differential calculus is used to determine values for the terms in the equation that minimize the distance between the observed data points and the values predicted by the regression equation. An example for the linear regression of systolic blood pressure on age is shown in Figure 1. In the example a single variable, age, is used to predict systolic blood pressure.

Multiple regression relates more than one predictor variable to a dependent variable. A multiple regression equation describes a surface in many dimensions rather than a straight line in two. As in linear regression, one attempts to minimize deviation between the observed data and the points that are predicted by the regression equation. Computer analysis using calculus and matrix algebra generally is used to calculate a multiple regression equation. The general form of a multiple regression equation is:

$$y = B_0 + B_1X_1 + B_2X_2 + \ldots + E$$

where $y$ is the dependent variable; the $X$s are a series of independent variables, the $B$s are the regression coefficients for each predictor variable, and $E$ is the error component. An example of multiple regression is the prediction of systolic blood pressure from the age and serum cholesterol of a given patient.

Multiple regression is closely related to other multivariate techniques. Typically, in a multiple regression equation, the dependent variable is a quantity on a continuous scale, such as blood pressure, serum cholesterol, or length of hospital stay. If one wishes to predict an outcome that has only two values, such as survival versus death, or hypertension versus no hypertension, one can use other mathematical models. The discriminant function is one such model. A computer program can calculate a discriminant function directly, or a multiple regression equation can be transformed mathematically into a discriminant function. The fundamental difference between the two methods is that the discriminant function is a more appropriate way to classify the dependent variable into two discrete groups. Some examples in which discriminant functions have been used include predicting patient survival after drug overdose, identifying gallstones dissolvable with chenodeoxycholic acid from their appearance on an oral cholecystogram, and predicting which patients with injured extremities need x-rays (Afifi et al. 1971; Dolgin et al. 1981; Brand et al. 1982).

One can classify the dependent variable into discrete groups using logistic regression, which depends on the mathematical properties of natural logarithms. Logistic regression is desirable when one wants to express the prediction of a dependent variable as a specific probability such as the probability (in percent) of a patient's having a myocardial infarction. As in multiple regression, the clinical characteristics and outcome are used to calculate the predictive model. The following case presentation demonstrates how logistic regression might be used to assist physicians in diagnosing acute ischemic heart disease.

### *Case Presentation – Part I: The decision to admit*

Mr. Smith, a 39-year-old accountant, arrives in the emergency room complaining of chest pain. For the past month, he has had sharp twinges of pain in the right side of his chest when walking up the three flights of steps to his office. Usually the discomfort subsides spontaneously when he sits at his desk, but sometimes it persists for 20 minutes. The pain most often occurs when he walks up the stairs, but has also occurred when he takes the elevator. At no other time does he experience the pain, although he does not exercise. He has come to the emergency room today because he does not have a personal physician and is worried that he might be experiencing serious heart disease.

The patient's past medical history is negative, except for an inguinal hernia repair when he was 25. He has two healthy brothers, whose ages are 45 and 41. One of the partners in his accounting firm had a myocardial infarction 2 months ago.

On physical examination, he is 5 feet 8 inches tall and weighs 165 pounds. His blood pressure is 138/84. His pulse is 84 and regular. He states that he feels short of breath, but his respiratory rate is 14. There is no evidence of peripheral vascular disease and no stigmata of hyperlipidemia. His chest radiograph, complete blood count (CBC), and cholesterol are normal. The electrocardiogram (ECG) shows nonspecific T-wave abnormalities.

Should this man be admitted to the hospital now? If he is admitted, should he be sent to the intensive care unit?

Both of these questions could be answered better if we knew the probability that the patient is suffering from acute ischemic heart disease. Pozen et al. (1980) developed a logistic regression model from a large group of patients with chest pain. There were nine important independent variables; if the variable was present it was assigned a value of 2, if absent, 1. The variables used as predictors were previous myocardial infarction, elevation or depression of the T-waves, dyspnea, S-T segment abnormalities, midsternal location of pain, chest pain as the patient's dominant symptom, history of angina, S-T segment elevation or depression, and T-wave abnormalities. When this patient is analyzed using the logistic regression equation of Pozen et al., the probability of acute ischemic heart disease is now 50 percent. It is decided to admit the patient to the coronary care unit.

### Advantages and limitations of multivariate techniques

Multivariate techniques are potentially valuable aids in medical decision making. They allow one to evaluate clinical information in a consistent, quantitative manner. The logistic regression model of Pozen et al. was tested in an emergency room. The probability of acute ischemic disease was calculated and given to the physician who was caring for each patient with chest pain. Use of the model resulted in a decrease in unnecessary admissions to the coronary care unit without an increase in the number of inappropriate discharges from the emergency room. Thus, the logistic regression model led to more appropriate utilization of resources.

The relative ease with which computers can generate multivariate equations makes it important to realize the limitations of the techniques. Most important is the need to validate predictive models by testing them on patients who are different from the patients used to create the model, although there are methods of partially validating models using only the original patients. A decline in accuracy may occur for many reasons. The patient population used to generate the equation might be unique to one geographic area or institution. The variables chosen for the analysis might be poorly defined or improperly selected. Few multivariate models have been subjected to external validation. When validation has been performed, decreases in the accuracy of the model can be observed (Rao 1973; Hyde 1973). Other limitations to the use of predictor models include the necessity for clinicians to remember which variables are important and what their coefficients are. The Pozen model requires the availability of a preprogrammed calculator.

In summary, multivariate techniques offer great promise for improved medical decision making (McNeil and Hanley 1981). Problems with validation and generalizability are being addressed. The increasing availability of programmable calculators and microcomputers may allow greater application of multivariate techniques. Quantitative models may enable physicians to make better decisions in utilizing expensive diagnostic and therapeutic technology.

DECISION ANALYSIS

## *Case Presentation – Part II: The decision to recommend coronary arteriography*

We used multivariate analysis to decide that Mr. Smith needed to be admitted to the hospital for his chest pain. A myocardial infarction has been ruled out by serial enzyme tests and ECGs. Nevertheless, Mr. Smith has symptoms of coronary artery disease, and wonders whether further diagnostic studies are necessary. He does not feel that the chest pain itself is troublesome, but he has talked to a friend who has had coronary artery bypass grafting (CABG) and wants to know if he is a candidate for the procedure.

### *Method*

Decision analysis is a technique that structures a problem in a defined manner and suggests an optimal choice (Weinstein and Fineberg 1980).

There are four steps in performing a decision analysis: (1) identify and bound the problem; (2) use a decision tree to identify explicit alternatives; (3) assign probabilities to chance events and values to different outcomes; and (4) choose the best strategy based on quantitative comparison of alternatives. We will use the case presentation to illustrate the method of decision analysis.

### Identify and bound the problem

We must choose, based on the information available, to wait, to order a diagnostic test, or to begin treatment. Mr. Smith wants to know whether he is likely to benefit from CABG. Pain relief is not an issue here; Mr. Smith wants to know if CABG will prolong his life. CABG has been shown to increase the 5-year survival only in patients with significant obstruction of the left main coronary artery or with significant obstruction in all three vessels (Second Interim Report by the European Coronary Surgery Study Group 1980). Coronary arteriography is required to determine if this pathology is present. One strategy is to perform coronary arteriography and recommend CABG if there is obstruction in the left main coronary artery or in all three vessels. We need to decide whether or not to recommend catheterization. Since data on CABG are available only for a 5-year follow-up period, we will consider survival at 5 years as the outcome of interest.

### Constructing a decision tree; assigning probabilities and values

When constructing decision trees, a square is used to represent a decision and a circle to denote chance events. We must analyze the consequences of the decision in an explicit manner. We will use a step-by-step process to construct a decision tree for the portion of the pathway catheterization (CATH). We will assign probabilities to chance events as we proceed.

*Chance event 1.* The first chance event reflects the risk of catheterization. There is a small but real chance of dying from the procedure, 0.001 (Braunwald 1968). The survival rate of catheterization is 0.999 (Figure 2).

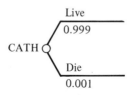

Figure 2.

*Chance event 2.* How many of the patients who survive catheterization will have coronary artery disease? In large series of patients similar to Mr. Smith, 0.78 have not had coronary artery disease (Diamond and Forrester 1979). Ninety-nine percent of these patients will survive for 5 years. The remaining 0.22 patients similar to Mr. Smith will have coronary artery disease (CAD) (Figure 3).

*Chance event 3.* Of the patients with CAD, 0.80 should not be operated on because they do not have disease in the left main coronary artery or in all three vessels; these patients have a 5-year survival of 0.90 (Principal Investigators of CASS 1981). The remaining 0.20 patients will have disease in the left main coronary artery or in all three vessels, and should have surgery performed (Figure 4).

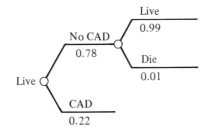

Figure 3.

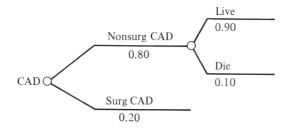

Figure 4.

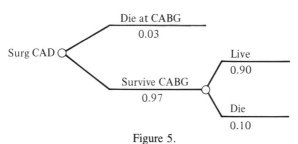

Figure 5.

*Chance event 4.* In the patients with surgical coronary artery disease, 0.03 will die at operation. The remaining 0.97 patients will have a 5-year survival rate of 0.90 (Figure 5).

The complete decision tree for the pathway CATH is shown in Figure 6.

### Choose a course of action

The final step in decision analysis is to calculate the expected value of the different pathways. We have assigned a value of 1.0 to survival at 5 years and a value of 0 to death at 5 years. This process of assigning values to different outcomes is known as *utility assessment*. It is easiest to perform when the outcomes are limited to two, such as life versus death. When multiple outcomes must be valued, utility assessment can be difficult to perform. To calculate the value of each chance node in the tree, we multiply the probability of the event by the

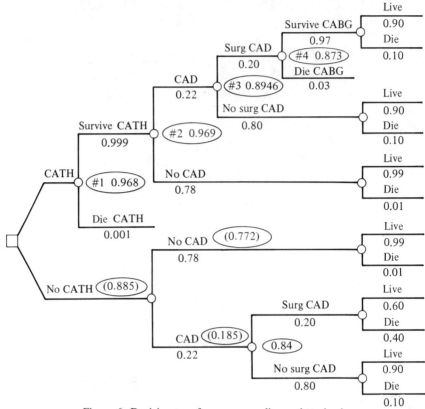

Figure 6. Decision tree for recommending catheterization.

value of the outcome. Since the value of death as an outcome is 0, we are left with a series of products that represent the probabilities for survival. The calculations for each branch are shown below and in Figure 6.

| Chance event 4 | 0.97 (survival rate of CABG) × 0.90 (5-year survival after CABG) | = 0.873 |
| | | |
| Chance event 3 | 0.20 (likelihood of SURG CAD) × 0.873 (value of chance node 4) = 0.1746 | |
| | + 0.80 (likelihood of no SURG CAD) × 0.90 (5-year survival of no SURG CAD) = 0.72 | = 0.8946 |

| | |
|---|---|
| Chance event 2 | 0.22 (likelihood of CAD) × 0.8946 (value of chance node 3) = 0.197 |
| | + 0.78 (likelihood of no CAD) × 0.99 (5-year survival of no CAD) = 0.772        = 0.969 |
| Chance event 1 | 0.969 (value of chance node 2) × 0.999 (survive CATH)        = 0.968 |

The process is repeated for the decision NO CATH. There is one new probability: The survival at 5 years of those with SURG CAD who do not receive CABG = 0.60. The entire tree with all probabilities and values is shown in Figure 6. The results of the decision analysis show that CATH, with the plan to operate on patients with left main or triple-vessel disease, is preferable to the decision NO CATH. There is a greater expected survival at 5 years for the decision CATH (0.968 compared with 0.885).

### Sensitivity analysis

We have assigned many probabilities at the different chance nodes. Although we have used the best information available in the literature, there is concern about its accuracy. *Sensitivity analysis* is a technique that demonstrates the importance of a given probability estimation to the overall decision analysis. For example, we might want to see how the estimate of mortality from catheterization affects the decision. We could substitute a series of different mortality rates into the decision tree and repeatedly calculate the expected value for the different strategies. For a catheterization mortality rate of 0.005, the value for the CATH strategy is 0.964; for a mortality rate of 0.010, the expected value for CATH is 0.959; for a mortality rate of 0.015, the expected value for CATH is 0.954. The first two mortality rates do not change the optimal strategy; the third mortality rate changes it to NO CATH. Alternatively, a technique called *threshold analysis* allows us to identify a critical value that changes the optimal decision. This means that there is a point of indifference at which the values of two strategies are equal. Any probability estimate deviating from the threshold value would change the optimal decision strategy. To calculate the threshold value of catheterization mortality, we need to find the point of indifference at which the value for the pathway CATH is equal to the expected value of the pathway NO CATH.

1. Set the pathways CATH and NO CATH equal to each other.
     0.969 (the expected value for SURVIVE CATH)
     × catheterization survival rate (threshold value)
     = 0.956 (the expected value for NO CATH)

2. Solve the equation for catheterization survival rate.
   Catheterization survival rate = 0.956/0.969
   = 0.987
3. This threshold value of 0.987 means that as long as the catheterization survival rate is 0.987 or greater, the decision CATH is preferred.

Although we were concerned about the accuracy of the survival data for catheterization, we are reassured that a 0.987 survival rate is lower than that of any published data. The same procedure of sensitivity analysis can be performed for any estimate of probability or valued outcome in a decision analysis.

### Advantages/limitations

Proponents of decision analysis point out its value in clarifying the communication of probabilities between individuals. Qualitative phrases such as ''not common'' and ''not infrequently'' have different meanings for different persons. Specifying a numerical range of probabilities facilitates communication between physicians and between patients and physicians (Schwartz 1979).

It is sometimes instructive to go through the process of structuring a decision, which forces one to consider explicitly the consequences of a decision. When there is a difference of opinion between physicians or authoritative recommendations, decision analysis can identify which components of a strategy are the sources of disagreement.

There are important limitations to decision analysis. In the case presentation, we considered only one outcome: survival at 5 years. We did not give different value to immediate deaths – those patients who die from catheterization or CABG, in contrast to those who die later in the 5-year follow-up period. We also did not take into account the pain and expense of catheterization and surgery.

Whose values should be used for the different outcomes, the physician's or the patient's? Methods for determining the value of outcomes have been an area of great concern.

Our case presentation involved CAD; the probabilities and estimates of morbidity and mortality are relatively accessible and accurate. In other situations, it is difficult to find reliable data. Although we can use sensitivity analysis to allow for ranges of probabilities, the calculations are time-consuming, as is the whole process of constructing a tree and valuing the branches. There are no published studies that demonstrate that the application of decision analysis results in better quality of care.

In summary, decision analysis has enormous potential to improve clinical decision making. Research is presently underway to gain a better understanding of valuing outcomes, to provide data bases for accurate probability estimation, and to use microcomputers to generate decision trees and perform sensitivity analysis.

## PATIENT DATA BANKS

In addition to providing help with computations, computers can be used to store enormous amounts of patient information. There are two leading examples of this approach. ARAMIS refers to the American Rheumatology Association's Medical Information System (Fries 1972). The ARAMIS data bank includes information on patients with a wide variety of diagnoses in rheumatology. The second data bank contains information on patients with ischemic heart disease and is located in the Division of Cardiology at Duke University Medical Center (Rosati et al. 1975). Each system contains comprehensive information on thousands of patients in a uniform format.

The principal use of the data bank is to perform studies that predict an individual patient's prognosis or response to therapy (Fries 1976). Data banks can be used to create groups of patients who have clinical characteristics that are similar to those of the patient in question. These groups can be observed to determine which therapy produced the best outcome. It is also possible to determine the prognosis of similar patients in the absence of therapy. When used this way, data banks serve the same function as the experienced consultant: They compare the individual patient with many other patients who have had similar problems.

For example, the data bank on ischemic heart disease at Duke University could be asked about Mr. Smith, the accountant with chest pain who was described earlier in this chapter. The data bank could identify all the patients in its files whose clinical characteristics were similar to Mr. Smith's. The data bank could then report the cumulative experience of all patients who had CABG and of all who were treated medically. With this information, Mr. Smith and his physician might be able to make a better decision about which therapy to choose.

Despite their great promise, data banks have not been widely used. One explanation is the need to accumulate large numbers of patients before the data banks can work effectively, and data collection and entry can be difficult and expensive. Even with large numbers, it is often difficult to find more than a few patients who match the patient in question. Rapid changes in medical practice can make the information on many patients unsuitable for solving current problems. Many clinicians are not familiar with the data banks or do not know how to access them. One way that data banks might be used more effectively would be to provide information on quantitative techniques such as decision analysis and multivariate analysis.

## ARTIFICIAL INTELLIGENCE IN MEDICINE

The quantitative techniques described previously may perform well in selected cases when compared with the judgment of experts. Yet many people believe that these techniques do not embody the same decision-making processes that the experts themselves use. Clinical judgment is based not only on detailed medical knowledge but also on a general understanding of medical problems that is gained through reasoning and experience. Experienced clinicians develop sophisticated (but as yet poorly understood) strategies for focusing on only the most relevant considerations, avoiding a detailed examination of all potential conditions that could explain the set of symptoms, signs, and laboratory abnormalities observed in a patient (Pauker et al. 1976; Elstein, Shulman, and Sprafka 1978). Since physicians have great difficulty in remembering exact numbers, and are obviously not as adept as computers in performing arithmetic calculations, it is likely that most clinicians' strategies do not utilize quantitative methods such as probabilistic calculations.

Increasingly successful efforts are being made to develop computer programs that can perform diagnostic tasks in a manner similar to that of experienced clinicians. Although none of these projects intends to reproduce exactly the logic used by clinicians, their goal is to develop "artificial intelligence" techniques that can accomplish the same tasks as the natural intelligence of the clinician. Physicians will interact productively with computer programs only when the programs become able to explain their reasoning on a level acceptable to clinicians.

There are distinct differences between the computer programs that strive for artificial intelligence and those that rely on the techniques described in the rest of this chapter (Duda 1983). Rather than calculating exact mathematical probabilities, or following a strict branching logic scheme in which the results of one test or decision strictly determine the remaining sequence of decisions to be made, artificial intelligence programs use symbolic reasoning. Such programs attempt to "understand" the context in which they are operating, and to apply context-specific guidelines in making decisions. The quantitative aspects of such programs' functioning are often greatly simplified compared with those of formal probability theory. As an example, INTERNIST-1, which is a program designed to make diagnoses in general internal medicine, measures the strength of association between a finding and a disease using a scale from 1 to 5 instead of assigning an exact probability.

In general, symbolic reasoning is accomplished by application of heuristic rules. Some systems are more dependent on rules than others. The best example of a rule-based medical program is the MYCIN program developed by Shortliffe and associates (1976) at Stanford University. Rule-based systems work from a set of decision rules of the form "If conditions X and Y are met, then conclude that conditions A, B, and C are true, and furthermore do procedures P, Q, and R." By linking such rules together, a production system can start with a small amount of initial information and proceed to derive hypotheses, obtaining additional information until the relevant conclusions are made. Such programs can provide detailed analyses of the logic (rules) used in making decisions.

By contrast, INTERNIST-1 uses a combination of probabilistic reasoning and rules in its decision making (Miller, Pople, and Myers 1982). INTERNIST-1 uses three simple quantitative values to represent the significance of diagnostic information. These values are (1) the evoking strength, which measures how strongly a piece of information (observed patient finding) suggests the presence of a particular disease; (2) the frequency with which a symptom, sign, or laboratory abnormality occurs in patients with a particular disease; and (3) the importance, or clinical relevance, of a finding (i.e., the degree to which one is compelled to explain the presence of the finding in a patient). INTERNIST-1 uses these values to calculate a score for each diagnosis under consideration. In the course of solving a diagnostic problem, INTERNIST-1 restricts its consideration to a relatively small set of possibilities by employing a heuristic rule called the *partitioning algorithm*. The partitioning algorithm defines a small set of competitors for the diagnosis with the highest score. INTERNIST-1 reaches a diagnosis when its score is sufficiently greater than the score of its next highest competing diagnosis. To paraphrase INTERNIST-1's logic, the program will conclude that a patient with chest pain has had a heart attack only when the likelihood of this condition is sufficiently greater than that of any other similar condition that is under consideration.

INTERNIST-1 avoids overlooking a potentially correct diagnosis because it tests hypotheses by requesting more information when it is not possible to reach the leading diagnosis. INTERNIST-1 reformulates the problem using alternative hypotheses when questioning does not confirm the original one. The program employs three basic strategies in asking for additional information. When there is a single leading diagnosis, INTERNIST-1 asks for pieces of information that tend to confirm that diagnosis – those pieces with high evoking strengths. When many competing diagnoses are being considered, the program asks for pieces of information that could eliminate some – those with high frequency values under the diagnoses. (The absence of such items in a patient would downgrade the status of hypotheses in which the items were expected to occur commonly.) If only a few diagnoses are being considered, INTERNIST-1 asks for discriminating information that can raise the score of one while lowering the scores of others.

To illustrate how artificial intelligence programs work, INTERNIST-1 was consulted about the case of Mr. Smith (Table 1), the accountant whose exertional chest pain was discussed from the perspective of multivariate analysis earlier in this chapter. Although all the information is not presented in Table 1, INTERNIST-1 concluded that the patient had angina pectoris. It further pointed out that either crescendo angina or a myocardial infarction could explain the recent increase in the duration/severity of the pain, but could not conclude which of the two was present. INTERNIST-1 does not make therapeutic recommendations, but presents the conclusion that the patient should be admitted to the hospital as a possible interpretation of the program's result.

The effort to develop programs with artificial intelligence in medicine is far from complete, but the partial success of programs such as INTERNIST-1 and MYCIN demonstrate that the effort may someday provide important benefits, especially in situations where access to human consultants is restricted. If such programs are to become widely used, it would be preferable for them to use

Table 1. *Edited transcript of INTERNIST's diagnostic evaluation of Mr. Smith. (Questions and information typed by INTERNIST are printed in* italics. *Responses by the person using the program are printed in standard upper and lower case. Explanatory information is in parentheses.)*

---

*Please enter findings.*

Sex male. Age 26 to 55. Chest pain substernal exertional. Chest pain substernal lasting less than 20 minutes. Chest pain radiating to neck and/or upper extremity.

*Considering: sex male, age 26 to 55, chest pain substernal exertional, chest pain substernal lasting less than 20 minutes, chest pain substernal radiating to neck and/or upper extremity.*

(INTERNIST explains that it is considering only diagnoses that explain all the symptoms.)

*Discriminate: angina pectoris, crescendo angina.*

(INTERNIST explains that because it is considering only these two diagnoses, it will ask for information that best discriminates between them.)

*Please enter findings of chest pain. Chest pain substernal relieved by nitroglycerin?*

Not available.

*Chest pain substernal recurrent nocturnal or morning only?*

Yes.

*Chest pain substernal paroxysmal increasing in duration and/or severity recently?*

Yes.

*Chest pain substernal at rest?*

No.

*Chest pain substernal unrelieved by nitroglycerin?*

Not available.

*Disregarding: chest pain substernal paroxysmal increasing in duration and/or severity recently.*

*Pursuing angina pectoris.*

(INTERNIST says that it will not attempt to explain the increase in the duration and/or severity of the chest pain, but will attempt to confirm the diagnosis of angina pectoris.)

*Chest pain substernal remote history?*

No.

*Chest pain substernal crushing?*

No.

*Chest pain substernal numerous attacks per day?*

No.

*Please enter findings of angiocardiography.*

Omit, not available.

*Please enter findings of EKG. EKG ST segment elevation with reciprocal depression?*

Yes.

*Pursuing angina pectoris. Conclude: angina pectoris.*

(INTERNIST announces that it has concluded that Mr. Smith has angina pectoris, which explains all the information except the increase in the duration and/or severity of the chest pain.)

*Considering: chest pain substernal paroxysmal increasing in duration and/or severity recently. Discriminate: acute myocardial infarction, crescendo angina.*

(INTERNIST says that it will now try to explain the increasing chest pain with the alternative diagnoses of acute myocardial infarction or crescendo angina. It will ask for information that best discriminates between the two diagnoses. This part of the transcript has not been included in the table because of space limitations.)

---

natural languages instead of computer-specific jargon to explain the logic behind their solutions to medical problems. The most stringent test for the use of artificial intelligence in medicine might be the Turing test: When we cannot distinguish between an artificial intelligence program and a human consultant seated at another console, we will know that we have a new colleague.

## CLINICAL ALGORITHMS

In addition to multivariate equations, decision trees, patient data bases, and artificial intelligence, clinical algorithms provide another way of guiding medical decision making. Clinical algorithms are flow charts that assist the clinician in pursuing a logical, step-by-step evaluation and treatment plan. They have been used to teach physicians about the appropriate way to care for patients with well-defined problems, to guide nonphysician clinicians (such as nurse practitioners) in the management of common problems, and to evaluate the quality of care that has been provided.

Few physicians were familiar with the word *algorithm* before it was applied to medical practice by innovative clinical scientists at Harvard and Dartmouth medical schools in the early 1970s (Komaroff 1982; Sox 1982). However, the word and its concept are ancient. As early as 1800 B.C., Babylonian mathematicians developed step-by-step rules for solving many types of equations. Around A.D. 825, the Persian mathematician al-Khowarizmi wrote an important textbook on arithmetic, and the word *algorithm*, derived from his name, remains as part of his legacy. More recently, algorithms have been popularized by advances in operations research and computer sciences. In these applications, as with the written medical algorithm, the emphasis has been placed on the branching aspect of algorithms, which allows them to guide the user in a sequential manner depending upon the conditions at that time (Wagner 1969).

## *What is a clinical algorithm?*

In its medical application, an algorithm is a branching logic diagram that explicitly illustrates the proper management of patients at various points in their care, depending upon the presence of certain findings or the occurrence of certain events (Eisenberg and Sussman 1981). The algorithm describes the appropriate steps to be taken in the care of a patient with a particular problem; it indicates the components of the history and physical examination that are needed and the diagnostic tests that should be obtained. Then the algorithm makes precise recommendations for further diagnosis. Alternatively, once enough diagnostic information has been acquired, it suggests a plan of treatment based on the data obtained (Komaroff 1982). Donabedian (1981) has described the clinical algorithm as ''a set of instructions, in the form of a logic flowchart, that leads the nonphysician practitioner through the necessary steps that are needed to begin the process of diagnosis and treatment.'' Although Sox describes the main synonym for clinical algorithm as *diagnostic protocol*, its branching logic often provides the clinician with guidance about treatment as well.

Elsewhere in this chapter, decision trees are described as branching diagrams that can guide the medical decision maker. How do decision trees differ from clinical algorithms? The most important difference is that decision trees provide the probabilities that certain events may happen (at chance nodes), and show the alternative choices for the clinician based upon those events (these choices are made at the decision nodes). Therefore, decision trees are probabilistic in nature, and the decision maker can exercise certain options based on the probabilities and his or her set of utilities. In contrast, clinical algorithms show what should be done in the event that a clinical situation does occur. No probabilities are expressed, and usually no choices are left to the clinician. Once the data have been gathered, the algorithm advises the appropriate next step, based upon the decision that has already been made by the algorithm's designer. Therefore, whereas the decision tree is probabilistic, the clinical algorithm is deterministic. In a sense, the clinical algorithm is a decision tree with the branches to be followed already determined, based upon the opinion of experts about the optimal strategy.

### Why use clinical algorithms?

Most clinical algorithms that have been developed guide decision making about common problems, and many clinicians feel that these problems are too simple to require a decision aid such as a clinical algorithm. There are at least two reasons why an algorithm may be useful.

First, clinical problems are rarely as simple as one may think. As Nobel laureate Peter Medawar has written, "What is wrong [about modern medicine] is the universally held belief that clinically mild diseases have simple causes while grave diseases are deeply complex and are proportionally difficult to discern the causes of or to cure. There is no truth in either; a common cold, caused by a multiplicity of upper respiratory illnesses and with an overlap of allergic reactivity, is an extremely complex ailment" (Medawar 1979).

Second, it is clear that medical decision making, particularly by inexperienced clinicians, is often flawed. Insensitivity to the prevalence of disease, distortion of many probabilities, a tendency to use irrelevant data to support hypotheses, resistance in giving up hypotheses even when there is convincing opposing information, greater ease of recalling more recent events, and altered judgment due to physical and emotional stress are some of the limitations of human judgment (Elstein 1976; Politser 1981; Kassirer 1982). These limitations can be offset by an explicit set of rules for decision making. Although the experienced clinician may override the rules of a clinical algorithm because of important information that the algorithm does not consider, the algorithm encourages the clinician to prove a clear reason for ignoring its recommendation. Wood et al.

(1980) point out that the explicit rules of the clinical algorithm can eliminate unnecessary steps in a diagnostic evaluation.

Sox (1982) has summarized the advantages of using clinical algorithms. He suggests that the algorithm (1) defines the types of patients that can be managed by the algorithm, since it establishes criteria for early referral of especially sick patients to a physician, (2) defines the data to be collected on an individual patient, (3) defines the criteria for obtaining consultation, (4) establishes which clinical findings should lead to diagnostic testing, and (5) defines the clinical findings that should lead to initiating treatment of a condition.

A number of examples of clinical algorithms that have been designed to guide clinical decision making have been published. The most common use of the clinical algorithm has not been by physicians to guide decision making, but rather by nonphysician clinicians, such as nurse practitioners and physician's assistants. Since these professionals are generally less experienced than physicians and have less knowledge of the pathophysiological and pharmacological aspects of diagnosis and treatment, they are more amenable to allowing their own clinical judgment to be bypassed and, therefore, to using clinical algorithms.

One of the most common problems seen in the walk-in clinic, where many of the new health professionals work, is acute upper respiratory illness. Thus, it is not surprising that many of the first algorithms guide the evaluation and treatment of this problem (Greenfield et al. 1974; Grimm et al. 1975; Vickery et al. 1975; Winikoff et al. 1977; Wood, Tompkins, and Wolcott 1980; Christensen-Szalanski et al. 1982). Figure 7 shows the algorithm designed by Wood et al. (1980) to guide army physicians' assistants in the evaluation of acute respiratory illness in adults. It provides several opportunities for consultation with a physician, but also enables the nonphysician to culture the throat, provide symptomatic relief, and treat patients with positive throat cultures. Numerous other protocols have been published for nonphysicians, and several medical publications have published series of algorithms to guide clinical decision making by physicians. It is clear that algorithms can guide the use of medical technology, particularly of diagnostic tests. However, Komaroff has found that few physicians use algorithms that have been developed elsewhere without some modification (Komaroff 1982).

In addition to the use of algorithms that have been described in this chapter – to train or direct nonphysicians in the care of patients with common problems, to standardize care, and to provide explicit guidelines for physicians – clinical algorithms have been used to assist patients in providing self-care, to remind physicians of important components of care that they may have overlooked, and to assess the quality of medical care (McDonald 1976; Komaroff 1982). It may be that the use of clinical algorithms to assess the quality of care will be their most important use for physicians, whereas nonphysician clinicians and patients will probably continue to use algorithms to guide care.

Let us imagine that the quality assurance committee of your hospital has asked you to serve as a member of the committee that will evaluate the care of patients

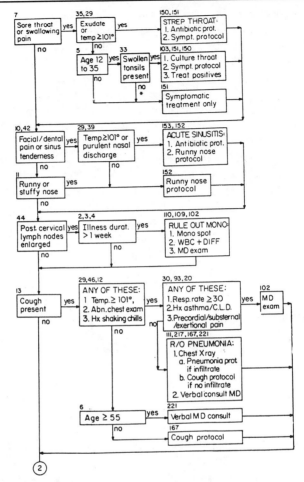

Figure 7. Clinical algorithm for evaluation of patients with acute upper respiratory illness. (From Wood et al. 1980).

presenting with chest pain in the emergency room, focusing particularly on the decision to admit these patients. This is the problem we encountered earlier in this chapter: whether to admit the 39-year-old accountant with chest pain. You and the other committee members meet to develop the criteria by which the quality of care will be evaluated. One member wonders if guidelines should be circulated to guide the decision on whether or not to admit patients with chest pain. What will you suggest?

One approach would be to list certain criteria that should be met for all patients. For example, one criterion might be that any emergency room patient with chest pain and more than 10 premature ventricular contractions per minute should be admitted to the hospital. Several other criteria would be listed, and patients not meeting these criteria would be considered to have received less than optimal

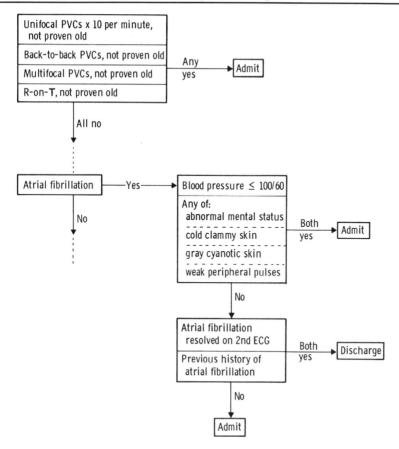

Figure 8. Criteria map algorithm for evaluation of patients with chest pain. PVC = premature ventricular contraction; R-on-T = R-wave on T-wave. (From Greenfield et al. 1977)

care. However, such a list is rarely designed to consider interactions among criteria, such as the importance of four premature contractions per minute in a 39-year-old man with chest pain, new atrial fibrillation, low blood pressure, and a change in mental status. Greenfield et al. (1975, 1977, 1978) have developed the "criteria map" as an application of clinical algorithms to assess the quality of care. Figure 8 shows part of the criteria map for chest pain and illustrates how the branching logic enables the reviewer to consider several related factors in determining whether appropriate care was rendered. Donabedian (1981) states that the criteria map solves a major problem in quality of care assessment – the potential conflict between inclusivity and specificity – because "the application of algorithmic criteria yields a stepwise increase of information that can be regarded as a progressive specification of both the referent and the criteria."

Greenfield et al. (1981) have shown that quality assessment based upon the criteria map is superior to that based upon lists of criteria.

## Evaluation of clinical algorithms

Sox (1982) has reviewed the evidence that the use of clinical algorithms to guide patient management can improve the quality of care. He points out that algorithms have been shown (1) to be effective educational tools for physician's assistants, (2) to improve the efficiency of care, (3) to improve the process of care given by nonphysicians, and (4) to reduce the cost of care of certain common complaints, particularly by altering the use of medical technology. In general, no difference has been noted between illness outcome and patient satisfaction when care by nonphysicians using algorithms has been compared with care by physicians without algorithms.

In one study of the use of clinical algorithms by physicians, Wirtschafter et al. (1979) showed that primary care physicians in Alabama used algorithms to provide cancer chemotherapy with disease-free intervals that were not distinguishable from those of patients treated at one of the state's major medical centers. Fleiss et al. (1972) have shown that the branched logic used in algorithms for recommending psychiatric therapy is superior to models using multivariate statistical equations. This may be, in part, because most multivariate models consider only about five independent variables, whereas algorithms may consider far more.

Despite these favorable results, the evidence that clinical algorithms are effective for purposes other than guiding nonphysicians is still inconclusive. Most studies, including those of nonphysicians, include small numbers of providers, and few studies have been large enough to detect small but important differences in outcome between protocol-driven care and standard care. Most of the reported literature has been published by developers and advocates of the clinical algorithm concept, and it is not yet clear how well their results can be generalized. Many other groups are using algorithms, and the absence of data from these practices raises the possibility that only favorable results are being published. Furthermore, the measures of patient outcome that are available are too insensitive to measure subtle but important differences, even in large studies designed to compare the use of algorithms by nonphysicians with standard care being provided by either nonphysicians or physicians. Wood et al. (1980) have questioned whether the apparent improvement in decision making by nonphysicians who use clinical algorithms is due to the flow chart's logic or to the structure that is forced on the clinician who needs to collect carefully and record certain information from the history, physical examination, and laboratory tests.

## Limitations of clinical algorithms

In addition to concerns about the quality of the evidence that clinical algorithms are generalizable and effective for providers other than nonphysicians, there are several important limitations of these logical flow diagrams.

One important limitation is that clinical algorithms are best suited for simple problems and cannot easily handle complex clinical problems. In using an algorithm, the clinician must start with the patient's presentation, yet few patients present with complaints that clearly fall into one symptom complex. Seldom can a single problem be described, and the algorithmic method, which is dependent on sequential logic, cannot handle multiple problems simultaneously. Perhaps the development of computer-based algorithmic models will remove the limitation of paper-based flow charts, but the sequential, step-by-step mode may continue to prevent the clinical algorithm method from dealing with complex problems. This topic is discussed in more detail in the section that deals with artificial intelligence.

Second, the branching logic of the clinical algorithm enables a clinical factor to be considered in light of other factors, but the steps are still considered independently. Therefore, several closely related factors must be considered in the same step (as Greenfield et al. have done with criteria mapping), or the fact that several variables interact must be ignored. For example, although each of these factors may not be clinically important, a combination of any two may be relevant, and the presence of all three may be essential in determining appropriate management. In addition to this inability to consider these interactions adequately, the clinical algorithm does not weigh the various clinical outputs, so that a very important factor may not be weighed more heavily than one that is less important.

Third, the algorithm is deterministic and suggests that certain actions be taken without indicating their importance or the level of confidence with which the recommendation is made. If the decision is a close call – what Kassirer and Pauker (1981) have described as a "toss-up" – the physician may want to consider factors other than those built into the algorithm. Sociocultural factors such as whether the patient has adequate home-care support or whether the patient can easily afford a certain diagnostic test are important examples.

Fourth, a limitation that is common to all explicit decision-making models is that the data needed for the decision may not be available. If the clinical and epidemiological data are not adequate to provide the probabilities of various outcomes at the branch points, then the designer of the algorithm must be less certain about the recommended course of action. When the data are questionable, the need for judgment by the individual decision maker becomes more important. Elstein (1976) and Politser (1981) have reviewed the debate in the clinical psychology literature between those who advocate the statistical, defined methods of decision making and those who favor a more "artful" clinical approach.

Fifth, the algorithm's design introduces another limitation. Although methods are being developed to enable computers to draw the algorithm's logical, step-by-step pathway of diagnostic and therapeutic reasoning, at present algorithms are generally designed by expert clinicians. Although a group of clinicians may reach a consensus and design an algorithm superior to one that any single member of the group could have designed, both of these methods (group and individual design) are limited by the nature of clinical judgment (which means that the human thought process has certain rules of reasoning, recall, and assembly of data that will influence the logic of the algorithm). These biases will also apply, at least to some extent, to computer systems that design algorithms, because humans will have programmed the computer.

Finally, as has been suggested, it may be that algorithms are useful only for minimally trained, inexperienced clinicians in caring for patients with single symptom complexes. In addition, Sox (1982) suggests that algorithms are most useful in practices with a high rate of personnel turnover, such as military medicine. These conclusions are supported by the finding of Christensen-Szalanski et al. (1982) that nurse practitioners and extensively trained physician's assistants may be less hesitant about violating the algorithm than are army medical corpsmen.

As more experience is obtained with clincial algorithms and their limitations become better understood, future algorithm design may make use of computer technology. Several investigators are currently developing flow diagrams by using computers to identify the optimal pathway of clinical care. Others are continuing to develop methods whereby patients enter historical information directly into the computer. Despite these advances, the clinical algorithms of the future will be only as good as the logic of the designer, the epidemiological data on the natural history of the disease, diagnostic test accuracy and therapeutic effectiveness, and the quality of the data from the history and physical examination.

## CONCLUSION

Because new medical technology has not always fulfilled its promise in practice, new evaluation methods have been developed to guide the clinician's use of technology. Some of these methods have been described in this chapter. Most of them are complex and difficult to master. Some, such as artificial intelligence and data banks, are not fully developed. Nevertheless, the clinician who seeks to use technology wisely will become increasingly dependent on the information it provides to make appropriate decisions about patient management. It is therefore important to understand its limits and advantages.

Some of the advantages are obvious. When properly performed in the appropriate setting, these methods can provide useful information that cannot be obtained by traditional means, and some of this information will lead to improved patient care. How this occurs may not be obvious. Although the results themselves are valuable, the evaluation process requires that the clinical problem be structured clearly and that critical information necessary to solve the problem be made explicit. Thus, the clear thinking imposed by the evaluation process may lead to improved decisions even before the final result is known.

An important limitation to keep in mind is that these methods provide information; they may not necessarily provide answers. The results must still be applied to the specific situation. Experience and intuition remain as important as ever in making final decisions about patient care. The information provided by these methods aids but does not replace clinical judgment.

## ACKNOWLEDGMENT

Randolph A. Miller, M.D., provided helpful advice about the section on artificial intelligence and supervised the use of INTERNIST-1 for the example in Table 1.

## SELECTED BIBLIOGRAPHY

Afifi, A. A., Sacks, S. T., Liu, V. Y., et al. (1971). Accumulative prognostic index for patients with barbiturate, glutethimide and meprobamate intoxication. *N. Engl. J. Med. 285:*1497–1502.

Brand, D. A., Frazier, W. H., Kohlhepp, W. C., et al. (1982). A protocol for selecting patients with injured extremities who need x-rays. *N. Engl. J. Med. 306:*333–9.

Braunwald, E. (1968). Mortality of coronary arteriography. *Circulation 37*(suppl. 3):17–26.

Christensen-Szalanski, J. J., Diehr, P. H., Wood, R. H., et al. (1982). Phased trial of a proved algorithm at a new primary care clinic. *Am. J. Public Health 72:*16–21.

Diamond, G. A., and Forrester, J. S. (1979). Analysis of probability as an aid in the clinical diagnosis of coronary-artery disease. *N. Engl. J. Med. 300:*1350–8.

Dolgin, S. M., Schwartz, J. S., Kressel, H. Y., et al. (1981). Identification of patients with cholesterol or pigment gallstones by discriminant analysis of radiographic features. *N. Engl. J. Med. 304:*808–11.

Donabedian, A. (1981). Using decision analysis to formulate process criteria for quality assessment. *Inquiry 18:*102–19.

Duda, R. O., and Shortliffe, E. H. (1983). Expert systems research. *Science 220:*261–8.

Elstein, A. S. (1976). Clinical judgment: psychological research and medical practice. *Science 194:*696–700.

Elstein, A. S., Shulman, L. S., and Sprafka, S. A. (1978). *Medical Problem Solving: An Analysis of Clinical Reasoning.* Cambridge, Mass.: Harvard University Press.

Eisenberg, J. M., and Sussman, E. J. (1982). Harder data for the soft science of quality assurance. *Med. Decision Making 2:*7–11.

Fleiss, J. L., Spitzer, R. L., Cohen, J., et al. (1972). Three computer diagnosis methods compared. *Arch. Gen. Psychiatry 27:*643–9.

Fries, J. F. (1972). Time-oriented patient records and a computer data bank. *J.A.M.A. 222:*1536–42.

Fries, J. F. (1976). A data bank for the clinician? *N. Engl. J. Med. 294:*1400–2.

Greenfield, S., Bragg, F. E., McCraith, D. L., et al. (1974). Upper respiratory tract complaint protocol for physician-extenders. *Arch. Intern. Med. 133:*294–9.

Greenfield, S., Cretin, S., Worthman, L. G., et al. (1981). Comparison of a criteria map to a criteria list in quality-of-care assessment for patients with chest pain: The relation of each to outcome. *Med. Care 19:*255–71.

Greenfield, S., Lewis, C. E., Kaplan, S. H., et al. (1975). Peer review of criteria mapping: criteria for diabetes mellitus. *Ann. Intern. Med. 83:*761–70.

Greenfield, S., Nadler, M. A., Morgan, M. T., et al. (1977). The clinical investigation and management of chest pain in an emergency department: quality assessment by criteria mapping. *Med. Care 15:*898–905.

Grimm, R. H., Shimoni, K., Harlan, W. R., et al. (1975). Evaluation of patient-care protocol use by various providers. *N. Engl. J. Med.* 292:507–11.

Hyde, T. A. (1973). Discriminant function in lung cancer. *Lancet 1*:107.

Kassirer, J. P. (1982). The clinical decision making process. In *Clinical Decisions and Laboratory Use* (D. P. Connelly, E. S. Benson, M. D. Burke, et al., eds.), pp. 29–38. Minneapolis: University of Minnesotta Press.

Kassirer, J. P., and Pauker, S. G. (1981). The toss-up. *N. Engl. J. Med. 305*:1467–9.

Komaroff, A. L. (1982). Algorithms and the "art" of medicine. *Am. J. Public Health* 72:10–11.

McDonald, C. J. (1976). Protocol-based computer reminders, the quality of care, and the non-perfectability of man. *N. Engl. J. Med. 295*:1351–5.

McNeil, B. J., Hanley, J. A. (1981). Statistical approaches to clinical predictions. *N. Engl. J. Med. 304*:1292–4.

Medawar, P. (1979). *Advice to a Young Scientist*. New York: Harper & Row, pp. 48–9.

Miller, R. A., Pople, H. E., and Myers, J. D. (1982). INTERNIST-1, an experimental computer-based diagnostic consultant for general medicine. *N. Engl. J. Med. 307*:468–79.

Pauker, S. G., Gorry, G. A., Kassirer, J. P., et al. (1976). Towards the simulation of clinical cognition: taking a present illness by computer. *Am. J. Med. 60*:981–95.

Politser, P. (1981). Decision analysis and clinical judgment. *Med. Decision Making 1*:361–89.

Pozen, M. W., D'Agostino, R. B., Mitchell, J. B., et al. (1980). The usefulness of a predictive instrument to reduce inappropriate admissions to the coronary care unit. *Ann. Intern. Med. 92*(Part 1):238–42.

Principal Investigators of CASS (1981). National Heart Blood and Lung Institute coronary artery surgery study. *Circulation 63*(suppl. 1).

Rao, L. G. (1973). Discriminant function based on steroid abnormalities in patients with lung cancer. *Lancet 11*:441–5.

Rosati, R. A., McNeer, J. F., Starmer, C. F., et al. (1975). A new information system for medical practice. *Arch. Intern. Med. 135*:1017–24.

Schwartz, W. B. (1979). Decision analysis: A look at the chief complaints. *N. Engl. J. Med. 300*:556–9.

Second Interim Report by the European Coronary Surgery Study Group (1980). Prospective randomized study of coronary artery bypass surgery in stable angina pectoris. *Lancet 11*:491–4.

Shortliffe, E. H. (1976). *Mycin: A Rule-based Computer Program for Advising Physicians Regarding Antimicrobial Therapy Selection*. New York: Elsevier.

Sox, H. C. (1982). Clinical algorithms and patient care. In *Clinical Decisions and Laboratory Use* (D. P. Connelly, E. S. Benson, M. D. Burke, et al., eds.), pp. 225–37. Minneapolis: University of Minnesota Press.

Vickery, D. M., Liang, M. H., Collis, P. B., et al. (1975). Physician extenders in walk-in clinics. *Arch. Intern. Med. 135*:720–5.

Wagner, H. (1969). *Principles of Operations Research*. Englewood Cliffs, N.J.: Prentice-Hall, pp. 96–102.

Weinstein, M. C. and Fineberg, H. V. (1980). *Clinical Decision Analysis*. Philadelphia: W. B. Saunders, pp. 3–8.

Winikoff, R. N., Ronis, A., Black, W. L., et al. (1977). A protocol for minor respiratory illness. *Pub. Health Rep.* 92:473–80.

Wirtschafter, D., Carpenter, J. T., and Mesel, E. (1979). A consultant-extender system for breast cancer adjuvant chemotherapy. *Ann. Intern. Med. 90*:396–401.

Wood, R. W., Tompkins, R. K., and Wolcott, B. W. (1980). An efficient strategy for managing acute respiratory illness in adults. *Ann. Intern. Med. 93*:757–63.

CHAPTER 11

# THE TECHNOLOGICAL TARGET: INVOLVING THE PATIENT IN CLINICAL CHOICES

HAROLD J. BURSZTAJN, ROBERT M. HAMM, and
THOMAS G. GUTHEIL

Involving the patient in medical decisions has, for good reasons, become a popular concept among both medical professionals and the general public. Nonetheless, physicians and patients who advocate patient involvement do not always grasp its full ramifications. They often assume that the patient is joining the physician in facing a situation of diagnostic and therapeutic certainty, a choice between a few clearly defined courses of action with known consequences. In fact, the medical situation is one of uncertainty regarding the available choices and their consequences (Burzstajn et al. 1981). To involve the patient in decision making, the physician must share the uncertainty with the patient and thereby come to terms with his or her own attitudes toward uncertainty. Such an acknowledgment of uncertainty, together with the patient's preexisting fear and anxiety, may lead the patient to make demands and express preferences that reinforce whatever tendency the physician may have to try to eliminate uncertainty; this may be achieved through the overuse of medical technology. The costs of this defensive strategy increase as technology becomes more expensive and invasive.

The explicit recognition of uncertainty brings to light anxieties that exist in medical situations, but that are experienced unconsciously rather than consciously. These anxieties, whether or not they are articulated, produce stress for both patient and physician, and may lead both to be less reasonable in making choices than they would be otherwise. Sharing the decision with the patient raises to a conscious level the universal clinical problem of how best to surmount the barriers to making reasonable decisions under conditions of uncertainty. Addressing this problem requires that both the patient and the physician subject their decision-making procedures to critical scrutiny. As an aid in the development of critical consciousness, we will consider the strengths and limitations of formal (decision analytic) and informal (heuristic) approaches to clinical decision making.

SHOULD THE PATIENT BE INVOLVED IN DECISION MAKING?

A number of considerations favor patient involvement in medical decision making. The factors can be divided into those that are extrinsic to the character of the decision itself and those that are intrinsic, in the sense that they affect directly the quality of the decision that is made. Although most nonmedical persons and a significant number of physicians make these arguments in favor of involving the patient, it must be noted that the same considerations can be and have been used to argue against such involvement.

### Pros and cons of involving the patient: extrinsic arguments

Much of the impetus for patient involvement comes from patients themselves, as stated in the literature of the patient's rights and holistic health movements (Boston Women's Health Book Collective 1973; Cousins 1979). Although this in itself does not justify accession to patients' demands on the grounds of "giving consumers what they want," it does warrant giving the question serious consideration. At the same time, patient demand is sometimes the reverse: The physician should take charge.

Traditionally, the role of the physician is a paternalistic one. The physician decides what is best for the patient. Today, however, our individualistic, consumer-oriented society decries paternalism in favor of honoring people's preferences. There is a presumption that involving patients in decision making is intrinsically worthwhile. Nonetheless, the paternalistic imperative is still maintained in the case of incompetent patients, and there are differences of opinion within the profession and the public about how far patient autonomy should go.

One of the disabling reactions in the face of uncertainty is a feeling of helplessness (Seligman 1975). The doctor's sharing of information and inviting participation can give the patient a greater sense of control over an uncertain fate. In addition to helping the patient maintain self-control in the face of an illness that threatens bodily integrity and decreasing the risk of a crippling depression, there is also some evidence that patient involvement may affect the progress of the illness. For example, Langer and Rodin (1976) found that increasing patients' decision-making opportunities in a geriatric setting increased longevity.

On the other hand, denial of uncertainty may be the most effective short-range remedy for the patient's anxiety. In one study, laboratory test results with no apparent diagnostic value were shown to have therapeutic benefit. Patients with chest pain who were given a routine electrocardiogram and serum creatine phosphokinase had a better recovery rate than those who did not have these tests, even though the tests were not clinically indicated for the patients in either group (Sox, Margulies, and Sox 1982). The implications of this study will be further explored subsequently. It should be noted, however, that the patient's anxiety may derive as much from uncertainty itself as from its disclosure. The distress that follows disclosure may simply be a manifestation of the underlying discomfort that preexists in patients who are hiding their anxiety about uncertainty even from themselves.

The patient's ability to make a decision can be increased by participation in decision making. For example, a patient who understands the rationale for taking a particular medication is more likely to be an active ally of the physician in carrying out the prescribed regimen and monitoring his or her response to the medication for signs of efficacy or iatrogenesis. Even so, those who hold that the physician's authority is an important element in the healing process may see this authority as being undermined by an egalitarian doctor–patient exchange.

Although the law in different jurisdictions is not entirely consistent on this matter, both case law and statute law recognize a patient's right to informed choice. In *Canterbury v. Spence* (1972), a District of Columbia circuit court, citing the fundamental legal premise that "every human being of adult years and sound mind has a right to determine what shall be done with his own body," ruled that "the patient's right of self-decision shapes the boundaries of the physician's duty to reveal. That right can be effectively exercised only if the patient possesses enough information to enable an intelligent choice." A New York State statute enacted in 1975 provides for disclosure of diagnostic and therapeutic alternatives and their "reasonably foreseeable risks and benefits . . . in a manner permitting the patient to make a knowledgeable evaluation."

The recognition that disclosure of information relevant to decision making may not always be good for the patient is built into the legal provisions that safeguard the patient's right to know. For example, the decision in *Canterbury v. Spence* acknowledges that "patients occasionally become so ill or emotionally distraught on disclosure as to foreclose a rational decision, or complicate or hinder the treatment, or perhaps even pose psychological damage to the patient." The New York State statute just cited provides that a physician may be justified in using "reasonable discretion" in disclosing alternatives and risks "because he reasonably believed that the manner and extent of such disclosure could reasonably be expected to adversely and substantially affect that patient's condition."

## Advantages intrinsic to the decision

Whereas the issues discussed so far have both positive and negative aspects, those that pertain directly to the decisions made give less ambiguous support to the notion of patient involvement. It can be argued plausibly that involving the patient improves decision making.

Any way of making medical decisions involves the patient either explicitly or implicitly. The subtleties of communication between patient and doctor, and vice versa, affect whatever decisions are made. As soon as the physician begins to explain anything to the patient, the physician must (to be honest) acknowledge the uncertainty that surrounds the clinical situation. Because sharing of the decision in this sense is inevitable, there are clear advantages in doing it consciously.

Uncertainty is easiest to bear in a context of mutual support. Involving the patient in the decision-making process makes it possible for physician and patient to share the uncertainty consciously, so that neither must bear the burden alone.

Formal decision theory requires that, in uncertain situations where the patient's values make a difference, the patient make a value assessment (Von Neumann and Morgenstern 1944; Pauker 1976). This formal requirement reflects a necessary step in informal decision making as well, one that entails the patient's active participation.

By discussing risks and benefits with the patient, the physician too becomes more fully aware of them. The collaborative process can enhance not only the patient's but also the physician's rationality, flexibility, and overall competence in decision making.

How conclusive these factors are, in and of themselves, is difficult to assess. The question, Should the patient be involved in decision making? cannot be separated from another question: How can the best decisions be made?

### Technology and the doctor–patient relationship

From the preceding discussion, two models of medical decision making emerge: paternalism and consumer preference. The one values doing what is in the patient's best interest; the other values patient autonomy and individualism. Both models can collapse into irrationality at their extreme – the irrationality of authoritarianism (rationalized as doing what is best for the patient) and the irrationality of honoring *any* preference, no matter how absurd and self-defeating, on the grounds that any wish expressed by a patient reflects a true preference rather than false consciousness engendered by the stress of illness, uncertainty, and the power of technology. Both models therefore leave the practitioner susceptible to the unwise use of technology. The use of technological aids (and technological mystification) to bolster the physician's authority is a commonly noted phenomenon. But as the previous examples show, the consumer satisfaction model, which is usually thought of as an impetus to greater patient involvement in decisions, may also be expressed as a clamor for technological placebos.

Involving the patient in decision making does not in itself resolve the choice between the two models. By providing explicit goals for decision making, however, it does present the choice openly to both parties. The question to be resolved is then no longer Should the patient be involved? but How can the patient best be involved? and finally, How can both the patient *and* the doctor stay involved rather than surrender the decision to purely technical considerations? Maintaining a critical consciousness of the implications of technology and keeping decision-making power in human hands are shared responsibilities.

It is tempting to invoke a simple rule to govern the use of medical technology. At present, as we shall see, there are many pressures dictating the use of as much technology as is available. In an ideal world, on the other hand, we would seek to decrease uncertainty without incurring the risks attendant upon technological procedures: "Above all, do no harm." But this rule is too simple. All of our actions in an uncertain world, including those designed to decrease uncertainty, run the risk of causing harm. Even so benign an act as giving a diagnosis of hypertension to male patients increases the risk of absenteeism from work (Haynes et al. 1978).

The next temptation we face is to seek a method for making decisions, including decisions about the use of technology. Indeed, a decision-making methodology has been devised. We will show, however, that this too, although useful in the appropriate context, is fraught with uncertainties. Like other methods, it cannot replace the process by which the astute clinician takes into account – and makes positive use of – the role of both doctor and patient in an evolving therapeutic alliance for decision making (Havens 1978).

### CLINICAL UNCERTAINTY THROUGH THE FILTER OF ILLNESS

In attempting to share uncertainty and involve the patient in decision making, special problems arise from the nature of the medical situation and the characteristics of the people involved in it. The difficulty of being rational in the face of uncertainty is intensified for those who are ill or who are engaged in treating those who are ill.

#### *Situational factors*

Illness may not only bring pain and physical disability, but may greatly constrict the scope of a person's existence, affecting work, personal relationships, and other aspects of daily life. Cassell (1982) lists the many losses that can contribute to the experience of suffering, as distinct from physical distress: "All the aspects of personhood – the lived past, the family's lived past, culture and society, roles, the instrumental dimension, associations and relationships, the body, the unconscious mind, the political being, the secret life, the perceived future, and the transcendent dimension – are susceptible to damage and loss." Suffering is associated with threats to the integrity of the person. These threats can arouse a range of emotions and bring about changes in self-esteem and values for both patient and physician.

The emotions aroused by illness – fear, anger, helplessness, hopelessness – can interfere with the patient's participation in decisions or influence the decisions reached by the patient. Moreover, they may prevent the physician from participating fully with the patient in decision making, because the physician may want to avoid experiencing these feelings either personally or in the patient.

Illness can reduce a person's self-esteem. Under the increased uncertainty brought on by the illness's threat to the integrity of the body, the patient can become more self-preoccupied, more narcissistic, more childish. Thus, the patient's expressed values may shift in the direction of emphasizing the more primitive, self-centered concerns associated with the experience of isolation in illness. Among these concerns may be the wish to bolster and gratify oneself with the best technological care money can buy, regardless of what resources are thereby used. An issue for the clinician is whether to honor the patient's normal, most mature, or "true" values (articulated by the patient's family or by the patient in better times) or the values expressed by the patient under the stress of illness.

The physician is not immune to the regressive changes experienced by the patient (McCue 1982). If being ill can make the patient feel fearful, angry, helpless, hopeless, worthless, and alone, a physician who is unable to provide a definitive diagnosis or a successful treatment may well go through this same set of emotions. When a case appears to be hopeless, when nothing can be done to help, the physician's self-esteem may diminish along with the patient's. The physician may then be susceptible to the appeal of face-saving technological procedures. A second mechanism of physician susceptibility to the loss of self-esteem comes from the human capacity not only to empathize with (i.e., understand) another's distress but to share it, actually feel it in the form of sympathy (Darwin 1965). A physician who has a patient whose self-esteem is plummeting may find his or her own self-esteem plummeting in sympathy.

### Personality factors

Kahana and Bibring (1964) list seven personality characteristics evoked by illness in hospitalized medical patients: (1) dependent, overdemanding; (2) orderly, controlled; (3) dramatizing, emotionally involved, captivating; (4) long-suffering, self-sacrificing; (5) guarded, querulous; (6) narcissistic, projecting feelings of superiority; and (7) uninvolved, aloof. Such personality characteristics may predispose the patient, in dealing with the emotions surrounding illness, to exhibit a cognitive style that is less well integrated and less helpful than the style this person is ordinarily capable of using. For example, the obsessive-compulsive personality, with its relentless search for objective data, may be predisposed to favor technological means of obtaining information (e.g., exhaustive diagnostic testing). The hysterical personality, on the other hand, tends toward emotional interpretations of reality and may therefore be receptive to intuitive judgments and nontechnological, holistic remedies. The obsessive deals with uncertainty by trying to control it, the hysteric by denying its existence (Shapiro 1965).

Medical training and the demands of medical practice select for the obsessive-compulsive personality, with its bias toward hard data. A related personality variable is intolerance of ambiguity. The lower the physician's tolerance of ambiguity, the greater the pull toward precise diagnostic indicators. Physicians who go into "soft" specialties such as psychiatry tend to be more tolerant of ambiguity than physicians in other specialties (Budner 1962).

Illness brings situation-specific personality changes, as noted by Kahana and

Bibring (1964). The obsessive personality may regress to paranoia. Clearly, such regression on the part of either doctor or patient can produce mistrust in their relationship. Mistrust is an obstacle to shared decision making, and may lead one or both parties to insist on objective verification of clinical judgments. The hysterical personality may regress to dependency, thereby relinquishing active participation in diagnosis and treatment.

### OVERRELIANCE ON TECHNOLOGY AS A RESPONSE TO UNCERTAINTY

Ideally, we wish to involve patients in making medical decisions under conditions of uncertainty. Unfortunately, the process of acknowledging and sharing uncertainty amid the stress of illness is fraught with tensions and evasions. Technology, to our wishful perception, offers an illusory escape from this dilemma with its promise that there is nothing left to bear, no decision left to make, because the uncertainty has already been removed or can be removed by pursuing the most technological of the available options. In fact, the complex decisions necessitated by the existence of technological options make it all the more vital to involve patients in making choices affecting their own well-being.

Decision analysis, a formal procedure for weighing the expected costs and benefits of alternate courses of action (the technology for making decisions, referred to earlier), has been described elsewhere in this book. It can be outlined briefly as follows:

> A simple and comprehensive rule for making decisions is the following. List all feasible courses of action. For each action, enumerate all possible consequences. For each consequence, assess the attractiveness or aversiveness of its occurrence, as well as the probability that it will be incurred should the action be taken. Compute the expected worth of each consequence by multiplying its worth by its probability of occurrence. The expected worth of an action is the sum of the expected worth of all possible consequences. Once the calculations are completed, choose the action with the greatest expected worth. (Fischhoff, Gotein, and Shapira 1982)

It should be added that enumerating all of the possible consequences of each action entails charting sequential pathways in a decision tree. One performs a diagnostic procedure, observes the result, institutes one treatment or another, sees whether it works, tries another test or treatment, and so forth. The decision tree includes both choice and chance, both value and probability.

Decision analysis brings the uncertainties of decision making into the open and allows one to verbalize one's attitude toward uncertainty rather than be driven by it. One may question, however, whether verbalization is the same thing as rationality and whether decision analysis can transcend the attitudes and heuristics it was designed to supplant. A case in point is that of Mrs. Pinelli, a 35-year-old bookkeeper with a history of surgically corrected renal artery stenosis who came to a family physician with a recurrence of severe hypertension. After reducing her blood pressure below immediately dangerous levels with medications, the physician went through a decision analysis with Mrs. Pinelli to evaluate the potential efficacy of continued treatment with drugs versus a diagnostic workup (intravenous pyelogram followed by arteriogram) to see if she should have another operation. The fact that the decision analysis (including the patient's value assessments) gave treatment with medications a higher expected value did not decrease Mrs. Pinelli's faith in a surgical cure or her concern that antihypertensive medications would make her too drowsy to work or take care of her children. She insisted on seeing a specialist, who agreed to hospitalize her. Against the specialist's better judgment and without her family doctor's knowledge, Mrs. Pinelli talked herself into a painful, costly hypertensive workup, which predictably revealed that she was not a candidate for surgery (Bursztajn et al. 1981).

What went wrong? At every step of the way there were lapses of communication among the patient, the family physician, the medical student who performed the decision analysis, and the specialist in hypertension, so that these well-intentioned individuals ended up working at cross purposes. The decision analysis procedure could not overcome normal discontinuities in personal relationships amid the pressures of the hospital milieu. A clinician can represent the data accurately, perform the calculations correctly, and gain the patient's compliance, but still not convince the patient. Once the patient leaves the office, the results of decision analysis, like those of psychoanalysis (Freud 1964), are diffused into the medium of the patient's continuing experience. Clinicians should heed the reasons that patients such as Mrs. Pinelli give for not taking decision analysis seriously.

The discussion that follows is a critical reconstruction of what patients experience in the course of being involved in formal decision-making procedures such as decision analysis.

### The return of the repressed

Decision analysis is used in an effort to avoid the untoward effects of personality, emotional, cognitive, and scientific (philosophical) influences on unaided human judgment. But can the use of a formal procedure eliminate these psychological and cultural tendencies, which seem to be rooted in the human condition? It appears, instead, that the same evasion of uncertainty and consequent overvaluation of technology may simply reappear in the guise of a structured approach to decision making. Here are some examples (the list is hardly exhaustive) of how the four kinds of predisposing factors can affect the three major decision-making functions: the structuring of options on a decision tree, probability assessment, and value assessment. These functions cannot be automated, and they have to be performed by the decision maker.

## Structuring options

Personality as evoked by the situation of illness takes on a different coloration from the personality that is normally observable. As used here, therefore, *obsessive* and *hysteric* should be understood as being tinged with the self-preoccupation brought on by illness. In structuring the decision tree, the obsessive personality will consider too many technological options (even irrelevant ones), the hysteric too few. The one will be constantly refining the data base, the other relying on global intuitions.

Even if the physician presents the options in an emotionally neutral light, the patient is likely to see them through an emotional filter. The optimistic person may see the choice as being between two opportunities for health promotion, whereas the pessimistic one will focus on the prevention of one terrible consequence or another. Usually the latter viewpoint will involve the use of more technology than the former.

A decision tree is structured according to people's attributions about causes and their consequences. For example, someone who sees hypertension as being caused by a chemical imbalance rather than a mind–body interaction is not likely to consider the option of lifestyle changes. In Mrs. Pinelli's case, the medical student eliminated at the outset the options of lifestyle change and "doing nothing" because she saw only drugs and surgery as potentially helpful. Another clinician – or Mrs. Pinelli herself – might have disagreed.

Someone who equates science with high technology will be more resistant to the idea of considering nontechnological options. One who believes that good science requires finding *the* cause of any illness either would resist accepting lifestyle as a contributing cause of hypertension or, having accepted it as a cause, might be susceptible to the idea of its being the only cause.

## Probability assessment

An obsessive person will order more and more tests and bolster probability assessments with closely reasoned arguments, whether or not these are relevant. A hysterical personality, on the other hand, runs the risk of confusing internal mood swings with actual changes in probabilities.

A person who is feeling optimistic will overestimate the probability of good consequences and underestimate the probability of bad ones. A person who is feeling pessimistic will do just the reverse. Although optimism focused on the natural course of an illness may lead to a feeling that less technological intervention is necessary, optimism can also generate a greater willingness to take chances with technological intervention itself.

Those who base probability estimates primarily on concrete information will attach comparable importance to the technological processes by which such information is obtained. Those who estimate probabilities on the basis of consistent sources of information may use technology redundantly. With blood cultures, for example, more is better up to a point, but one can rapidly reach a point of diminishing returns in terms of accuracy, if not confidence. Yet the illusion persists that the best workup for suspected bacterial endocarditis is the one with the most blood cultures.

If certainty is conceived as the touchstone of knowledge, then one will use technological methods yielding findings that have an appearance of certainty, and will also tend to overestimate the probabilities of the predicted consequences so as to validate the scientific form of the information – one that *ceteris paribus* approaches certainty. The paradigmatic case here is the move from "There is an irreducibly small chance that you might have a heart attack" to "There is no chance in the world that you might have a heart attack." The latter, said in the emergency room to reassure the anxious patient with chest pain, can lead to tragic consequences, as when the patient delays in returning to the physician in the face of a crescendo of chest pain, denial buoyed by a certainty guaranteed in the name of science. Conversely, one who is comfortable working with probabilities as a form of scientific knowledge will show more flexibility and discrimination in estimating them.

### Value assessment

It is hard to pin down an obsessive person to a clear preference. The person's values may be so enmeshed in rational arguments and universal rules as not to be easily elicited for the purposes of decision analysis. Any preferences the obsessive person may express will tend to favor technological approaches, which lend themselves to justification by articulated reasons. The hysteric's value judgments, on the other hand, tend to be vague and global: "This is what I want; I'm not sure why, but I know it." The hysteric may express indiscriminate, all-or-nothing value judgments about technological options.

One's overall frame of mind affects the value one places on health. Optimism may lead one to minimize the impact of illness, and thus to undervalue those things (including technology) that are involved in preventing and curing illness. By the same token, when pessimism sinks into depression, one may undervalue what one normally values, including health and what is necessary to maintain or recover it.

The procedure by which values are elicited shapes people's understanding of the choices and the issues at stake, and thereby affects the values expressed. People make clearer choices about things with which they are familiar. The less familiar the technological option under consideration, the more susceptible the patient is to the influence of the person using the elicitation procedure. The technical nature of the elicitation procedure itself may cue the patient to overvalue technology (Fischhoff, Gotein, and Shapira 1982).

A world view that grants "scientific" status only to objective data and methods of investigation will predispose people to overvalue those data and methods that yield user-independent results – that is, to overvalue technology.

### *Decision analysis reconsidered*

In addition to the fact that the limitations of human decision-making capacities are not removed by the use of a formal procedure for decision making, we must ask whether the procedure itself introduces a bias toward technology into the choice of technological versus nontechnological options. There would at least appear to be a gap between the apparent precision of the results obtained through decision analysis and the uncertain information processed at the various stages of the analysis. Thus, decision analysis can bias the implementation of decisions by confusing confidence in the method with confidence in the answers it produces (Hammond 1982). Moreover, the decisions themselves may be biased by resort to this ''technology'' of decision making.

The bias toward technological options begins in the structuring of the decision tree, in which one may overlook nontechnical options whose consequences may be difficult to quantify. This happened not only in the case of Mrs. Pinelli, but also in the study reported earlier in which clinically useless laboratory tests were found to be therapeutically beneficial (Sox, Margulies, and Sox 1982). There the patients who were given the tests were compared with those who received no intervention, rather than with patients who received a nontechnological intervention such as psychotherapy or simply a physician's reassurance. ''No technology'' was equated with ''no action,'' as if the reduction of uncertainty through the doctor–patient relationship would not constitute action. A bias toward technology can also be introduced into the decision tree when the patient and family are not consulted in structuring options that make sense in the context of their lives. Patients and families often can suggest and help carry out nontechnological, cost-saving options that would not occur to the physician, such as caring for a dying patient in the home (Bursztajn et al. 1981).

The use of a formal calculation procedure does not obviate the need for subjective probability assessment, because in many cases the frequency data base needed for objective probability estimates is lacking. Moreover, even when frequency data are available, their application to the particular case requires a judgment that they are a relevant reference population. For on some level each case is unique, and one must therefore decide whether and to what extent the ''objective'' data base is relevant in *this* case (Edwards 1972). In what is usually called the use of objective probability, one has to make subjective *similarity* judgments, whereas in using subjective probabilities, one must make subjective *probability* judgments (Bursztajn and Hamm 1977). Thus, one no more escapes judgment and its vicissitudes when one uses objective data bases than when one uses subjective ones. But the mind set encouraged by the formal procedure is one of overconfidence in the statistical basis of the probabilities plugged into the formula.

People have mixed feelings and contradictory values. Eliciting a patient's values is as sensitive a task as taking a history, in that it must take into account the possible effects of fear, repression, and concealment (Havens 1978). Formal approaches to value assessment such as the "lottery method" (Raiffa 1968) not only lack this sensitivity but may also make the doctor–patient relationship more emotionally distant and thereby reduce the trust necessary for patients to express their most deeply held values (Bursztajn and Hamm 1982). Values are formed and expressed in social contexts; the doctor–patient relationship is one such context, as are relationships with family and friends. A patient who is isolated from these formative, supportive contacts during the value elicitation procedure may be more likely to express self-centered, individualistic values rather than altruistic or communal ones (Bursztajn and Hamm 1979).

Formal decision analysis is useful as an abstraction and simplification of the decision-making process. Its purview is limited to a series of anticipatory calculations culminating in a decision, which is comparable to limiting the concerns of psychoanalysis to what goes on in the office between the patient and the analyst. Decision analysis is best used as the "training wheels" of a bicycle, as a provisional substitute for the internal balance that one develops with experience. To remain dependent on this learning tool is comparable to using psychoanalysis for self-analysis only when lying on the psychoanalyst's couch.

### SHARING UNCERTAINTY IN A THERAPEUTIC ALLIANCE

A tradition in negligence law holds that having done what a reasonable and prudent practitioner would do in the same circumstances is a defense against malpractice. Instead of subjecting a given case to the judgment of others or to a mathematical calculation, it accepts the uniqueness of the individual case and allows the practitioner to fit the decision to the context. Of course, the "reasonable and prudent" tradition contains elements of professional custom and cost–benefit calculation. It is further disciplined by science, because the place of medicine in society is predicated on its being a scientific discipline. Thus, in answering the question of whether a decision is reasonable and prudent, this tradition addresses the issue of whether the clinician's behavior is akin to the behavior of that paragon of reason and prudence, the laboratory scientist.

Science is the authoritative source of many of the cognitive heuristics that we use without thinking, instead of thinking, or as a way of thinking in daily life. Science stands for the "right" way to find out what to do. Our conception of science is a mechanistic one, derived from the classical (Newtonian) physics of the seventeenth century and adapted for the teaching and practice of experimental medicine in the nineteenth century by Claude Bernard (1957). The mechanistic paradigm, which to this day constitutes the scientific foundation of medical education, is defined by three main criteria. First, it seeks a single, unchanging cause or set of causes that can be known with certainty. Second, it discovers causal relationships by means of decisive experiments in which the observer has no effects on the observed other than those intended in the context of experimental manipulations. Third, it separates objective and subjective knowledge and excludes the latter from science (Bursztajn et al. 1981). All three of these criteria reinforce the overvaluation of technology in medical decisions.

The science practiced by the reasonable and prudent physician is not, however, the mechanistic science of Newton. Rather, it parallels the probabilistic science of twentieth-century quantum physics. In place of the three criteria of the mechanistic paradigm, which are (in effect) technologically oriented, the criteria of the probabilistic paradigm allow technological and nontechnological approaches to be used as appropriate. In this emerging paradigm of physics, the first criterion acknowledges an inherent uncertainty in causal relationships. For support in overcoming the anxiety that might prevent this acknowledgment of uncertainty, a trusting relationship between doctor and patient is required. The second criterion recognizes that the process of observation cannot help but affect what is observed in ways unintended by the observer. In place of confident experimental manipulation with all available technology, this criterion implies the need for ongoing awareness of the doctor–patient relationship that is formed in the course of the investigation – the history taking, physical examination, testing – as an important influence on the illness and its prognosis, as well as on the diagnostic and treatment decisions. The third criterion accepts the continuity of objective and subjective knowledge and admits the latter to scientific consideration. Not only laboratory reports, x-rays, and electrocardiograms, but also the feelings of the patient and physician are important data (Bursztajn et al. 1981). Under the probabilistic paradigm, it is legitimate and necessary to pay attention to personal motives, including those generated by the prevailing economic ethos.

This new scientific world view, which is itself more conducive to the critical, discriminating use of technology than was the mechanistic paradigm, also makes possible a different approach to the personality, emotional, and cognitive factors that play such a large, though unacknowledged role in medical decisions. The probabilistic paradigm allows for recognition of the interplay of the observers' personalities (criterion 2) and emotions (criterion 3) as an unavoidable part of scientific investigation. Instead of being ignored, denied, or dismissed as corruptions of pure science, these influences can be observed and consciously managed. The cognitive heuristics by which patients and physicians think, make judgments, and take actions no longer need be derived from experience that is poorly understood and unconsciously mediated by the mechanistic paradigm. To the extent that the rules of thumb used in making decisions can be subjected to conscious examination, they can be critically evaluated in terms of the three criteria of the probabilistic paradigm. They can then be used selectively in contexts where they are more likely to bring about improved outcomes (Bursztajn and Hamm 1982). No one can have perfect self-awareness as a thinking being or make perfect discriminations between the appropriate and inappropriate use of heuristics. Nonetheless, the probabilistic paradigm, as a consciously held philosophy rather than a historical and cultural holdover (held over, as it were, in the unconscious), can aid patients and physicians in being more aware of their heuristics and examining their use critically within a trusting relationship.

Heuristics consistent with the probabilistic paradigm are those that foster acceptance rather than denial of uncertainty. They constitute what has been called *principled gambling*, which grows out of a conviction that, because in the pursuit of truth in the service of health one must take chances anyway in an uncertain world, one may as well do so consciously, with an appreciation of the stakes and the odds (Bursztajn et al. 1981). The conscious acceptance of uncertainty, which is often avoided out of anxiety, becomes possible when it is shared in a context of mutual trust, so that no one must bear the psychological burden alone. This is the crucial importance of a supportive therapeutic alliance in which doctor and patient (and, where possible, the patient's family) can make the most reasonable and prudent decisions of which they are capable (Gutheil and Havens 1979). A trusting alliance does not come ready made. It requires shared experience and some effort on both sides. Sometimes even to achieve it requires some technology. Here, as in other areas of medicine, the physician may be at an advantage in knowing more about the relevant technology than the patient does. Havens (1978) delineates some of this "technology" when he speaks of the therapeutic approaches used to work through a patient's fear, repression, or concealment in order to take a medical history. He concludes, "We need to use these new tools as efficiently as the stethoscope and ophthalmoscope. They are not very difficult tools and their edge is often surprisingly keen."

## CONCLUSION

Medical decisions made by both patients and physicians are in many ways unconsciously biased toward greater use of technology, even when inappropriate. Formal decision-making techniques, although sometimes useful in helping patients and physicians to articulate their reasons for overvaluing technology, do not reveal the source of this systematic preference and may indeed be undermined by it. The choice of decision-making methods, formal or otherwise, in particular medical situations should be guided by an up-to-date scientific world view such as that embodied in the probabilistic paradigm of modern physics. The choice should reflect not only which method gives the "best" answers, but also which method helps both physician and patient deal with the psychological ramifications of uncertainty. Through a trusting alliance, physician and patient can support each other in working with uncertainty, rather than pressure each other to use technology as an escape from uncertainty.

## SELECTED BIBLIOGRAPHY

Bernard, C. (1957). *An Introduction to the Study of Experimental Medicine*. New York: Dover.

Boston Women's Health Book Collective. (1973). *Our Bodies, Ourselves*. New York: Simon & Schuster.

Budner, S. (1962). Intolerance of ambiguity as a personality variable. *J. Pers. 30*:29–50.

Bursztajn, H., Feinbloom, R. I., Hamm, R. M., et al. (1981). *Medical Choices, Medical Chances: How Patients, Families, and Physicians Can Cope with Uncertainty.* New York: Delacorte/Seymour Lawrence.

Bursztajn, H., and Hamm, R. M. (1977). Behavioral decision theory: a research framework for studies in probability and value assessment with selected applications to primary care medicine. Unpublished manuscript, Harvard Medical School, Boston.

Bursztajn, H., and Hamm, R. M. (1979). Review of Crane, D. The sanctity of social life: physician treatment of critically ill patients. *Biosciences 29*:112.

Bursztajn, H. and Hamm, R. M. (1982). The clinical utility of utility assessment. *Med. Decision Making 2*:161–5.

*Canterbury v. Spence*, 464 F.2d 772, D.C. Cir. 1972.

Cassell, E. J. (1982). The nature of suffering and the goals of medicine. *N. Engl. J. Med. 306*:639–45.

Cousins, N. (1979). The holistic health explosion. *Sat. Rev. 6*(7):17–20.

Darwin, C. (1965). *The Expression of the Emotions in Man and Animals*, 2nd authorized ed. Chicago: University of Chicago Press. (Originally published 1872.)

Edwards, W. (1972). N = 1: diagnosis in unique cases. In *Computer Diagnosis and Diagnostic Methods* (J. A. Jacques, ed.), pp. 139–51. Springfield, Ill.: Charles C. Thomas.

Fischhoff, B., Goitein, B., and Shapira, Z. (1982). The experienced utility of expected utility approaches. In *Expectations and Actions: Expectancy-Value Models in Psychology* (N. T. Feather, ed.), Hillsdale, N.J.: Erlbaum.

Freud, S. (1964). Analysis terminable and interminable. In *The Standard Edition of the Complete Psychological Works of Sigmund Freud* (J. Strachey, ed.), vol. 23, pp. 235–43. London: Hogarth Press and the Institute of Psychoanalysis.

Gutheil, T. G., and Havens, L. L. (1979). The therapeutic alliance: contemporary meanings and confusions. *Int. Rev. Psychoanal. 6*:467–81.

Hammond, K. (1982). Unification of theory and research in judgment and decision making. Unpublished manuscript, University of Colorado, Boulder.

Havens, L. L. (1978). Taking a history from the difficult patient. *Lancet 1*:138–40.

Haynes, R. B., Sackett, D. L., Taylor, D. W., et al. (1978). Increased absenteeism from work after detection and labeling of hypertensive patients. *N. Engl. J. Med. 299*:741–4.

Kahana, R., and Bibring, G. (1964). Personality types in medical management. In *Psychiatry and Medical Practice in a General Hospital* (N. E. Zinberg, ed.), pp. 108–23. New York: International Universities Press.

Langer, E., and Rodin, J. (1976). The effects of choice and enhanced personal responsibility for the aged: a field experiment in an institutional setting. *J. Pers. Soc. Psych. 34*:191–8.

McCue, J. D. (1982). The effects of stress on physicians and their medical practice. *N. Engl. J. Med. 306*:458–63.

New York Public Health Law §2805-d 1975.

Pauker, S. G. (1976). Coronary artery surgery: the use of decision analysis. *Ann. Intern. Med. 85*:8–18.

Raiffa, H. (1968). *Decision Analysis.* Reading, Mass.: Addison-Wesley.

Seligman, M. E. P. (1975). *Helplessness: On Depression, Development, and Death.* San Francisco: W.H. Freeman.

Shapiro, D. (1965). *Neurotic Styles.* New York: Basic Books.

Sox, H. C., Margulies, I., and Sox, C. H. (1982). Psychologically mediated effects of diagnostic tests. Unpublished manuscript, Stanford University School of Medicine, Palo Alto, California.

Von Neumann, J., and Morgenstern, O. (1944). *Theory of Games and Economic Behavior.* Princeton, N.J.: Princeton University Press.

CHAPTER 12

# DOES TECHNOLOGY WORK?
# JUDGING THE VALIDITY
# OF CLINICAL EVIDENCE

RALPH I. HORWITZ, ALVAN R. FEINSTEIN, WILLIAM B. CREDÉ,
and JOHN D. CLEMENS

Clinical decision making in medicine has become a complex exercise that balances potential benefits from efficacious diagnostic and therapeutic procedures against the inherent risk and cost of these technologies. The armamentarium of potent measures available to physicians today far exceeds the expectations of almost any practitioner 10 to 20 years ago. Confronted with this impressive array of technological developments, clinicians have struggled to evaluate the evidence of their efficacy and to develop strategies for their appropriate application.

The evidence needed to evaluate the clinical efficacy of these technological developments requires an appreciation of the diverse purposes of diagnostic tests in clinical medicine. The same technological procedure, when ordered for patients with the same clinical condition, may be used in making many different decisions. For example, in a patient with classical angina pectoris, an electrocardiogram may be ordered to establish a diagnosis of coronary disease, to determine whether antiarrhythmic therapy is needed, to note the consequences of antecedent antiarrhythmic therapy, or to reassure the physician or the patient that no changes have occurred since the previous tracing.

The assessment of tests used for establishing a diagnosis is a particularly complex procedure. The evaluation must include provision for both the role of the test and the degree of clinical suspicion with which the test is ordered. In terms of their role, certain tests can be definitive, contributory, or surrogates for the diagnosis. For example, the glucose tolerance test is definitive for the diagnosis of diabetes mellitus; the serum creatinine phosphokinase (CPK) test is contributory for the diagnosis of acute myocardial infarction; and the exercise stress test may be a surrogate for the diagnosis of coronary artery disease. Definitive tests, which are the procedures that may be used to establish the presence of a disease, are rarely evaluated for their capacity to make correct diagnoses. We may worry about the standards for glucose ingestion, specimen

193

Table 1. *Results of diagnostic tests*

|  | Confirmed disease state | | |
| --- | --- | --- | --- |
| Test result | Present | Absent | Total |
| Positive | $a$ | $b$ | $a + b$ |
| Negative | $c$ | $d$ | $c + d$ |
| Total | $a + c$ | $b + d$ | $N$ |

timing, and chemical measurement when a laboratory performs a glucose tolerance test, but we are seldom concerned that the test itself is misleading.

It is the surrogate tests that create the main difficulty in evaluating technological procedures, because these tests do not identify the disease, but rather something that we hope will denote the disease. We often use surrogate tests because they are simpler, less expensive, safer, and more convenient than the corresponding definitive test.

Diagnostic tests, regardless of whether they are definitive, contributory, or surrogate, are applied in at least three circumstances of differing clinical suspicion. First, healthy volunteers from the general population may be tested, as when the members of a college alumni organization are invited to have a free exercise stress test. Testing apparently healthy people from the general population is called *screening* (Sackett and Holland 1975). Second, patients who come to a physician's office because of an illness (e.g. urinary frequency and burning) may take a routine stress test regardless of the tests that are ordered to assess their chief complaints. Testing for disorders that are unrelated to the reason for the patient's visit is called *case finding* (Sackett and Holland 1975). Third, an exercise test may be specifically ordered to explain the cause of a patient's presenting illness (e.g. chest pain); this process is called *diagnosis*. The remainder of this chapter will focus largely on the use of surrogate tests for the diagnosis of a patient's illness.

## STATISTICAL INDEXES AND METHODS FOR ASSESSING DIAGNOSTIC TESTS

The efficacy of a diagnostic test is its ability to indicate the presence or absence of a disease, and is usually calculated from the arrangement shown in Table 1. In this table, the column headings denote the patient's confirmed disease status; the row headings denote the result of the test; and the four interior cells denote whether the patient has been correctly or falsely diagnosed. The sensitivity of the test, which is $a/(a + c)$, answers the question: If the disease is present, how likely is the patient to have a positive test? Specificity, which is $d/(b + d)$, answers the question: If the disease is absent, how likely is the patient to have

Table 2. *Test results in 400 patients*

| Test result | Confirmed disease state | |
|---|---|---|
| | Present | Absent |
| Positive | 180 | 20 |
| Negative | 20 | 180 |

a negative test? These vertical indexes of sensitivity and specificity, which are the test's stable, inherent properties, are sometimes called *nosologic* because they determine the presence or absence of the disease.

In clinical practice, however, when we attempt to diagnose a patient's illness, we do not know the confirmed disease status of the patient. The clinical questions that a physician asks are: If the patient has a positive test, how likely is the patient to have the disease? Or, if the patient has a negative test, how likely is he or she not to have the disease? The indexes that answer these questions are two horizontal indexes: the predictive value of a positive test result, which is $a/(a + b)$, and the predictive value of a positive test result, which is $d/(c + d)$.

If a diagnostic test's predictive value is our focus of clinical interest, why do we even bother considering the indexes of sensitivity and specificity? The answer to this question is readily perceived by considering the following illustration. Suppose an investigator has studied a test using 200 patients known to have the disease and 200 patients known not to have the disease. Assume that the sensitivity and specificity of the test are 90 percent, so that the fourfold table of results is as shown in Table 2. In this arrangement of the data, the test's predictive value is quite high: The predictive value of a positive result is 90 percent (180/200), and the predictive value of a negative test result is 90 percent (180/200).

Suppose, however, that another investigator studies the same test using 20 patients known to have the disease and 200 patients known to not have the disease. Because, as noted earlier, the sensitivity and specificity of the test are its stable, inherent properties, they would presumably remain unchanged at 90 percent each. After the test was performed, the fourfold table would be as shown in Table 3.

In these data, the sensitivity (18/20) and the specificity (180/200) are each 90 percent. But a dramatic change has occurred in the test's predictive value. The positive accuracy rate has declined to only 47 percent (18/38), and the negative accuracy has increased to 99 percent (180/182).

We now recognize that the predictive value of a test depends both on the test's sensitivity and specificity and on the prevalence of the disease among all of the patients tested. Regardless of the sensitivity and specificity of the test, by altering the proportion of cases in the test population, an investigator can arrange

Table 3. *Test results in 220 patients*

| Test result | Confirmed disease state | |
| --- | --- | --- |
| | Present | Absent |
| Positive | 18 | 20 |
| Negative | 2 | 180 |

for the results to show almost any desired value for positive or negative predictive accuracy (Vecchio 1976).

As a consequence of changes in disease prevalence, a test of high sensitivity and specificity evaluated in a hospital setting may be used in customary clinical practice with distressing results. Suppose an investigator describes a new diagnostic test for cancer with a sensitivity of 95 percent and a specificity of 85 percent. When we apply this test to patients seen in normal clinical settings out of the hospital, the cancer prevalence might be 150 per 100,000 patients. By developing our fourfold table, we can determine that the predictive value of a positive result for the test is 0.9 percent. Thus, whenever the test gives a positive result, the chances are less than 1 percent that the patient actually has cancer.

A method for adjusting the predictive values of diagnostic tests or procedures for the effects of disease prevalence is based on a mathematical equation, derived by the Reverend Thomas Bayes (1963), describing the conditional probability of two or more events. In contrast to ordinary probability involving the prediction of a single event, conditional probability involves at least two events, with the prediction of the second event depending on the previous occurrence of the first. See Appendix A for a more detailed discussion.

## ROC ANALYSIS

Values for positive and negative predictive accuracy for a given diagnostic test vary according to the disease prevalence. Although values for test sensitivity and specificity are independent of disease prevalence, they do depend on the choice of a test cutoff point. The test cutoff point is the value of the diagnostic test used to separate positive from negative test results. Using the cutoff point, each member of the study group will be classified as having one of four possible test results: true positive (TP), true negative (TN), false positive (FP), and false negative (FN). The particular choice of a cutoff point can influence the proportion of the population that falls into each of these four categories, and thus create shifts in test sensitivity and specificity.

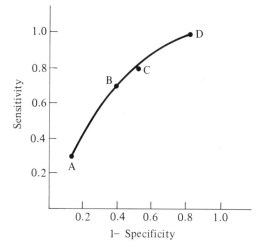

Figure 1. Example of an ROC curve.

## CONSTRUCTION OF THE ROC CURVE

*Receiver-operating characteristic* (*ROC*) analysis is used to select cutoff points and to evaluate test performance (McNeil, Keeler, and Adelstein 1975). The ROC curve plots true-positive rates (sensitivity) against false-positive rates (1 − specificity) for the entire range of potential test cutoff values. The term *receiver-operating characteristic* refers to the ability of these curves to describe the nosologic characteristics (sensitivity and specificity) of the test, and to the ability of the *receiver* of the test information to *operate* at any point on the curve by selecting a given test cutoff value. An example of an ROC curve is given in Figure 1. In this curve, a cutoff point with high sensitivity (point D) also increases the false-positive rate (which decreases the test's specificity). Alternatively, selecting a cutoff point that enhances the test's specificity (point B) reduces its sensitivity. Such a curve might describe a value of exercise stress test in diagnosing coronary artery disease. Using the exercise test, one could vary the cutoff value for ST segment depression from 0.5 to 2.5 mm. Thus, when test results larger than those corresponding to the value at point A (e.g., 2.5 mm) are considered abnormal, the test has very high or 90 percent specificity (10 percent false-positive results) but poor sensitivity (0.3). When test results greater than those corresponding to point C (e.g., 1.5 mm) are considered abnormal, the sensitivity increases to 80 percent, but the specificity decreases to 50 percent. A very low test value (e.g., 0.5 mm) can be used to designate abnormal results at cutoff point D, identifying all of the diseased patients (sensitivity = 100 percent) but reducing the specificity to 20 percent. The operating position is the location of a cutoff point along an ROC curve. See Appendix B for more details.

### METHODOLOGIC ISSUES IN ASSESSING DIAGNOSTIC TESTS

Regardless of the mathematical strategies employed to calculate the various indexes used for describing the efficacy of a diagnostic test, the clinician who uses the tests must be aware that the values attained for these indexes can be distorted by three types of problems: the spectrum of patients included in a study; bias in interpreting the test result; and bias in determining the confirmed presence or absence of the disease (Ransohoff and Feinstein 1978). In the evaluation of a diagnostic test, the assessment often proceeds sequentially. In the first phase of nosologic assessment, the investigator establishes the values for the test's indexes of sensitivity and specificity; in the second phase of clinical assessment, the focus is on the accuracy for positive and negative prediction (Credé and Horwitz 1982). Information about the test's possible benefit in various settings may be presented to the clinician at any time during this process of test evaluation. In the section that follows, we shall present the information needed to evaluate the validity of claims for the efficacy of a diagnostic test.

### NOSOLOGIC ASSESSMENT

The initial methodologic requirement of the nosologic assessment requires an independent "blind" comparison with an accepted "gold standard" of diagnosis. In studying the value of exercise testing in the diagnosis of coronary artery disease, this methodological requirement demands that the diagnostic test be studied in a group of patients with confirmed coronary disease (by application of a gold standard test such as coronary arteriography) and a second group of patients without the disease (using the same gold standard test). Furthermore, to avoid bias that occurs when the test is interpreted with knowledge of the diagnosis, the diagnostic test (e.g., the exercise stress test) must be interpreted by physicians who are unaware (blind) of the patient's confirmed condition (test-review bias) (Ransohoff and Feinstein 1978). To avoid bias that occurs if the result of the test affects the subjective review of the data that establish the diagnosis, the interpretation of data from the definitive test must be made without knowledge of the surrogate test (diagnostic-review bias) (Ransohoff and Feinstein 1978). Finally, to avoid the bias that occurs when the test result is incorporated into the evidence used to diagnose the disease, the criteria for diagnosing the confirmed condition must not include the test being examined (incorporation bias) (Ransohoff and Feinstein 1978).

A second requirement in the nosologic assessment of the diagnostic test is the need for a broad spectrum of diseased and nondiseased patients that is comparable to the population in which the test will be used. A perfect test would have 100 percent sensitivity and 100 percent specificity. However, false-negative and false-positive results commonly occur, and thus interfere with a clinician's major diagnostic goals. In ruling out disease, a test needs to have nearly perfect accuracy for negative prediction (i.e., close to 100 percent, as in the lung scan for diagnosing pulmonary embolism). Using the algebraic symbols noted earlier, this type of accuracy requires a relatively small value for $c$ (false-negative results), and thus a high sensitivity. Similarly, to rule in a disease, a test needs to have nearly perfect accuracy for positive prediction, requiring a small value for $b$ (false-positive result) and a nearly perfect index of specificity. To rule out a disease effectively, a test's sensitivity must be examined in a broad spectrum of diseased patients; to rule in a disease, the test's specificity must be studied in a broad spectrum of nondiseased patients (Ransohoff and Feinstein 1978).

The concept of a broad spectrum of study patients includes the pathological, clinical, and co-morbid components of the illness. Each component must be examined separately for the diseased and nondiseased groups. In the diseased group, the challenge is to discover whether the test is perfectly sensitive (which it rarely is), or whether and in which patients the test yields a false-negative result. Extensive, typical disease usually presents a much smaller diagnostic challenge than the same disease in an atypical, less extensive form; the real value of a new diagnostic test often lies in its predictive value among commonly confused disorders. For example, in studying exercise stress testing for coronary artery disease, the test might be positive in a patient with three-vessel disease but negative in a patient with single-vessel disease (pathological component); positive in patients with typical angina pectoris, but negative in patients with atypical chest pain (clinical component); and falsely negative in patients with co-morbid condition, such as intermittent claudication, that limits the patient's ability to exercise.

The challenge in the comparative group of nondiseased patients is to discover whether the test is perfectly specific (which it rarely is), or whether and in which patients it yields false-positive results. By contemplating the features of a disease that make a test positive, and by looking for similar features in patients without that disease, it is often possible to challenge the test's specificity. For example, if a disease is characterized by certain clinical features (e.g., left ventricular hypertrophy, which may make the test falsely positive in patients with ischemic coronary disease), nondiseased patients with these associated symptoms (e.g., left ventricular hypertrophy in patients with hypertension) should be included in the comparative group. Similarly, co-morbid ailments should be included if they are also likely to yield false-positive results.

### DEFINITION OF NORMAL

A commonly ignored aspect in assessing the clinical efficacy of diagnostic tests is the definition of a normal or abnormal test result. Several different definitions of normal are used in clinical medicine, but we shall briefly discuss only those definitions that are often employed in diagnostic test studies.

The most common definition of normal is obtained by assuming that the test results of a presumably disease-free group of people will conform to a special theoretical distribution called the *Gaussian* or *normal distribution* (Sackett 1978).

One of the attractive properties of the Gaussian distribution is that 95 percent of the test results are contained within the mean plus or minus ($\pm$) approximately two standard deviations (sd). The remaining 5 percent of the test results are in the upper and lower 2.5 percent of the distribution. Consequently, the mean $\pm$ 2 sd is a frequently used definition of normal.

Unfortunately, this common definition of normal may be used to lead to conclusions that are clinically inconsistent. For instance, using the Gaussian distribution to define normal ensures that many nondiseased patients will be erroneously considered diseased. This occurs because 5 percent of the patients already known to be disease-free under the study are classified as having abnormal tests (Haynes 1981).

Recognizing that diagnostic test results may not fit in a Gaussian distribution, many laboratories have substituted the percentile method to define normal. Using this approach, the shape of the distribution of test results is ignored, and the inner (or lower) 95 percent of values is classified as normal. The same clinically inconsistent conclusions that were described for the use of the Gaussian method also apply to the use of the percentile method, because in both instances the 5 percent abnormal test results were established on disease-free patients.

A third definition of normal, called a *diagnostic definition* (Haynes 1981) identifies a range of test results that are associated with the confirmed presence or absence of a disease. Using this approach to study the diagnostic value of exercise testing in coronary artery disease, the disease is established by a gold standard method such as coronary arteriography, and certain values of the test result (e.g., 1 mm of ST segment depression, 2 mm, 3 mm, etc.) are classified as abnormal. One of the consequences of this approach is that the quantitative indexes of efficacy (sensitivity, specificity, and predictive accuracy) will vary according to the change in the definition of abnormal (selection of the cutoff point). If we wanted to maximize a test's sensitivity, we would simply lower the threshold for classifying the result as abnormal (e.g., 0.5 mm of ST segment depression); and if we wanted to enhance the test's specificity, we would raise the threshold for an abnormal test (e.g., 3 mm of ST segment depression). Notice, however, that as the criteria for an abnormal test result are made less stringent, the sensitivity increases at the expense of an increase in false-positive results (lower specificity); and as the criteria are made more stringent, the specificity increases at the expense of an increase in false-negative test results (lower sensitivity).

## INDETERMINATE TEST RESULTS

Regardless of the method chosen and the criteria used to classify a test result, there are often instances in which the result cannot be called either positive or negative. For example, an exercise stress test may be considered positive if there is at least 1 mm of ST segment depression; and the test may be considered negative if the patient reaches a predetermined level of exercise without the associated change in the ST segment of the electrocardiogram. When the test is performed, there may be 1 mm of ST segment depression, but the cardiologist is unable to interpret the test as positive because the baseline cardiogram showed an abnormal depression of the ST segment; or the patient has left ventricular hypertrophy or was using digitalis medications, either of which may have contributed to the abnormal cardiogram. Conversely, the test may be performed and the ST segment remains unaltered, but the test cannot be interpreted as negative because the patient never reached the predetermined level of exercise, or was taking a medication (e.g., propanolol) that limited the heart rate response to exercise.

The problem of indeterminate test results occurs often. In a recent survey that we conducted of about 200 consecutive exercise stress tests, the results of nearly 40 percent of the tests were classified as indeterminate (Philbirck et al. 1982). Thus, regardless of the sensitivity and specificity of the test in patients with a definite positive or negative result, the clinical usefulness of any diagnostic test will be affected by the occurrence of indeterminate results. The way in which these indeterminate test results are handled can have major effects on the calculation of sensitivity and specificity.

If the indeterminate tests are all classified as negative, the sensitivity of the test will be decreased; and if all the tests are classified as positive, the specificity of the test will be decreased. If the test results are discarded altogether, as apparently is frequently done, the statistical indexes of efficacy may be artificially inflated. In addition, the test evaluator will have failed to report an important piece of information that influences the clinician's assessments of the test's utility: how frequently the test result fails to provide a clinically distinctive element of diagnostic evidence. Perhaps the most cogent way to handle the dilemma of indeterminate test results is by separately reporting and analyzing the indeterminate findings. Because few studies provide this separate analysis, the clinical reader must beware of the inflated claims of test efficacy that ignore the problem of indeterminate results.

## CLINICAL ASSESSMENT

After completing the nosologic assessment, the investigator is ready to perform a clinical assessment of the diagnostic test. The clinical assessment requires an analysis according to the purpose for which the test was ordered, the clinical setting in which the test is applied, and a comparison of the test with already existing diagnostic procedures.

A diagnostic test is usually ordered for any of several reasons. First, the physician may have a strong suspicion that the disease is present, and orders the test to confirm this suspicion. For example, suppose we saw a 65-year-old man with substernal chest pain that is initiated with exercise and relieved by rest or nitroglycerin. Because we have a strong suspicion from the history that the patient has clinically significant coronary artery disease, we would want to rule in the diagnosis by selecting a *confirmation* test that has high accuracy for positive prediction (or high specificity).

In other clinical circumstances, we might include a disease among a comprehensive list of disorders that could explain the patient's complaints, even though we think it is unlikely that the disease is present. For instance, in a 35-year-old woman with a history of nonpleuritic chest pain, we may consider the diagnosis of a pulmonary embolism. If the patient has no other clinical characteristics to suggest that diagnosis, we may want to rule out the diagnosis by selecting an exclusion test that has high accuracy for negative prediction (or high sensitivity). In the first example (the patient with angina pectoris), we might select a thallium stress test to confirm the diagnosis of coronary artery disease; in the second example (the woman with nonpleuritic chest pain), we would choose a pulmonary ventilation-perfusion scan to exclude the diagnosis of pulmonary embolism.

Our clinical assessment of diagnostic tests must consider not only the purpose of the test but also the clinical setting in which the test is ordered. Diagnostic tests, such as lung scans, are often studied in hospitalized patients in whom pulmonary embolism occurs with considerable frequency. Since the indexes of positive and negative prediction depend on the disease prevalence, the test will have disappointing results when applied to ambulatory patients in customary clinical practice. Hospitalized patients frequently differ from ambulatory patients in other ways that may influence the apparent efficacy of the test. If a test is more likely to yield positive results in cachectic rather than well-nourished patients, hospitalized diseased and nondiseased individuals may have a larger number of positive test results. Similarly, if co-morbid clinical disorders affect the results of the test, studies of hospitalized patients may not be applicable to ambulatory patients with minimal co-morbid disease.

Even among ambulatory patients, there is considerable variability in clinical settings that may affect the assessment of diagnostic tests. Ischemic coronary artery disease is likely to occur more commonly in the elderly population of a retirement community than in the younger patients of a university health service, and hepatitis infection may be considerably more frequent among health workers in a dialysis center than among people working in an automobile assembly plant. In each of these settings, the test evaluation may be affected by the prevalence of the disease as well as the distinctive demographic and clinical features of the study groups.

### THE USE OF COMBINATION TESTING

If a single diagnostic test were both perfectly sensitive and perfectly specific, the disease under study could always be diagnosed by that single diagnostic procedure. However, because few surrogate tests have sufficiently high sensitivity and specificity for this purpose, two or more tests are often used to evaluate a diagnostic possibility. To illustrate the combined operating characteristics of multiple tests, consider the problem of a middle-aged man with atypical chest

Table 4. *Combination testing for patients with chest pain*

|  | Index of | |
|---|---|---|
|  | sensitivity (%) | specificity (%) |
| Exercise test (A) positive | 60 | 75 |
| Thallium test (B) positive | 70 | 85 |
| Both tests positive[a] | 42 | 96 |
| Either test positive[b] | 88 | 64 |

[a]When both tests are positive: sensitivity (A and B) = sensitivity A × sensitivity B; specificity (A and B) = 1 − [(1 − specificity A) × (1 − specificity B)].
[b]When either test is positive: sensitivity (A or B) = sensitivity A + sensitivity B − sensitivity (A × B); specificity (A or B) = 1 − [(1 − specificity A) + (1 − specificity B) − (1 − specificity A) (1 − specificity B)].

pain in whom the physician suspects the diagnosis of coronary artery disease. As frequently occurs in this setting, the physician may order both an exercise stress test and a thallium perfusion scan. Using typical data for the sensitivity and specificity of each test alone, and assuming that the test results are statistically independent, we can calculate the results of the combined use of these tests.

In Table 4 the exercise stress test is considered to have a sensitivity of 60 percent and a specificity of 75 percent; the thallium scan has corresponding values of 70 and 85 percent. The consequences of the tests' outcome for the physician's clinical decision will depend to a certain extent on whether the physician requires a positive result on both tests or either test to rule in the diagnosis of coronary artery disease.

If the physician is willing to make the diagnosis of coronary artery disease only if *both* tests are positive, then the combined sensitivity is 42 percent. In this circumstance, the combined specificity is calculated as 96 percent. Requiring a positive result on *either* test leads to quite different sets of indexes of sensitivity and specificity for the two tests. The combined sensitivity in this circumstance is 88 percent, and the combined specificity is 64 percent (methods for combining probabilities are outlined in Table 4). The simple probabilities in Table 4 are summarized as follows: When the physician requires both tests to be positive, the sensitivity is lower than it is for either test alone, and the specificity is higher; when a positive result on either test is accepted, the sensitivity is increased at the expense of a lower specificity. When two tests such as these have moderate specificity, their combined use can result in a good strategy for ruling in coronary disease.

Although an occasional test has been evaluated in this manner by thoughtful clinical epidemiologists (Hull et al. 1977), most tests continue to be studied as though they were ordered in isolation. Clinical readers contemplating the use of tests in a pragmatic clinical strategy of sequential application will need to consider the altered test performance that results when a new test is given to a patient who has already been tested and was negative.

## CLINICAL SUSPICION AND THE USE OF DIAGNOSTIC TESTS

To use a diagnostic test for the full range of its clinical applications, the test must be evaluated in groups of people who suitably represent the different diagnostic challenges. The patients studied should not be chosen merely according to whether they were shown to have the disease in question. Because the physician's preceding clinical suspicions will affect the choice of a test and thus the evaluation of the test's performance, the study population must at least be divided according to the existence of clinical suspicions.

Suppose, for example, that a positive test result depends on the disease having produced a certain level of pathological involvement (e.g., multivessel coronary disease). When this level of involvement occurs, the diseased persons almost always develop symptoms that are typical of the disease (e.g., typical angina pectoris). In such suspected persons with typical symptoms, the test will have high sensitivity. On the other hand, if the disease is present without having reached the prerequisite level of pathological involvement, the patient may be symptomless or have atypical symptoms of chest pain. In such a population, the diagnostic test may have lower sensitivity. This phenomenon is illustrated by an analysis conducted by the Coronary Artery Surgery Study, in which the sensitivity of the exercise stress test varied according to the characteristics of the patients' symptoms (Weiner et al. 1977). The sensitivity was 85 percent for men with definite angina pectoris, 75 percent for men with probable angina, and 53 percent for men with non-ischemic chest pain.

When the test results are correlated with the patients' actual clinical condition, we would calculate several sets of values for sensitivity and specificity: one set for patients with typical symptoms in whom the physician has a high suspicion of the disease; a second set for patients with atypical symptoms in whom the physician has only a moderate suspicion of the disease; and a final set for patients who may be symptomless and in whom the physician considers the diagnosis unlikely.

## SUMMARY

In applying a diagnostic test to clinical practice, a physician must consider the effects of three distinctive features on the test's performance: the clinical suspicion of the physician; the clinical characteristics of the patient; and the clinical setting in which the test is ordered. When a patient has typical clinical features of a disease and the physician has a strong suspicion that the disease is present, tests are ordered to rule in (or confirm) a diagnosis. For this purpose, the test must have high prediction for a positive test result. In this clinical setting, the physician would select a test with excellent specificity and a low rate of false-positive test results.

In other circumstances, the patient may have very few of the features typical of a particular disease, and the physician's suspicion will be very low. To rule out (or exclude) a diagnosis, the test must have high prediction for a negative test result. Thus, the physician would select a test with excellent sensitivity and a low rate of false-negative test results.

As we noted earlier, distinctive clinical features of patients may affect the sensitivity and specificity of the test. When evaluating a patient with chest pain, the physician must adjust the interpretation of a stress test result according to the patient's clinical symptoms. Thus, if the patient has typical angina pectoris, false-negative tests will be uncommon, but will occur frequently among patients with atypical chest pain. Because the test's predictive accuracy depends in part on the indexes of sensitivity and specificity, the predictive accuracy will also vary according to the distinctive clinical features of the patient.

Finally, the clinical setting in which a test is ordered will also influence the clinician's interpretation of a test's usefulness. As we pointed out previously, if a disease occurs uncommonly in the ambulatory setting, even tests with high sensitivity and specificity will have disappointing accuracy for positive and negative prediction. In this circumstance, the clinician must be especially alert to avoid misinterpreting a test result. Even in a hospital setting, if a disease has only a moderate prevalence, the predictive accuracy may be considerably lower than reported during the initial development of a test.

With increasing advances in technology, clinicians will increasingly have to evaluate the costs, risks, and diagnostic discrimination of new tests. In order to make appropriate decisions, the clinician must understand the methods and results of studies evaluating this new technology. If these evaluations are to contribute to a rational clinical science for guiding the use of these new tests, the subtleties and complexities of the clinical setting must be acknowledged and incorporated into the plans for choosing the patients who are tested and for expressing the results.

### APPENDIX A. FORMULATION OF THE BAYES THEOREM

We can arrive at the formulation of Bayes' theorem by considering the groups of patients illustrated in Figure 2. In this example, we have a total population of $N$, containing some individuals with coronary artery disease (group $S$), and a second group who have an abnormal exercise stress test (group $A$). Patients without coronary disease can be designated as $\bar{S}$, and those with a normal stress test as $\bar{A}$. The intersection designated $A \cap S$ represents persons who have an abnormal stress test and coronary artery disease.

If we consider $N$ as the total number of people studied with exercise stress tests, the constituent groups will be enumerated as $n(A)$, $n(\bar{A})$, $n(S)$, $n(\bar{S})$, $n(A \cap S)$, etc. The probability of having an abnormal stress test $(A)$ is $P(A) = n(A)/N$; $P(S) = n(S)/N$; $P(A \cap S) = n(A \cap S)/N$. By definition of conditional probability,

$$P(S|A) = \frac{n(A \cap S)}{n(A)}$$

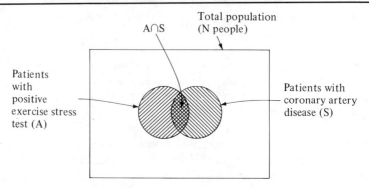

Figure 2. Venn diagram showing the intersection of sets of patients with coronary artery disease (S) and positive exercise stress test (A).

expressed as "probability of S, given A." Dividing both the numerator and the denominator by N, we get

$$P(S|A) = \frac{P(A \cap S)}{P(A)}$$

Algebraic rearrangement leads to $P(A \cap S) = P(S|A) \times P(A)$. Similarly, by definition of conditional probability

$$P(A|S) = \frac{n(A \cap S)}{n(S)}$$

By analogous transformation and rearrangement, $P(A \cap S) = P(A|S) \times P(S)$. Because we now have two things equal to $P(A \cap S)$, we can set them equal to each other, and $P(A|S) \times P(S) = P(S|A) \times P(A)$. Solving this equation for the right-hand term, we get

$$P(S|A) = \frac{P(A|S) \times P(S)}{P(A)}$$

which is the mathematical expression of Bayes' formula.

The formula just cited is a noncontroversial algebraic relationship that is always true regardless of the data being examined. Although there is considerable controversy regarding the usefulness of Bayes' formula as a guide to differential diagnosis or therapeutic decisions (Feinstein 1977), there is agreement that Bayes' formula can be used to adjust for the impact of disease prevalence on a test's predictive accuracy. The value we seek for the accuracy of a positive prediction is $P(S|A)$. Because we know the sensitivity of the test, which is $P(A|S)$, and the prevalence of the disease, $P(S)$, we need only find $P(A)$ in order to calculate $P(S|A)$. To get $P(A)$, however, we need to find the sum of the values corresponding to a and b in the four tabular cells of a, b, c, and d (Table 1).

The value of a is $P(A|S) \times P(A) \times N$, and the value of b is $P(A|\bar{S}) \times P(\bar{S}) \times N$. The probability for the sum of $a + b$ will be $P(A)$, which is $P(A|S) \times P(S) + P(A|\bar{S}) \times P(\bar{S})$. Substituting the latter expression for $P(A)$ in the denominator of Bayes' formula, we get:

$$P(S|A) = \frac{P(A|S) \times P(S)}{P(A|S) \times P(S) + P(A|\bar{S}) \times P(\bar{S})}$$

Using the same illustration as before, we can assume that sensitivity $[P(A|S)] = 0.9$, $1 - $ specificity $[P(A|\bar{S})] = 0.1$, and prevalence $P(S) = 0.09$, so that the positive accuracy is:

$$P(S|A) = \frac{(0.9) \times (0.09)}{(0.9) \times (0.09) + (0.1) \times (0.91)} = 0.47$$

Although we have obtained the same estimate of positive accuracy using this method, compare the complexity of this computation with the simplicity of the direct computation of positive predictive accuracy ($a/a + b$) noted earlier.

## APPENDIX B.   LIMITATIONS OF ROC CURVES IN COMPARING DIAGNOSTIC TESTS

Comparisons of ROC descriptions are often conducted to assess the relative effectiveness of diagnostic tests. The closer an ROC curve is to a straight line with a slope of 1, the less efficient the test is in distinguishing between diseased and nondiseased individuals. The farther to the left that a curve is placed, the more discriminating the test is. Despite these distinctions, there are several important limitations to the use of the ROC curves.

First, ROC curves for different diagnostic tests can be compared only if they are derived from test results on patients with similar clinical characteristics. Most reports evaluating diagnostic tests provide inadequate descriptions of the types of patients studied. Since the ROC curves are estimated from the data assembled in these studies, it is often difficult to know whether the resulting curves are comparable. Second, statistical tests are not well developed for determining whether the different locations of the curves could have arisen merely by chance, and not by actual distinctions in the performance of the compared tests. Third, ROC curves are applicable only to the nosologic features of the test (sensitivity and specificity), and do not reflect the test's predictive accuracy. Finally, since the tests do not incorporate any of the other information about the costs or benefits of test performance, the simple comparison of ROC curves is inadequate for making clinical decisions about the usefulness of a specific test for various test purposes (e.g., screening or disease confirmation).

## SELECTED BIBLIOGRAPHY

Bayes, T. (1963). Essay towards solving a problem in the doctrine of chances. *Phil. Trans. R. Soc. 53*:370–418; reprinted 1958 in *Biometrika 45*:293–315.

Credé, B., and Horwitz, R. I. (1982). New phased approach for assessing diagnostic technology. *Clin. Res. 30*:234A.

Feinstein, A. R. (1975). On the sensitivity, specificity, and discrimination of diagnostic tests. *Clin. Pharmacol. Ther. 17*:104–16.

Feinstein, A. R. (1977). The haze of Bayes, the aerial palaces of decision analysis, and the computerized Ouija board. *Clin. Pharmacol. Ther. 21*:482–96.

Haynes, R.B. (1981). How to read clinical journals: II. To learn about a diagnostic test. *Can. Med. Assoc. J. 124*:703–10.

Hull, R., Hirsch, J., Sackett, D. L., et al. (1977). Combined use of leg scanning and impedance plethysmography in suspected venous thrombosis. An alternative to venography. *N. Engl. J. Med. 296*:1497–1500.

McNeil, B. J., Keeler, E., and Adelstein, S. J. (1975). Primer on certain elements of decision making. *N. Engl. J. Med. 293*:211–15.

Philbirck, J. T., Horwitz, R. I., Feinstein, A. R., et al. (1982). The limited spectrum of patients studied in exercise test research: Analyzing the tip of the iceberg. *J.A.M.A. 248*:2467–70.

Ransohoff, D. F., and Feinstein, A. R. (1978). Problems of spectrum and bias in evaluating the efficacy of diagnostic tests. *N. Engl. J. Med. 299*:926–30.

Sackett, D. L. (1978). Clinical diagnosis and the clinical laboratory. *Clin. Invest. Med. 1*:37–43.

Sackett, D. L., and Holland, W. W. (1975). Controversy in the detection of disease. *Lancet 2*:357–9.

Vecchio, T. J. (1976). Predictive value of a single diagnostic test in unselected populations. *N. Engl. J. Med. 274*:1171–3.

Weiner, D. A., Ryan T. J., McCabe, C. H., et al. (1979). Exercise stress testing. Correlations among history of angina, ST segment response and prevalence of coronary artery disease in the Coronary Artery Surgery Study (CASS). *N. Engl. J. Med. 301*:230–5.

# CASE STUDIES

Each case in this section is directed at an issue involving the use of contemporary health care technology. We believe that these cases as a whole epitomize the scope of key questions surrounding the application of these technologies. Every case is accompanied by a set of questions to facilitate discussion and a selected bibliography of important sources. Some cases are based upon an actual medical event, while others are composite portraits drawn from the authors' diverse experiences in health care.

# DILEMMAS OF INTENSIVE CARE

# THE PATIENT WHO WANTS TO FIGHT

ROBERT BAKER

Mr. C was a 51-year-old broker who had suffered from emphysema (a severe, chronic, and irreversible lung disease) for over 20 years. Throughout, he saw himself engaged in a desperate and unremitting struggle. His personal physician, Dr. S, reported that Mr. C had actually attempted to jog with an oxygen tank strapped to his back. Whether or not the story is true, it certainly captures the spirit of Mr. C – a man who had chosen to rage against the empty night. He was determined to fight for his own life as aggressively as he fought for his clients in the marketplace. In May 1982, Dr. S informed Mr. C that his lung condition was approaching the end stage, and that death within the next few months was quite likely. Characteristically, Mr. C responded by volunteering to serve as a subject in the still experimental total heart-lung transplant program at a large university medical center. Unfortunately, the center's protocol excluded subjects who were over 50 years old, so Mr. C's application was denied.

During the course of the next 2 years, Mr. C's lungs degenerated to such an extent that he needed hospitalization. He chose to go to a public service university medical center, a large private medical center patronized by upper middle class residents of the metropolitan city in which Mr. C lived. Once he had settled into one of the private rooms on the internal medicine ward of the hospital, Mr. C transformed it into a second law office. Briefcase-toting assistants in pin-striped suits scurried in and out, clients consulted him regularly, the phone was constantly ringing, secretaries came in for dictation, and but for the presence of nurses – and the labored nature of Mr. C's breathing – one could easily have imagined that this was Wall Street.

Mr. C was able to maintain this situation for about 3 months. Then, despite a number of experimental and aggressive attempts to reverse his condition, it worsened to the point where he was beginning to become oxygen impoverished. When Dr. S noticed this, he asked whether Mr. C wished to be transferred to the intensive care unit (ICU). Mr. C replied that he wanted everything done that could be done. Upon inquiry, however, Dr. S learned that it was against ICU policy to admit terminal patients, except when ICU technology offered some hope of reversing the disease processes or palliating their effects. Because Mr. C's condition was irreversible and terminal, his admission would require special permission. Dr. S arranged to have Dr. K, one of the attending physicians in charge of the ICU, meet with Mr. and Mrs. C and explain the ICU's policy to them.

The meeting was arranged for 6:30 P.M. on a Friday evening. Before the meeting, however, Mrs. C sought Dr. K for a private interview. At the interview Dr. K discovered that "although Dr. S, I am sure, had talked to her...he had not understood...that she had *not* wanted [her husband] to be aggressively treated; on the contrary, she was, at that time, very concerned that we would treat him too aggressively." Dr. K then explained that, although he shared her concerns, he could not make any decisions without her husband's knowledge. After the conversation Dr. K recalls musing to himself that this "was the kind of situation that brings out the best and the worst in an intensive care unit."

At 6:30 the two physicians met with Mr. and Mrs. C in the patient's room. They explained to Mr. C that he would soon lose the ability to breath without assistance. Although mechanical intervention could halt this process temporarily, it would involve inserting a tube via the mouth into the windpipe (intubation) through which a mechanical ventilator would pump oxygen. The process would be painful and undignified; it would deprive him of the power of speech, and would serve no medical purpose because the disease process would shortly make the device useless. Mr. C replied, "I don't want to lose any chances that I might have of prolonging my life; and if you are telling me that the ventilator will keep me from dying at that time, and might give me a chance to live, that I wouldn't have to die and might have a chance to live, then I want to take it no matter how small it is."

According to the two physicians, what happened next was that "the three of us looked at each other and it was very clear the message that he was giving. And the decision was made at that point that we would be very aggressive with him and that we would treat him the way that he wanted." Dr. K then admitted Mr. C into the ICU and noted on his chart that he and the patient had agreed he was to be intubated when this treatment became necessary.

IN THE ICU

The world of the ICU has three foci: the crisis, the conference, and rounds. Rounds are the primary mechanism of coordination. A mechanism for coordination is essential because a typical 16-bed respiratory surgical ICU like Dr. K's has a staff of 2 or 3 attending physicians, who direct the unit; 2 or 3 fellows (physicians taking advanced training); 2 to 4 residents (physicians 2 or 3 years beyond medical school); 2 to 4 interns (physicians in their first year out of medical school); 2 to 4 medical students; 60 to 70 nurses; respiratory therapists, and physical therapists, and one or more social workers, plus secretaries, aides, and assistants. Somehow, all these different people must work together to care for 16 patients and to implement a cohesive and complex treatment program that is different for each patient. One tool of coordination is, of course, the patient's written medical record (which is actually a series of records, notes, treatment plans, and charts kept between one set of covers). But the record is more a formalization of interactions, decisions, and results than a primary mode of medical communication. The appropriate forum for discussion and decision making – and hence for the coordination of care – in an ICU is house staff rounds, in which, each morning, the staff reviews the condition of each patient and determines what changes, if any, are to be made in the treatment plan.

Monday morning rounds were particularly important at Dr. K's ICU because the attending physicians rotated on a weekly basis. Thus, Dr. K not only had to present the case of Mr. C at rounds that morning, but also had to turn over the care of Mr. C to Dr. A, because it was A's turn to take charge of the ICU. This was awkward not only for Dr. K (who had admitted Mr. C in violation of ICU policy) but also for Dr. A. As Dr. A put it when he was interviewed a week later, when he came on duty that morning, "I found myself in the unique position of being involved in a contract that I was only involved in because it was made by the person in whose stead I was operating."

Mr. C was the last patient discussed that morning. His nurse, G, reported that Mr. C was deteriorating rapidly and would require intubation by early afternoon. She also reported that the family had visited that weekend, that "the wife" had appeared quite troubled, distancing herself from the event, but taking a great interest in the conversation and interaction between her husband and their children at the bedside.

The wife also seemed fascinated and repelled by the Bear ventilator. She kept staring at it and continually asked if that was "the *machine*," italicizing the word as she spoke. Sometimes the wife called the machine the "monstrosity."

Dr. K concurred with Nurse G's observations about Mrs. C. She had expressed to him her dislike of the machine and had repeatedly asked him not to put her husband on the ventilator. But over the weekend, Dr. K had become increasingly comfortable with the decision to intubate Mr. C. "It was obvious that this philosophy of his – this attitude – was very compatible with how he lived his life. I mean . . . he . . . fought against the disease, he was working on a bond issue . . . in the hospital before he came to the IC ward. It was obvious that he . . . did want to keep up the fight; and I felt increasingly comfortable with a decision that I was *medically* uncomfortable with. Because I knew that all the evidence was that this man's lung disease was terminal and hopeless." Dr. K had told Mrs. C that "it wouldn't be fair to him to go back on it [our agreement], even though all the evidence suggested that it was hopeless." But Dr. K said that because he was going off duty, he would put the question to the entire staff.

There was further discussion, and each of the eight staff members voted for or against intubation. Four voted against: Dr. A, Nurse G, the anesthesiology fellow, Dr. N, and the surgery fellow, Dr. S. Dr. A argued against intubation because it was medically senseless and painful to the family. Nurse G, echoing Mrs. C's words, said, "We couldn't help to make him any better by putting him on the monstrosity." Dr. S said, "We really are concerned with two sets of patients here, a wife and three children, and Mr. C. We couldn't do anything more for Mr. C, but we could help the wife and children. So I voted not to intubate him."

The most eloquent voice in opposition to intubation, however, was the anesthesiologist, Dr. N. "I am not in agreement with the decision to put him on the ventilator...this case is as clear-cut as can be imagined in terms of the inability of us to contribute medically in any way to reversal of the disease or to a meaningful prolongation of his life...this is not even a gray area in this particular case.... You have to respect the patient's wishes – and yet – the patient's wishes, in effect, involve him getting ineffective medical therapy. And in this particular case...it is medical therapy that is *outrageously* expensive.... This is a major intervention. I am not willing to do it simply to cater to the patient's wishes...beds are scarce and are needed for the most viable patients possible...and not only rooms, but ventilators, especially Bears."

The resident and two interns who voted with Dr. K did so on the grounds that although it was "noble" to honor someone's deathbed wishes, acting on this last desire to joust with death, the primary reason for intubating Mr. C was that Dr. K had made a contract with him, and the unit was bound to honor it. This last sentiment won the day; the unit agreed that Mr. C should be intubated.

### THE INTUBATION

Dr. A was in charge of the intubation, and was assisted by anesthesiologist N, Nurse G, and Dr. K. They reported that the procedure was quite complicated, involving tubes of two different sizes, two different pressures, and so on, each designed to cope with the markedly different disease processes affecting Mr. C's two lungs. Although Mr. C could not speak, he cooperated with Dr. A completely, responding to his commands and giving information by squeezing Dr. A's hand once for yes and twice for no. Dr. K agreed with Dr. A that "it was a very difficult, technically complicated maneuver...but once the decision was made, it became a challenging technical and medical exercise...to do this to someone with this degree of lung disease...we did...we finally accomplished it – putting him on the ventilator."

When they were finished, Nurse G attempted to clean up Mr. C in order to make him more presentable to his family. It was only then that she realized what he must look like to someone who did not think of him as having successfully completed an intricate technical process. "He looked really kind of rumpled. He hadn't been shaved and he had tape all over his face. The double tube that he had in his...it was sort of like a double barrel coming out of his mouth.

One blue tubing was coming out one way, the other had tubing to the ventilator that was moving quite rapidly. And there were all these tubes coming out. One was full of water, the other was filled with. . .it was just a mess. . . .I mean, I don't think he looked like anything. . . .I mean, very emaciated, very thin. We tried to spruce him up a little bit.'' Then his family came into the room. His wife talked to her husband, but he did not respond. Then she whispered, ''I can't stand looking at him this way. And I can't stand that thing. I can't stand that thing.'' She was pointing at the ventilator.

### RENEGING ON THE CONTRACT

On Tuesday, Mrs. C and her children were in the unit all day. Nurse G encouraged her to talk to him. (''I never want to come right out and say that hearing is one of the last things that people lose. . .people that come back always say that they could hear.'') Mrs. C also talked to Dr. K and persuaded him to modify the ''contract'' slightly by writing a ''Do Not Resuscitate'' order in the chart, so that if her husband did suffer a potentially fatal episode, no one would attempt to resuscitate him.

At Wednesday's rounds (two days after ventilation had been started), Mr. and Mrs. C were again the major topic of discussion. The house staff (fellows, interns, and residents) were virtually unanimous in suggesting that Mrs. C's feelings be respected and that a ''compromise'' with the contract be effected by decreasing Mr. C's oxygen from 90 to 50 percent, to ''hurry matters up a bit.'' A note could then be written in the chart that ''in order to minimize oxygen toxicity, concentrations were turned down to 50 percent.

Dr. A objected. ''What we were really talking about was something that would result in this man's dying. . .just turning the oxygen down to 50 percent in a man with a good heart would prolong this experience for everybody. Whether or not he would suffer. . .his family would suffer, his wife and sons would suffer. They wanted us just to remove the mechanical ventilator and cut his oxygen down to 21 percent and let him pass on in peace. And so what I did was. . .over a period, as the day went by, give him more and more morphine. . .until he was at a point where I would have to stimulate him vigorously to get him to squeeze my hand when I talked with him. The family came and talked with him several times. They were there when I disconnected the ventilator (I turned it from 90 percent to 21 percent; with a turn of the knob I turned it all the way off). And they stayed with him until he expired 15 minutes later.''

### REFLECTIONS AND QUESTIONS

That Mr. C died when the machine was turned off is, in a way, fitting, for his case is very much the story of a machine. Mr. C's illness became a *case*, in fact, when he asked to be put on the machine. The request initiated a debate about whether to allow him access to the machine, whether to put him on the machine, and finally, whether to turn the knob on the machine down to 50 or 21 percent. For Mr. C the machine was a symbol, an icon of technological salvation. He seemed to see physicians as priests of the body who somehow, despite all their protestations to the contrary, could prevail on providence with their marvelous machines to change his fate – if only he were willing to sacrifice his body at the altar of the machine. Mr. C also seems to have insisted on intubation as part of a personal, existential struggle with death, a struggle in which his cause would be abetted by technology. Mr. C, jogging with an oxygen tank strapped to his back, presents just such a picture – humans, running against death, using technology to overcome the infirmities of the flesh. Intubation, for Mr. C, was merely another way of continuing the struggle, only in this case, the ventilator would replace the oxygen tank.

In the eyes of Nurse G and Mrs. C, however, the ventilator was not as innocuous as the oxygen tank. The idea of jogging with an oxygen tank reaffirms the transcendance of the human being, for here technology serves merely as an aid to a human purpose. The ventilator, however, did not so much serve as dominate. It transmogrified Mr. C from an existential hero into a mere appendage of the ventilator. Mr. C, who had triumphantly conquered the hospital ward, transforming this way station to death into a place for carrying on his everyday life, was now merely an object of the action of a machine. The machine moved, and C was inanimate; symbolically, the machine even robbed C of his face, replacing it with blue and white plastic double-barreled tubes.

Each member of the C family had a different conception of the relationship of Mr. C to the ventilator. Perhaps the most important question generated by the case is, which of them was the most perceptive?

The case of the Cs also generates more specific questions. Why, one wonders, did Dr. S even suggest the ICU to Mr. C as an option? Dr. S knew that the therapeutic modalities available in the ICU could not prevent, palliate, control, or cure Mr. C's disease. Why, then, did he bring up the subject with Mr. C? Was Dr. S perhaps hiding behind the myth of technology? Was he holding out the hope of a miracle because, after all these years, he could not face telling a patient like Mr. C that there was no more hope?

Once raised, however, the issue of transfer generates fundamental questions about the physician's role. The physicians in this case were unanimous on only one point: Transferring Mr. C to the ICU and intubating him would serve no medical purpose whatsoever. Yet it was Mr. C's dying wish to be transferred. Should physicians respond to a patient's wishes, or should they treat only his medical needs? Some might argue that Mr. C had a right to be intubated. Patients have a right to express their autonomy; the attempt to deny Mr. C his wishes is merely medical paternalism.

The consensus among contemporary ethicists and lawyers is that physicians must respect the autonomy of competent patients (and no one ever suggested that Mr. C was anything but competent). Paternalistic medical interventions, it is generally agreed, abrogate fundamental moral and legal rights and should not be countenanced. But does this imply that Mr. C had a right to be admitted to the ICU and intubated? The consensus that has formed around patients' rights was generated by a group of cases in which the medical profession insisted upon treatment against the wishes of the patient and/or the patient's family. The most famous of these cases is, of course, that of Karen Ann Quinlan. Karen's father, Joseph, it will be recalled, wanted her taken off the MA-1 ventilator, but her physicians refused to do so, insisting that she remain on the machine. Ultimately, Joseph won the case, and Karen's right to refuse treatment was affirmed. The Quinlan case has since become the symbol of patient autonomy.

The case of Mr. C, however, is the reverse of that of Karen Ann Quinlan. Mr. C wanted treatment; his physicians wanted to refuse. The question raised by the case of the Cs, therefore, is not whether patients have a right to *refuse* treatment insisted upon by their physicians, but rather whether patients have a right to *insist* on being treated in the manner they choose, against the advice of their physicians. The case of Mr. C raises the question of whether *physicians* have a right to refuse to treat, or at least to refuse to give medically unnecessary treatments. Has a patient the right to request an invasive medical intervention for essentially symbolic ends? Do dying patients who desire what might almost be thought of as medical mutilation, a sort of technological immolation in search of immortality, have a right to such treatment? Can they enforce these demands over the objections of their physicians? Are there moral or legal grounds for compelling physicians to intubate?

If patients have a right to treatment that serves no medical purpose, have they the right to deprive other patients of scarce resources in order to obtain this treatment? That, after all, was anesthesiologist N's objection to admitting Mr. C to the ICU. There were only two Bear ventilators for a 16-bed unit. One was being used. If Mr. C were admitted, there would be no ventilator available if a potentially viable patient (with difficult respiratory problems) were also admitted. Mr. C was, in effect, asking for the last of the ICU's sophisticated ventilators, and he was doing so in order to make a futile gesture of defiance in the face of death. Dr. N thought it irresponsible, almost outrageous, that the unit acceded to this request. Was Dr. N right? Should the staff of the ICU have permitted Mr. C to use their last ventilator? Did Mr. C have a right to jeopardize others in order to make a gesture against death?

In fact, Mr. C's use of the Bear ventilator for 3 days did not harm any other patient. One reason, of course, is that the ICU reneged on its contract with Mr. C by turning his oxygen down to 21 percent (the percentage of oxygen in room air). Their reversal, it should be noted, was not in response to any change in Mr. C's physiological state. They seemed to have changed their minds because of Mrs. C's evident distress and because of her iterated insistence that the ventilator be removed. Mrs. C had objected to the ventilator from the very first. On what grounds, then, could the ICU justify acceding to her wishes now, but not while her husband had still been articulate? What had released the ICU from its contract with Mr. C? Were they justified in overriding his express wishes?

The last issues posed by this case concern the therapeutic decisions to administer morphine and turn the ventilator knob to 21 percent. Mr. C died 15 minutes after the knob was turned down. One way to describe these actions was that Dr. A was following the family's wishes, and, by turning off the machine he let nature take its course; Dr. A merely let Mr. C die naturally. From the standpoints of ethics and philosophy, what perspectives can be introduced to examine this type of situation?

## ACKNOWLEDGMENT

This case was recorded as part of the Moral Methodologies of Intensive Care Units Study, which is funded by Ethics and Values in Science and Technology (EVIST), a joint program of the National Endowment for the Humanities (NEH) and the National Science Foundation (NSF). Taped interviews with nine participants were conducted the week after Mr. C's death.

## SELECTED BIBLIOGRAPHY

Unfortunately, there is very little literature on the relations between people and machines in ICUs. The information that does exist focuses on ethical dilemmas, especially those that arise with respect to infants born with congenital defects. One of the few studies of ICUs in general is Diana Crane's first-rate book *The Sanctity of Social Life* (New York: Russell Sage, 1975). A. Jonsen and M. Garland's *The Ethics of Newborn Intensive Care* (Berkeley: Institute of Governmental Studies, 1976) is an excellent study of the moral problems faced by newborn intensive care units (NICUs). Recent reviews of the cost and benefits and cost effectiveness of these units have been done by the Office of Technology Assessment, Background Papers Series No. 2, *Case Study No. 10* (NICUs), August 1981, and *Case Study No. 12* (AICUs), July 1981.

A number of professional organizations and ICUs have developed guidelines for determining when not to resuscitate a patient. The American Medical Association's recent statement on the subject is "Standards and guidelines for cardiopulmonary resuscitation (CPR) and emergency cardiac care (ECC)," *J.A.M.A. 244* (5), 453–509, 1980 (see especially Part IV). A number of individual units have published policy statements, the most frequently cited of which are the two that appeared in the August 12, 1976, issue of the *New England Journal of Medicine*, pp. 362–6. The protocol that most clearly typifies practice in adult ICUs, however, is found in Ake Grenvik et al., "Cessation of therapy in terminal illness and brain death," *Critical Care Medicine 6* (4): 284–91, 1978.

John Ladd's *Ethical Issues Relating to Life and Death* (New York: Oxford University Press, 1979) is perhaps the best introduction to the recent philosophical literature on the moral problems of terminating life support.

CASE 2

# THE TRIAGE DECISION

ALBERT G. MULLEY, JR.

## INTENSIVE CARE AS A CONSTRAINED RESOURCE

The high and rapidly rising costs of health care have focused increased attention on clinical decisions that influence expenditures on health care. Particular scrutiny has been directed at decisions to use technology-intensive, expensive interventions with doubtful or unproven effectiveness. Much of the technology-intensive care within hospitals is concentrated in medical and surgical intensive care and coronary care units. The costs of care provided in such units have been rising more rapidly than the costs associated with any other hospital activities. It is not uncommon for intensive care units (ICUs) to account for as much as 20 percent of total hospital costs. The mean number of hospital beds dedicated to intensive care is 5 percent; rarely does this proportion exceed 10 percent.

These high costs are incurred despite the unproven effectiveness of intensive care. The conviction that ICUs decrease morbidity and mortality is supported only by uncontrolled or poorly controlled studies and by the enthusiasm for the specific diagnostic and therapeutic modalities that have emerged since the establishment of such units. Physicians, however, are less likely to consider the effectiveness of intensive care than the effectiveness of the individual diagnostic and therapeutic interventions that are made in the ICU. The common denominator of intensive care, in different settings and for different patients, is closer attention to the patients' condition and therapy. Although the potential for patient discomfort and iatrogenic disease in the ICU is well recognized, it is difficult to deny the potential benefit of more attention rather than less for many patients with or at risk for critical illness. Following this reasoning, those who make intensive care allocation decisions for individual patients view the benefits as unmeasured rather than uncertain.

The presumed benefit of being in an ICU is rarely weighed explicitly against

221

the added cost of intensive over conventional care, when the decision is made to admit a patient to the ICU. Rationing ICU resources is, however, an inevitable part of clinical decision making. Life-threatening illness and the need for intensive care is a stochastic event. There is often a wide variation in occupancy rates of intensive or coronary care units. Even the largest units are at least sometimes full. When this happens, a critically ill patient presenting to the emergency ward must be turned away, must be admitted to a conventional care bed, or must displace a patient from the ICU who would otherwise have had the presumed advantage of a longer ICU stay.

How are such rationing decisions made? How does the physician decide which of two patients should be admitted to the ICU when only one bed is available? Which patient should be displaced when a critically ill patient with acute reversible disease needs an ICU bed and the unit is already full? The theoretical answer is that the bed is allocated to the patient most likely to benefit from intensive monitoring. Practical difficulties when applying this principle are illustrated in the following case study.

### CASE STUDY: ICU TRIAGE DECISIONS

You are responsible for authorizing all admissions to a 10-bed medical ICU. It is 8 P.M. when you are called down to the emergency room to evaluate for possible admission to the ICU each of three patients.

The first patient is a 22-year-old female who is comatose and apneic, presumably secondary to an intentional overdose of barbiturates. She has been intubated and will require mechanical ventilation at least overnight. You know very little about the circumstances surrounding her drug overdosage, but scars on her wrists suggest that she has a past history of depression and impulsive behavior.

The second patient is a 68-year-old female with a long history of chronic obstructive pulmonary disease who was intubated in the emergency room after presenting with apparent cyanosis and rapidly increasing somnolence. Her hospital chart is available, and you quickly locate her baseline pulmonary function tests, which are consistent with very poor pulmonary function. Based on these test results, you estimate that she has a 90 percent chance of dying within 2 years.

The third patient is a 44-year-old male who, until hours ago, had never been sick in his life. He presented with chest and left arm pain suggestive of a heart attack. His electrocardiogram is consistent with coronary artery disease but is not diagnostic of an acute myocardial infarction.

### CLINICAL QUESTIONS

Under normal circumstances, all three of these patients would be admitted to ICU as quickly as possible. However, it has been a busy day, and 8 of the 10 beds are occupied. What characteristics of each patient must be considered in

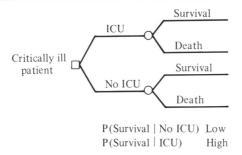

P(Survival | No ICU)  Low
P(Survival | ICU)     High

Figure 1. Decision analysis tree for patient with a good prognosis with ICU intervention.

deciding which two of them should be admitted immediately? What clinical information is most relevant? What clinical predictors or probability assessments must be made?

After weighing the relative indications for intensive care for each patient, you consider the eight patients who are already in the ICU. Among these is a 40-year-old man who was admitted 20 hours earlier with a suspected heart attack. So far, his course has been stable, and tests for myocardial infarction have been negative. Would you transfer him out of the ICU at this point to make room for one of the new patients? Again, what clinical predictions or probability assessments must be made? Try answering the questions before reading the discussion.

ISSUES FOR DISCUSSION

The allocation of ICU resources is determined by the kinds of decisions illustrated by the case study – decisions to admit a patient to an ICU, to maintain the patient there, or to transfer the patient at some point. The clinical predictions (or probability assessments) that provide a basis for such decisions can be better understood by using decision analysis constructs (Figures 1, 2, and 3).[1]

The first patient presents a relatively simple decision (Figure 1). Her acute illness is life-threatening but entirely reversible. Without continuous ventilatory support, she will die. With it, she will almost certainly survive. The clinical decision to admit this patient is straightforward because there is a reasonable expectation that ICU intervention is efficacious, and that the probability of a good outcome given ICU intervention is greater than the probability without such intervention.

The decision regarding the 68-year-old woman with acute respiratory failure superimposed on chronic pulmonary disease can be represented by the same decision tree. However, although the probability of survival without ICU care is low, so is the probability of survival with this care (Figure 2). This decision tree represents the kind of ICU decision that has attracted the most attention

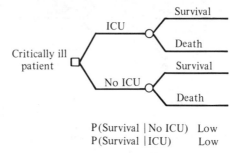

P(Survival | No ICU)   Low
P(Survival | ICU)         Low

Figure 2. Decision analysis tree for patient with a poor prognosis despite ICU intervention.

from those concerned about the financial and human costs of intensive care. Although hospital committees have established guidelines for classifying such patients and have sanctioned the withholding of therapy from patients with extremely poor prognoses, the criteria are so stringent that they are rarely applicable and have little clinical utility.

The decision regarding the third patient is illustrated by a more complex decision tree (Figure 3). The patient would be admitted not because he is in need of the kind of life-support intervention characteristic of intensive care, but because he is at risk of suddenly developing such a need. The crucial issue is how certain we are that the third patient's blood pressure and heart rhythm would remain within satisfactory ranges and that no other complications would occur. It is the probability of a life-threatening complication, which is more likely to occur when an infarction is taking place, rather than the diagnosis itself, that determines the need for ICU admission. An improved ability to assess such probabilities might improve ICU decision making.

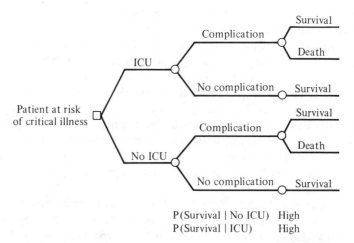

P(Survival | No ICU)   High
P(Survival | ICU)         High

Figure 3. Decision analysis tree for patient with a good prognosis regardless of ICU intervention.

The transfer decision regarding the fourth patient who has been in the ICU for 20 hours without evidence of myocardial infarction illustrates the importance of reassessing over time the risk of a major complication and thereby the potential benefit of remaining in the ICU. Can patients at low risk be identified early? Equally important, can patients who remain at high risk despite a period of intensive monitoring in the ICU be identified?

Additional specific points that should be addressed include the following:

1. Clinical decisions that effectively ration intensive care among individuals are inevitable. The frequency with which difficult rationing decisions must be made depends on local availability of ICU resources.
2. There are no necessarily correct answers to triage questions. Our ability to predict the patient's outcome with or without intensive care is limited.
3. The efficacy of intensive care for a particular acute condition (which can be considered as the difference in probability of a good outcome with and without intensive care) is not the sole basis for triage decisions. More subjective variables are often considered implicitly. The potential for conscious and unconscious discrimination in rationing ICU resources on the basis of implicit consideration of age, diagnosis, or social position should be appreciated.

NOTE

1 A number of simplifications should be noted in this model. First, intensive care is treated as if it were a single intervention when, in fact, it is a composite of interventions about which individual decisions can be made. For example, the overdose victim may be intubated and given ventilatory support even if other components of usual intensive care are unavailable. Second, the model is static. It does not adequately reflect the time dimension of ICU decision making unless it is viewed as one in a series of snapshots. The relative probability of survival with intervention may change from day to day or even from moment to moment. The decision to continue an intervention is reassessed as the clinical course evolves and new prognostic information becomes available. The third simplification regards outcomes, which in reality are not dichotomous. Intermediate outcomes, including survival of varying duration and various degrees of morbidity, would be included in a more realistic decision model.

SELECTED BIBLIOGRAPHY

Cullen, D. J., Ferrara, L. C., Briggs, B. A., et al. (1976). Survival, hospitalization charges and follow-up results in critically ill patients. *N. Engl. J. Med.* 294:982–7.

Detsky, A. S., Stricker, S. C., Mulley, A. G., et al. (1981). Prognosis, survival, and the expenditure of hospital resources for patients in an intensive care unit. *N. Engl. J. Med.* 305:667–72.

Griner, P. F. (1973). Medical intensive care in the teaching hospital: costs versus benefits: the need for assessment. *Ann. Intern. Med.* 78:581–5.

Knaus, W. A., Wagner, D. P., Draper, E. A., et al. (1981). The range of intensive care services today. *J.A.M.A.* 246:2711–16.

Mulley, A. G., Thibault, G. E., Hughes, R. A., et al. (1980). The course of suspected myocardial infarction: the identification of low risk patients for early transfer. *N. Engl. J. Med. 302*:943–8.

Shepard, D. S., and Ghanotakis, A. J. (1979). *Hospital Costs in Massachusetts: A Report of the Massachusetts Funds Flow Project* (HRP-0029335). Springfield, Va.: National Technical Information Service.

Singer, D. E., Mulley, A. G., Thibault, G. E., et al. (1981). Unexpected readmissions to the coronary care unit during recovery from acute myocardial infarction. *N. Engl. J. Med. 304*:625–9.

Thibault, G. E., Mulley, A. G., Barnett, G. O., et al. (1980). Medical intensive care: indications, interventions, and outcomes. *N. Engl. J. Med. 302*:938–42.

# SURVIVAL OF THE STAFF

THEODORE A. STERN

Although the psychological experience of being a seriously ill patient has been the focus of a great deal of attention, the psychological reactions of medical personnel in intensive care units (ICUs) have only recently been described. Tension levels run high in the presence of pain, delirium, and death. Potential emergencies lurk behind every curtain, and the unexpected becomes the expected. The sights and sounds of new technologies, with the attendant buzzers, lights, whooshes, and alarms of cardiac monitors, infusion pumps, and ventilators, bombard one's consciousness. The atmosphere is pierced by painful moans, gasps for air, and sobs of grief. Rarely is the situation emotionally neutral. In this environment, with its endless demands and stress, it is no wonder that reports of anxiety, hostility, and depression among staff are common. For physicians, who often see the world through sleep-deprived eyes, irritability is increased and judgmental functions are hampered.

It should be understood, however, that all happenings in the ICU are not acute and dramatic. Much of the fatigue and strain felt by ICU personnel comes from daily routine. Lifting heavy patients, living with unpredictable schedules, feeling the weight of personal responsibility, dealing with overwrought and anxious families, having poor avenues of communication with other staff members, and coming to grips with the severity of the patient's illness and prognosis have been shown to be the main concerns of ICU nurses. Repetitive routines abound, especially for the nursing staff. Vital signs and central venous pressures are measured and charted as frequently as every 15 minutes. Patients are suctioned, urimeters are emptied, intravenous flow rates are calculated and adjusted, and electrocardiograms are taken. Each of these functions is performed under the ever-present pressure of time. Moreover, constant vigilance and alert readiness need to be maintained in preparation for the sudden crisis that will undoubtedly arise.

Yet, technical skills alone are insufficient for ICU staff. They must be prepared to provide reassurance and comfort to the distressed. A middle-aged man becomes hypotensive; a subclavian line must be inserted. His face is covered by a towel to provide a sterile field in which to work; he panics, and comfort must be given. The histrionic young woman with diabetic ketoacidosis must be reassured that she will not be left alone and abandoned. The obsessive, controlling, and demanding engineer admitted to rule out a myocardial infarction needs to be provided with detailed explanations of his current situation. When therapeutic strategies are developed based upon an understanding of the patient's dynamics, patient care is facilitated by decreasing tension and fear.

The following case example should help to identify the psychological problems faced by physicians, nurses, and other health care staff in dealing with each other and with patients in the setting of intensive care.

## CASE EXAMPLE

J, a 20-year old, previously healthy, solidly built single male, the owner of his own small business, was transferred to our medical ICU from another hospital. His pulmonary function was deteriorating. He was polite, cooperative, quiet, and somewhat apprehensive. His chest x-rays showed progressive bilateral pulmonary infiltrates, which were consistent with his worsening clinical status. Repeated samples of arterial blood gases drawn over the next few days confirmed his downward spiral.

His lungs were not getting the oxygen they needed. As a result, a nasotracheal tube was placed to ensure that his organs received enough oxygen and to maintain adequate ventilation. A machine was provided to breathe for him. However, this alone did not help his condition. He began fighting the respirator by trying to breathe on his own, making it impossible for the ventilator to do the work of breathing deeply enough for him. The nurses tried desperately to calm him down but were unsuccessful. He was extremely uncomfortable with the tube down his throat, and felt that he was suffocating. Repeatedly, he tried to remove the tube. In order to prevent this, his arms were restrained. Agitation was a major problem, but more importantly, better oxygenation was required.

To facilitate better oxygenation, the patient was paralyzed for the next 3 days with curare. This prevented him from resisting the ventilator but made it impossible for him to move any of his muscles. At the same time, a morphine drip was instituted; it prevented him from being awake, frightened, and in pain, but also left him unable to tell anyone how he was feeling or what he was thinking. He was helpless, totally dependent on the machine that breathed for him and on the staff who cared for him.

In response to this increase in responsibility, the nurses became visibly more tense. They listened more closely for the sound of alarms because he was unable to give them any signal of distress.

Although he no longer needed to be paralyzed, his illness progressed over the next 2 weeks, and additional invasive procedures were required. A sense of impending doom pierced by rays of optimism settled around his bedside. He developed bilateral pneumothoraxes and had chest tubes inserted bilaterally to reexpand his lungs. The upper half of his body became markedly swollen with subcutaneous emphysema (air under his skin), which distorted his face and made him unrecognizable, almost porcine. Still, he remained awake and alert. To monitor his pulmonary and cardiac functions more accurately, both pulmonary artery and radial arterial lines were placed. This necessitated tying his arms to the sides of the bed. For infusion of fluids and antibiotics, numerous intravenous lines were placed in his arms, neck, and feet. His bladder was catheterized so that urine output could be continuously monitored. A rectal tube was placed to collect stool. His temperature frequently spiked to 104°F, and he was intermittently placed upon a cooling blanket. Although the shivering caused by the cooling blanket was uncomfortable, it brought down his temperature. Two separate lung biopsies were performed in the hope of establishing a diagnosis.

After 2 weeks in the ICU, a tracheostomy was performed to prevent the possible development of tracheal stenosis from prolonged intubation. Still unable to talk, he was using a letter board to indicate his needs letter by letter. He became septic, developed a toxic megacolon, and was taken to surgery once again.

He returned to the ICU after abdominal surgery with a subtotal colectomy and an ileostomy. It suddenly became clear to the nurses that he would not leave the ICU unchanged. Part of him was gone. They became discouraged and depressed. Because he was not much younger than they, they readily identified with the problems ahead of him. They could no longer believe that all would be well once again. Complications continued to arise. Next came the development of a severe myopathy, leaving him with only limited strength in his right arm.

After 4 weeks in the ICU, still without a diagnosis, he slowly began to improve. At the end of 5 weeks he regained the ability to talk (with the placement of a talking tracheostomy tube). He began to demand constant attention. Yet, instead of asking the nurses to "fix my feet," "fix my pillow," or "get my juice," he would insist upon spelling out his demands on the letter board he had been using for the past few weeks. The nurses became irritated. For weeks he had been too sick to do anything for himself, but now he was at the point where he could help with his own care. Speaking, not pointing, would make things easier for everyone. They wanted to tell him to ask for what he needed and wanted, but they didn't want to be cruel. He had been through so much already. They felt guilty about being angry with him.

Suspecting that he was depressed, they requested a psychiatric consultation. As his use of denial as a psychological defense wore thin, his neediness increased. It was no longer easy for anyone involved in his care to remain optimistic. Exhausted by their dealings with him, the staff developed a feeling of aversion to him and his needs. Even walking into his room became a chore. The staff members' recognition of their own feelings allowed them to identify the onset of his depression. Brief psychotherapy, which supported his use of denial and set limits on his demands, was started. He began to exercise while still in bed and took more responsibility for his care. Both his physical condition and his mental outlook continued to improve. Caring for him, although time-consuming, was far less emotionally draining than it had been.

Suddenly, after 7 weeks in the ICU, he had a cardiopulmonary arrest, the result of a massive pulmonary embolus. One nurse froze from the shock of it. Another felt as if she was torturing him while continuing to pump on his chest. The resuscitative effort was stopped after 2 hours. He was dead.

Afterward, the feelings of helplessness, loss, shock, depression, and relief were discussed in order to prevent future conflicts. It was noted that death is never easy, but that it is especially painful when one has worked closely with someone for a long period of time and has gotten to know him well. There were still nine other patients in the unit to be cared for, and J's bed would shortly be filled by someone else. Everyone needed to keep functioning.

### ISSUES PERTAINING TO THE ICU EXPERIENCE

As demonstrated by this case, it is clear that a wide range of emotions are experienced by ICU personnel. One thing that does remain constant in such a unit, however, is the presence of serious illness. In the face of such illness patients regress, and frequently manifest increased dependency and anger. When these behaviors are added to the constant threat of loss (death), it makes one wonder how long staff resources will endure. If not dealt with satisfactorily, burnout, with its familiar anxiety, irritability, depression, and need to change jobs, will result.

### QUESTIONS FOR DISCUSSION

1. How can staff remain sane, efficient, and at the same time nurturant?
2. Does it simply become a matter of dealing only with the numbers (e.g., blood urea nitrogen, creatinine, arterial oxygen pressure, hematocrit) involved in patient management while avoiding the patient?
3. How can one balance technological care and empathic caretaking?

### SELECTED BIBLIOGRAPHY

Adler, G. (1972). Helplessness in the helpers. *Br. J. Med. Psychol. 45*:315–26.

Cassem, N. H., and Hackett, T. P. (1975). Stress on the nurse and therapist in the intensive-care unit and the coronary-care unit. *Heart Lung 4*:252–9.

Groves, J. E. (1978). Taking care of the hateful patient. *N. Engl. J. Med. 298*:883–7.

Hay, D., and Oken, D. (1972). The psychological stresses of intensive care nursing. *Psychosom. Med. 34*:109–18.

Kahana, R. J., and Bibring, G. L. (1965). Personality types in medical management. In *Psychiatry and Medical Practice in a General Hospital* (N.E. Zinberg, ed.), pp. 108–23. New York: International Universities Press.

Maltsberger, J. T., and Buie, D. H. (1974). Countertransference hate in the treatment of suicidal patients. *Arch. Gen. Psychiatry 30*:625–33.

Messner, E. (1979). Autognosis: diagnosis by the use of the self. In *Outpatient Psychiatry: Diagnosis and Treatment* (A. Lazare, ed.), pp. 230–8. Baltimore: Williams & Wilkins.

Stern, T. A. (1980). Autognosis rounds for medical housestaff. Submitted for publication. Initially delivered at the APA Symposium, Consultation-Liaison Psychiatry in the 1980s, San Francisco.

Vreeland, R., and Ellis, G. L. (1969). Stresses on the nurse in an intensive-care unit. *J.A.M.A. 208*:332–4.

# TECHNOLOGY AND THE HOSPITAL

# COMING TO TERMS WITH THE COMPUTER

EDWARD H. SHORTLIFFE

You are asked to assist a major teaching hospital in the assessment of a large computer system that was installed 3 months ago to help with doctors' orders, laboratory test reporting, nursing schedules, and bed control. Because of mixed reviews of the system's effectiveness, the hospital has decided to bring in outside experts to assess the computer's strengths and weaknesses.

The computer system was installed by a vendor of large-scale hospital information systems (HIS). The company had developed the programs over several years, but this is its first major commercial installation. The HIS has several capabilities that, taken as a whole, have had an impact on almost all aspects of the hospital's operation. Because most of the concerns that have been raised have come from those who are involved with patient care, you have decided to focus your analysis on features of the system that are designed for clinical use. Every nursing unit in the hospital has video display terminals for use by medical and paramedical personnel. There are also printers on each unit so that the computer can generate reports for the patient charts and worksheets for use by nursing and paramedical staff. The system is dependent on a large dedicated computer housed in the hospital complex and staffed by several full-time personnel.

Several system capabilities are particularly pertinent to your analysis:

1. The pharmacy system. This component of the HIS allows physicians to order drugs for their patients and to have the request immediately displayed in the hospital pharmacy. Pharmacists then fill the prescriptions and affix a computer-printed label to the bottle. The drugs are delivered to the ward by a pneumatic tube system. The computer keeps a record of all drugs administered to each patient and warns the physician about possible drug interactions at the time that a new prescription is ordered.
2. The laboratory system. Like the pharmacy component, this system permits the physician to order laboratory tests for a patient. The request is displayed

in the clinical laboratory, and worksheets are created to assist laboratory personnel in planning their blood-drawing schedule as well as the actual performance of the test. When results are available, they can be called up on the screen of any system terminal. Paper summaries are also printed on the wards for inclusion on the patients' charts.

3. The bed control system. The admissions office of the hospital, in conjunction with the various ward administrators, uses the system to keep track of the location of patients within the hospital. When transfers occur, the computer is notified so that physicians, telephone operators, and others can locate patients easily. The system is also used to identify patients who are ready for discharge; this helps the admissions office plan the bed assignments of new patients.

4. The diagnosis system. To help physicians reach correct diagnoses regarding their patients, the system includes a clinical consultation program. Physicians can enter the signs and symptoms, laboratory abnormalities, and x-ray results for their patients, and the system will suggest a list of likely diagnoses.

Although the HIS has several other components not mentioned here, you decide to focus on these four when interviewing hospital staff. After a few days of conducting taped interviews, the following responses are among those that you choose to have transcribed.

## STAFF RESPONSES TO HIS

### From a nurse on a medical floor

"I like the system a lot. It was hard to get used to at first (I never have been a very good typist), but once I got the hang of it, I found that it simplified much of my work. I use it to chart medications when I have given them, and also to log nursing notes. The worst problem has turned out to be dealing with doctors who don't like the system; when they get annoyed, they tend to take it out on us, even though we're using the system exactly as we've been trained to do. For instance, I can't log on the computer as a physician verbal orders in someone else's name, and that makes some of the doctors furious. The only time I personally get annoyed with the computer is when I need to get some work done and the other nurses are using all the ward terminals. As for how much I use it, I guess I might spend a total of 45 minutes at a terminal during an 8 hour shift."

### From a medical resident

"I wish they'd rip the darn thing out! It is totally unrealistic in the kinds of things it asks us to do or won't allow us to do. Did the guys who built it have any idea what it is like to practice medicine in a hospital like this? For example, the only thing that used to keep our morning ward rounds efficient was to bring the chart rack with us and write orders at the bedside. With the new system, we have to keep sending someone back to the ward terminal to log orders for a patient. What is worse, they won't let the medical student order drugs, so we have to send an intern. Even nurses aren't allowed to log orders in our name (something to do with the 'legality' of having all orders entered by a licensed physician, but that was never a problem with paper order sheets so long as we eventually countersigned the orders!). Some of the nursing staff are following everything by the book so much now that they seem to be obstructing efficiency rather than aiding it. And the designers were so hung up on patient confidentiality that we have a heck of a time cross-covering patients on other services at night. The computer won't let me write orders on any patient that isn't 'known' to be mine, so I have to get the other physician's passwords from them when they sign out to me at night. And things really fall apart when the machine is down unexpectedly for some reason. Everything grinds to a halt, and we have to save our management plans on paper and transcribe them into the system when it finally comes up. I should add that the system always seems to be about 3 hours late in figuring out about patient transfers. I'm forever finding that the computer still thinks a patient is on the first floor when I know he's been transferred to somewhere in the intensive care unit.

"In addition, the 'diagnosis system' is a joke. Sure, it can generate lists of diseases, but it doesn't really understand what the disease processes are, can't explain why it thinks one disease is more likely than another, and is totally unable to handle patients with more than one simultaneous disease. I suppose the lists are useful as memory joggers, but I no longer even bother to use that part of the system.

"And by the way, I still don't really know what all those buttons on the terminal keyboard mean. We had a brief training session when they first put the system in, but now we're left to fend for ourselves. Only a couple of the house staff really seem to know how to make the system do what they want reliably. As for the best part of the system, I guess it is the decrease in errors in drugs and lab tests and the improved turn-around time on those orders – but I'm not sure they're worth the hassle. How much do I use the system? As little as possible!''

### From a third-year medical student

"I've enjoyed using the system most of the time, although I've noticed that some of the house staff seem more grouchy now compared to before the system was installed. I don't think they're really very eager to learn about it or to adapt to it; all they know is that it has disrupted their usual routine. Personally I can see it will have a lot of real advantages once they get some of the bugs ironed out. I particularly like the diagnosis system. Before I do a 'student writeup' for a new patient, I always run his data through the system to see what I might be missing. A couple of times the computer has changed my entire assessment of a case. I can't hope to remember all the stuff they're trying to teach me, so it is nice to know that we may be able to turn to computers for help with keeping track of all this medical knowledge in the future. As for the frequency with which I use it, I guess I sit at a terminal for an hour or so a day while I'm on a ward rotation. That varies, of course, depending upon whether I can find a terminal free or can avoid getting booted off by an intern in a hurry. They ought to have a few more terminals scattered around.''

### From a hospital pharmacist

''The HIS has been a real boon to our pharmacy operation. Not only can we fill new orders promptly because of the improved communication, but the system prints labels for the bottles and has saved us the step of typing them ourselves. Our inventory control is also much improved; the system produces several useful reports that help us anticipate shortages and keep track of drugs that are soon to expire. The worst thing about the system from my point of view, though, is the impact it has had on our interaction with the medical staff. We used to spend some of our time consulting with the ward teams about drug interactions, for example. You know, we'd look up the relevant articles and report back at ward rounds the next day. Now our role as members of the ward teams has been reduced by the system's knowledge about drugs. Currently a house officer finds out about a potential drug interaction at the moment he is ordering a treatment, and the machine even gives references to support the reported incompatibility.''

### From a member of the HIS computing staff

''Frankly, I think the doctors have been too quick to complain about this system. It has only been here for 3 months, and we're still discovering problems that will take some time to address. What bothers me is the gut reaction many of them seem to have; they don't even *want* to give the system a chance. Every hospital is a little different, and it is unrealistic to expect any HIS package to be immediately right for a new institution. There has to be a period of 'breaking in.' We're trying hard to respond to the complaints we've heard through the grapevine. Hopefully, they'll be pleased as the new features are introduced and they see that their complaints are being attended to.''

### QUESTIONS FOR DISCUSSION

1. What problems would be the focus of your report to the hospital?
2. Do you feel that the benefits of the HIS outweigh the problems that have been cited? What are the principal advantages of the computer system de-

scribed? Are there equally good noncomputer solutions to the problems with which the HIS was designed to help?

3. It is clear that the physician quoted is the most strongly opposed to the new system. How would you summarize this doctor's chief complaints? Can you propose design changes that would overcome some of the problems outlined? Try to compile a list of physician concerns that you feel must be addressed in the design of an acceptable hospital computing system. Why do you think the physician is less tolerant of the system than the other persons who were interviewed?

4. In addition to the hospital staff already noted, you interview a patient, and an attending physician practicing largely outside the hospital, about their reactions to HIS. What do you think they might say about the system?

5. Consider the psychological barriers to successful implementation of computer systems in clinical environments. What are their roots? Do you believe they can be overcome?

6. Discuss the impact of the computer system on relationships among physicians, nurses, and other paramedical personnel.

7. How would you change the system? Among the topics you might address are hospital staff training, computer staff training, computer reliability, effect on hospital routine, terminal availability, and the role of diagnostic aids.

8. Are there ways in which courses in medical school, nursing school, or training programs for paramedical personnel could help alleviate some of the problems that occur when hospital staff encounter computer systems for the first time? What effects might the increasing availability of computer-based clinical tools, especially those designed to help with decision making, have on the quality and content of medical education?

### SELECTED BIBLIOGRAPHY

Barnett, G. O. (1968). Computers and patient care. *N. Engl. J. Med. 279*:1321–7.

Croft, J. D. (1972). Is computerized diagnosis possible? *Comput. Biomed. Res. 5*:351–67.

Fox, J. (1977). Medical computing and the user. *Int. J. Man–Mach. Stud. 9*:669–86.

Friedman, R. B., and Gustafson, D. H. (1977). Computers in clinical medicine: a critical review. *Comput. Biomed. Res. 8*:199–204.

Lindberg, D. A. B. (1979). *The Growth of Medical Information Systems in the United States*. Lexington, Mass.: Lexington Books.

Schwartz, W. B. (1970). Medicine and the computer: the problems and promise of change. *N. Engl. J. Med. 283*:1257–64.

Shortliffe, E. H. (1979). Knowledge engineering for medical decision making: a review of computer-based clinical decision aids. *Proc. IEEE 67*:1207–24.

Shortliffe, E. H. (1983). Medical consultation systems: designing for doctors. In *Designing for Human Computer Communications* (M. E. Sime and M. J. Coombs, eds.), pp. 209–38. London: Academic Press.

Teach, R. L., and Shortliffe, E. H. (1981). An analysis of physician attitudes regarding computer-based clinical consultation systems. *Comput. Biomed. Res. 14*:542–58.

CASE 5

# RESOURCE ALLOCATIONS AND IMAGING OF THE BODY

ANN A. JONES  and  ROBERT M. HEYSSEL

You are chief of radiology at a major academic medical center. Your department is internationally renowned, not only for its clinical excellence but also for its contributions to radiology research and development. Maintaining excellence in patient care, teaching, and research are your highest priorities. Within your hospital, the other clinical departments also enjoy international reputations and have similar commitments to excellence.

Each department's quest for excellence, to some extent, requires high-technology capital equipment to stay at the cutting edge of the field. Hospital resources for the development of highly technological clinical and research facilities are limited, and fierce competition exists among the departments for funding of new technologies and programs. Each department receives hospital funds for new capital equipment by submitting an annual long-range plan outlining departmental growth over the next 5 years. Through a series of negotiations focused on the goals of each department's long-range plans, administrators and clinicians divide up the available funds for technological development. The result is a budget – essentially a price tag for the plan – that determines each department's spending on the long-term development of high technology.

You are currently faced with the task of allocating your budgeted funds for the next 5 years. You have been advised by the hospital's chief financial officer that your spending should not exceed $10.8 million. Your desk is swamped with memos from members of your department requesting large expenditures on new equipment. Each request convincingly argues in favor of high-technology development. Furthermore, you must adhere to a replacement schedule for routine equipment. Your dilemma is to respond to these requests and allocate the available funds.

Excerpts from several memos follow:

Subject: PETT Scanning
From: Nuclear Medicine

241

Within the last few years computed tomography (CT) and ultrasound procedures have reduced the need for some nuclear medicine anatomical studies. There has been increasing emphasis on imaging dynamic events. With improved resolution and increased use of computer components, these dynamic studies will continue to grow. The major piece of equipment we would like to acquire is the positron emission transverse tomography (PETT) scanner. The PETT scanner is an integral part of a major study we are conducting on "Neuroreceptor Binding in Man." By employing radiotracers produced by the cyclotron (already available in Nuclear Medicine), the PETT scanner will be used to quantitate and image the distribution of radiotracer in the brain. It is this ability to image in three dimensions, analogous to CT scanning, and to provide quantitative data that make the PETT scanner so powerful when compared with conventional nuclear medicine imaging devices. We anticipate much clinical demand for the PETT scanner, and this demand may offset some current use of nuclear medicine imaging. The PETT scanner can be obtained for $950,000, with an initial down payment of $500,000, and the payment of $150,000 per year for the following 3 years. After the first year, maintenance would cost $100,000 per year.

Entirely new developments will be introduced with the acquisition of a PETT scanner. The cyclotron-generated radioisotopes will be used in conjunction with the PETT scanner to pursue National Institutes of Health (NIH)-supported research in conjunction with the Departments of Neuropharmacology, Neurology, Neurosurgery, and Neurophysiology. This research will be conducted under a multiyear grant totaling $2,900,000. It is not predictable at this time what the hospital costs or benefits will be. The PETT scanner is expected primarily to complement the functioning of the Neurosciences Department. The NIH grant will offset 50 percent of the purchase price of the PETT scanner and 50 percent of the maintenance costs for 2 years.

Subject: CT scanning
From: Neuroradiology

Currently, we have one head scanner, purchased in 1975, and one full body scanner, bought in 1979. The head scanner requires replacement because the updated models are far more efficient and will increase the number of patients we can see by at least 25 percent. We have received approval from the health planning agency to purchase another head scanner because we are the designated regional CT scanning center. The number of requests we currently receive for CT scanning far exceeds our capabilities with one scanner. A second head scanner would allow us to eliminate our backlog of patients. Decreased waiting time for scanning would shorten the length of hospitalization for many patients. Furthermore, by adding a second scanner, many more patients could be admitted to the hospital for diagnostic workups.

Each new scanner costs $1.2 million, and annual maintenance costs after the first year are $50,000 each. With 50 percent down in the first year, the balance could be paid off in the following 2 years. If we buy both scanners at the same time, we would get a break of $200,000, and maintenance costs would drop to $75,000 for both machines. If we delay a decision on the second machine, purchasing costs are certain to increase by at least $150,000 each year. In addition, the hospital animal research group would like to purchase a CT scanner dedicated to animal research. The manufacturer would sell this scanner at a considerable discount, a one-time cost of $250,000, and free maintenance as long as the machine is used for animal research.

Subject: Nuclear Magnetic Resonance Scanning
From: Nuclear Medicine

Nuclear magnetic resonance scanning (NMR) is a new field attracting considerable attention at the moment because the technology does not utilize ionizing radiation, and has the potential to provide a considerable amount of supplemental data by a noninvasive technique. It is ultimately expected to provide new information on disease localization and disordered metabolism in an anatomical and biochemical framework. There is a feeling among pioneers in this area that clinical applications will occur within the jnext few years. Because we are leaders in this field, we propose first purchasing a resistive magnet NMR with an option to upgrade to a superconductive magnet later without penalty. The NMR equipment costs $1.1 million, and maintenance costs are $135,000 per year after the first year. With $250,000 down, no further payments are due for 2 years. We would then have 2 years to pay the balance.

In addition to these memos, you have other considerations. Your own project is cardiac and coronary angiography. You are the recognized leader in this field and have published extensively in these areas. Recently, the cardiac and coronary angiography done in the old laboratory was moved to a new radiology area. There are now four major diagnostic rooms and one minor room. With the move, new equipment for adult cardiac catheterization and pediatric cardiac catheterization is needed. The minor room has been supplied with secondhand equipment.

The additional digital angiography equipment needed costs $550,000, with annual maintenance of $20,000. Two clinical research fellows are coming to the hospital to work under your supervision, and you are anticipating taking more time for research next year. Therefore, funding this project is one of your highest priorities.

Ultrasound is another of your concerns. The head of the ultrasound division is an old friend who has made a substantial contribution to the department. You have committed $2 million over the next 5 years for ultrasound, but you wonder if these funds will be sufficient. From a very small beginning less than 10 years ago, the ultrasound program has increased by approximately 20 percent per year, outpacing planning. This has proved to be an important development because of improved imaging without radiation hazard, especially in its application in pediatrics, obstetrics and gynecology. Ultrasound has replaced a number of other examinations that use ionizing radiation.

You have also committed $3 million over the next 5 years for numerous pieces of small equipment such as a portable $\gamma$-ray camera ($200,000), portable x-ray units ($120,000), processors, and other miscellaneous items. You have estimated an additional $800,000 per year for maintenance, repair, and replacement of the present equipment. This figure concerns you somewhat, because planning for replacement involves the assumption that the same types of procedures will be performed and the same types of equipment used over the next 5 years. However, you know from experience that this is not the case; new technologies frequently replace old ones. Furthermore, the life span of radiology equipment is very short, and the new technologically sophisticated radiology equipment carries a much higher price tag than the more traditional x-ray equipment. The amount of money allocated for replacement is not sufficient to replace any equipment on a desired 10-year cycle due to inflation, advanced and more expensive technology, and the obsolescence of some equipment in less than 10 years. Fortunately, some equipment remains functional beyond 10 years, and CT and ultrasound have reduced the need to replace all existing equipment. Equipment used less frequently lasts longer and can remain useful if it is not technologically outdated. However, timely replacement of routine equipment has been a problem at the hospital for the last 25 years.

In summary, the demand exceeds your $10.8 million budget by about one third. Not only must you balance the budget, you must also consider the ramifications of any changes brought about in clinical practice as a result of new technologies.

Using the available information, prepare a 5-year budget for radiology capital equipment expenditures.

## QUESTIONS FOR DISCUSSION

1. What factors do you take into consideration for budgeting? Should the case mix of the hospital influence your allocation of technology and staff? Do these factors support rational decision making? Discuss the problem in terms of making decisions in the face of uncertainty.
2. Is there a possibility that some of the functions of your department will be decentralized and taken over by other departments? How does this possibility affect your decision analysis? Which functions are most likely to be affected?
3. What are some of the potential effects on the rest of the hospital due to the planned technological changes in radiology? How will these effects, in turn, influence the Department of Radiology?

SELECTED BIBLIOGRAPHY

Fineberg, H. V., and Hiatt, H. H. (1979). Evaluation of medical practices: a case for technology assessment. *N. Engl. J. Med. 301*:1086–91.

Friedman, E. (1981). Imaging technology approaches the frontiers of physics. *Hospitals 1*:76–108.

Goldschmidt, P. G. (1977). Future of medical care technology. Paper presented at the National Association of Blue Shield Plans, National Professional Relations Conference, Chicago, May 24.

Harris, J. E. (1977). The internal organization of hospitals: some economic implications. *Bell J. Econ. 8*:467–82.

Heyssel, R. M. (1981). The need for strategic planning. Paper presented at the annual meeting of the National Association of Children's Hospitals and Related Institutions, Norfolk, Virginia, September.

Heyssel, R. M. (1980). The role of the clinical department chairman in hospital management. The Organization and Governance of Academic Health Centers – Position Papers. *Assoc. Acad. Health Centers 3*:207–14.

Moloney, T. W., and Rogers, D. E. (1979). Medical technology: a different view of the contentious debate over costs. *N. Engl. J. Med. 301*:1413–19.

Rogers, D. E., and Blendon, R. J. (1978). The academic medical center: a stressed American institution. *N. Engl. J. Med. 298*:940–50.

# CONSIDERING AN ARTIFICIAL HEART PROGRAM

DEBORAH P. LUBECK and JOHN P. BUNKER

Coronary heart disease is responsible for over half of the deaths that occur annually in the United States. However, many of these deaths might be averted by innovative surgical procedures. Approximately 30,000 to 75,000 persons with end-stage heart disease or patients who are unable to resume normal circulation after open heart surgery might have their lives extended by cardiac replacement. But donor hearts are not plentiful, and the shortage limits the number of heart transplants that might be done to no more than 1,000 per year, and closer to 500 a year when existing surgical teams are performing at full capacity (two operations a month). However, the artificial heart, a totally implantable mechanical device intended to replace an ailing natural heart, surmounts the problems of donor shortage and immunological rejection associated with heart transplants. Nevertheless, both procedures require a large amount of hospital resources and are very costly.

To date, only a limited number of artificial hearts have been implanted worldwide, but the head of surgical services of your community hospital has proposed that a cardiac replacement program specializing in artificial heart implantation be initiated during the next 5 years. You are a member of the board of trustees of this hospital and have to make a decision on this request at the next meeting. To provide background information, there is a report on the artificial heart, recently prepared by an ad hoc panel of physicians, lawyers, economists, and ethicists for the National Heart, Lung, and Blood Institute (NHLBI), which is summarized below.

## THE DEVICE AND THE SURGICAL PROCEDURE

Artificial hearts are composed of two ventricles made of plastic and aluminum that are attached to the atria, aorta, and pulmonary artery after the patient's own ventricles have been removed. They may be powered by thermal or electrical sources. Electrical energy converters utilize power from an electrically charged external battery pack. These batteries may be implantable in the future, and the prototypes must be recharged after several hours and replaced every few years. Systems currently in use rely on an external power source of compressed air or electricity. Plastic tubes lead to a console that controls the rate and pressure required to stimulate the pulsation of the heart. This console is linked to the power source. Although work is proceeding on the fabrication of smaller and lighter implantable converters, they will be external for at least the next decade.

The surgical procedure, personnel, and postoperative care are similar to those for heart transplants performed today. At a minimum, a chief surgeon, assistant surgeon, heart-lung technician, cardiologist, and two anesthesiologists will be required for the 6-hour procedure. A patient can expect to be hospitalized for 4 weeks to 2 months, with at least 1 week in the coronary intensive care unit. Continuing medical surveillance, including periodic visits to the attending physician, is required for the patient's lifetime because there is a chance of infection and mechanical failure. At a minimum, twice monthly monitoring of the heart's electrical system will also be necessary.

Patients who are tethered to air compressors have an even greater risk of infection in the tissue along the air hose lines, and should remain under close medical supervision. They will be required to maintain living quarters on a single floor, with space available for all the support equipment, such as the compressor and tanks of compressed air for emergency use. These conditions will require that patients lead a sedentary existence. For all artificial heart recipients, rehabilitation programs will be a critical aid in adjusting to the inconvenience and anxiety related to such restricted mobility, the daily recharging of batteries, the potential mechanical or electrical failure, and the total reliance on an implanted device.

## RECIPIENT SELECTION

The yearly pool of potential recipients includes 114,000 new candidates of all ages who have end-stage heart disease with a poor prognosis for survival without the surgery, and who have no other life-threatening systemic illness. If medical selection criteria restrict heart implantation to those persons under the age of 65 who have the greatest probability of survival, there are an estimated 34,300 candidates each year. However, as the artificial heart becomes available, it might be difficult to impose such age restrictions, and the candidate pool might include eligible persons under the age of 70, increasing the number to 68,000. Success might also bring pressures to accept patients who might otherwise be rejected on the basis of psychosocial factors or co-morbid conditions, because the artificial heart will be their only chance for survival. All hospitals will be faced with the need to limit the number of procedures performed each year through established criteria for patient selection. These criteria might be determined by each facility's

Table 1. *Effect of the number of implants per year on total societal costs*
*($1,000s)*

| Implants per year | Per person implantation costs ($) | | |
|---|---|---|---|
| | 25,000 | 29,000 | 84,000 |
| 16,000 | 400,000 | 464,000 | 1,344,000 |
| 34,300 | 857,500 | 994,700 | 2,881,000 |
| 68,000 | 1,700,000 | 1,972,000 | 5,712,000 |

implantation team, or by a broader cross section from the hospital, community, or federal government.

## COSTS AND BENEFITS

Cost estimates for an individual surgical procedure and the device range from a low of $25,000 to a high of $84,000 (1980 figures). An average cost of $29,000 assumes a 4-week hospital stay, professional fees equivalent to those of major open heart surgery, and a $12,000 device. The higher figure assumes an 8-week hospital stay and professional fees equal to those of heart transplantation. Total annual cost estimates are summarized in Table 1 for a range of patient pools. These projections cover only the first year and do not take into account continuing medical surveillance, which may be as low as $1,500 per year or as high as $6,200 per year. We need more experience with the surgical procedure, continuing medical care, and projected survival rates before these cost figures can be narrowed.

The annual benefit of artificial heart implantation is the change in life expectancy due to the postponement of premature death from coronary heart disease. Life tables have been used to give a set of "best case" and "worst case" projections regarding delaying death from heart disease. Under the best case conditions, the average increase for the general population is 0.0697 year (about 25 days). Under the worst case condition, the average increase is 0.0106 year (4 days). For those persons destined to develop ischemic heart disease, the average increase in life expectancy is considerably greater: about 163 days under the best conditions and 34 days under the worst conditions.

## INSURANCE COVERAGE

Cost and patient selection are inextricably linked with payment and insurance coverage. Even the minimum cost estimates for an artificial heart would be a severe burden on most families. Some insurance policies may reimburse the costs for part of the procedure, but only to the limit of coverage; the Health Care Financing Administration has made no statement on whether it will approve future coverage for Medicare patients. It is unclear if state control over Medicaid eligibility includes the right to deny cardiac replacement surgery to a patient. If most third-party payors are unwilling to cover the high costs of this treatment, we will be faced with a serious dilemma: to allow those who cannot afford to pay for the surgery to go without a potentially lifesaving device, or to guarantee payment by the federal government through special Medicare coverage similar to that now provided for renal transplant patients. Such a commitment cannot be taken lightly because it may mean an investment of several billion dollars annually.

The situation before you at the next trustees' meeting represents a great responsibility, and a number of decisions are necessary. You have been provided with a list of the critical issues that will be discussed at that time before a vote is taken.

1. The hospital is concerned that resources not be diverted from other forms of medical care, such as routine open heart surgery. The chief of surgery, in presenting his proposal, asked that five beds be set aside to provide care for only 30 artificial heart patients each year. Some members of the hospital staff contend that to do so will deprive 150 patients of the opportunity for other forms of care, such as total hip replacement, microsurgery of the ear to correct deafness, and correction of birth defects in children. How will you respond to this contention?

2. The ad hoc team has noted that it is quite likely that the hospital will be faced with a greater demand for the surgery than it can meet. Thus, selection criteria will be necessary if the hospital decides to go ahead with artificial heart implantation. What should these criteria be? What should be the composition of the committee to establish the particulars? Would you yourself accept the task?

3. The federal government has stated that it cannot implement special coverage of heart implantations because of the funding that would be lost for prevention programs. Do you agree with this argument? Would you be willing to work toward compromise legislation to ensure equal access through payment for all eligible patients? If a local subsidy were required to ensure that the legislation passes, would you be willing or able to develop an artificial heart program at the hospital? If access through equal payment is limited after all attempts have failed, do you think the hospital should still go ahead with the surgical procedure for those patients who can afford to pay for the implantation?

SELECTED BIBLIOGRAPHY

Ad Hoc Task Force on Cardiac Replacement. (1969). *Cardiac Replacement: Medical Ethical, Psychological and Economic Implications*. Washington, D.C.: U.S. Government Printing Office.
Annas, G. (1978). Rationing health technology: legal and ethical issues. In *Technology*

*and the Quality of Health Care* (R. H. Egdahl and P. M. Gertman, eds.). German-town, Md.: Aspen Publications.

Artificial Heart Assessment Panel. (1973). *The Totally Implantable Artificial Heart.* DHEW Publication (NIH) 74-191. Washington, D.C.: U.S. Government Printing Office.

Calabresi, G., and Bobbitt, P. (1978). *Tragic Choices.* New York: Norton.

Cardiology Advisory Committee. (1977). *Mechanically Assisted Circulation.* Washington, D.C.: Department of Health, Education and Welfare.

Charles, E. D., and Kronenfeld, J. J., eds. (1980). *Social and Economic Impact of Coronary Artery Disease.* Lexington, Mass: Lexington Books.

Christopherson, L. K., Griepp, R. B., and Stinson, E. B. (1976). Rehabilitation after cardiac transplantation. *J.A.M.A. 236*:2082–4.

ERDA Artificial Heart Program Workshop. (1976). *Final Report.* Contract No. E (11-1) 2815–1. Washington, D.C.: U.S. Energy Research and Development Administration.

Havlik, R. J., and Feinleib, M., eds. (1979). *Proceedings of the Conference on the Decline in Coronary Heart Disease Mortality.* DHEW Publication No. (NIH) 79–161. Washington, D.C.: U.S. Government Printing Office.

Hittman Associates. (1966). *Final Summary on Six Studies Basic to Consideration of the Artificial Heart Program.* Contract No. Ph 43-66-99. Washington, D.C.: National Institutes of Health.

Jarvik, R. (1981). The total artificial heart. *Sci. Am. 244*:74–80.

Jonsen, A. (1973). The totally implantable artificial heart. *Hastings Center Rep.* 3:1–4.

Kolff, W. J., and Lawson, J. (1975). Status of the artificial heart and cardiac assist devices in the United States. Presented at the Workshop on the International State of Artificial Internal Organs.

Kolff, W. J., and Lawson, J. (1979). Perspectives for the total artificial heart. *Transplant. Proc.* 11:317–24.

Lubeck, D. (1981). An application of benefit–cost analysis: heart disease research and prevention. Ph.D. dissertation submitted to the University of California, Berkeley.

Lubeck, D., and Bunker, J. P. (1982) *The Artificial Heart: Costs, Risks and Benefits.* Washington, D.C.: Office of Technology Assessment.

National Heart and Lung Institute. (1982). *Totally Implantable Nuclear Heart Assist and Artificial Heart Devices.* Washington, D.C.: U.S. Government Printing Office.

Sapolsky, H. M. (1978). Here comes the artificial heart. *Sciences 18*:25–7.

U.S. Department of Health and Human Services. (1980). *Circulatory Assistance and the Artificial Heart.* NIH Publication No. 80-2032. Washington, D.C.

*Editor's note*: For a discussion by participants and other commentators of clinical and social issues posed by the first implantation of a total artificial heart, and the 112-day survival of its recipient, Barney Clark, see the *New England Journal of Medicine*, vol. 310, no. 5, Feb. 2, 1984.

# TECHNOLOGY AND THE SCREENING AND PREVENTION OF DISEASE

# THE PRENATAL STATE: SCREENING AND TREATING NEURAL TUBE DEFECTS

JOHN C. FLETCHER

Physicians, nurses, and their co-workers in health fields often feel uncomfortable about the legal risks and ethical issues created by new technologies. Screening of genetic and other disorders in the fetus is a prime example of a controversial innovation about which practitioners can hardly afford to be neutral or to avoid discomfort. Practitioners are fully involved in the social and ethical consequences of prenatal diagnosis whether they like it or not. Further, practitioners take on the role of moral counselor when the patient and family want guidance and turn to them for help.

Prior to 1968, when amniocentesis (AM) was first used for genetic diagnosis, parents who knew or suspected that they were at risk had only two choices: (1) prepare for the birth of a possibly affected child, or (2) abort every pregnancy. Prenatal diagnosis results in a negative finding more than 95 percent of the time. In 4 to 5 percent of positive diagnoses, parents have the option of abortion, waiting for birth with whatever therapy is available, and, in a very small number of cases, therapy for the fetus in utero.

### THE TECHNIQUES

AM is a needle puncture of the uterus and amniotic cavity through the abdominal wall that allows amniotic fluid to be withdrawn by syringe. AM is done optimally at 16 to 18 weeks of pregnancy. Laboratory workers then culture fetal cells for study, and also examine amniotic fluid in certain diseases. Chromosomal abnormalities and many other disorders can now be diagnosed before the third trimester.

Chorion villus sampling (CVS), currently being studied in many nations, may surpass AM as the preferred method of obtaining fetal cells for study. By guiding a catheter through the vagina to the chorionic villi, small amounts of tissue can be obtained by syringe. Direct methods of karyotyping fetal cells without previous in vitro culture make a diagnosis possible within hours of sampling, at between 8 and 10 weeks gestation. Controlled clinical trials of CVS compared to AM have not yet been conducted, although a study of the safety and accuracy of these two techniques will soon be sponsored by the National Institute of Child Health and Human Development in a multicenter cooperative trial.

Physicians insist that ultrasound (UL) examinations accompany AM and CVS to locate the placenta and fetus and to guide the procedure. UL machines direct high-frequency, low-intensity sound waves through the mother's abdomen via a transmitter. The same transmitter receives the returning signals reflected from the fetus. The signals are transposed visually onto a screen. Real-time UL involves a special transducer by which fetal movements and physiological events can be observed and measured. Physicians readily study the structure of fetal organs, even the beating heart. When necessary, they use portable UL machines at the bedside. In obstetrical practice, in addition to the assistance of AM, UL helps to date gestation, to determine fetal position when the mother has vaginal bleeding, and to identify multiple gestation. UL can also detect significant defects in the fetus, such as anencephaly.

The use of UL has grown rapidly in routine obstetrical care. A Consensus Development Conference of the National Institutes of Health on the use of diagnostic ultrasound imaging in pregnancy was convened in February 1984. Concern about the safety and efficacy of UL prompted this conference. Data were presented that estimated that between 15 and 40 percent of pregnant women are exposed to at least one UL examination. The panel concluded that UL for pregnant women improves patient management and pregnancy outcome only when there is an accepted medical indication. The panel noted, on the one hand, that a number of epidemiological studies tend to support the safety of UL in humans and, on the other hand, that some animal studies using higher levels of energy caused teratological effects and other biological changes that might be suggestive of harm. More animal and other laboratory studies were recommended.

Physicians now accept AM and UL as routine practice in the management of a pregnancy at risk for genetic abnormalities. The risk of fetal death from infection or other reasons following AM is less than 0.5 percent (1 fetal death in every 200 procedures) and much less in the most experienced hands. This risk of AM is 0.5 percent higher than the known risk of fetal death in everyday life. The risk of fetal death from CVS is higher than from AM, currently between 3 and 5 percent. In 1981, the costs of a routine prenatal diagnosis with counseling, AM and UL, and laboratory work, were $750 to $1,000.

Fetoscopy (FE) is still in the research stage of the technological process. FE permits visualization of the fetus by an endoscope equipped with fiberoptic lenses. Physicians can obtain fetal blood or skin samples for diagnosis of disorders that the study of fetal cells alone will not (now) readily disclose, such as sickle cell disease and β-thalassemia. Risks of fetal death are slightly higher following FE than with AM, and the financial costs are also higher.

Fluorescence-activated cell sorting (FACS) deserves mention as a promising technique in the experimental stage of development for prenatal diagnosis. Fetal cells (erythrocytes and leukocytes) enter the maternal circulation. If such cells were separable from maternal blood, having been stained for identification, it might be possible to use them for prenatal diagnosis. A commercially available FACS machine separates various cell populations on the basis of different factors, including staining with fluorescent antisera. If FACS were feasible for prenatal diagnosis, the higher risks and costs of AM could be virtually bypassed. At this time, however, no investigator has employed FACS for prenatal diagnosis.

The cutting edge of research in prenatal diagnosis is in studies of new methods that will reduce risks and produce new forms of fetal therapy. The ideal accompaniment to diagnosis is a safe and effective therapy. Physicians can now offer fetal therapy for only a few disorders, but research will likely add more. In 1980–1, surgeons successfully operated on fetuses with congenital defects of the urinary tract. Others placed an intracranial shunt in a fetus with hydrocephalus. Researchers employing recombinant DNA techniques moved closer in animal experiments that promise, if successful, to lead to experimental gene therapy in humans. The 1980s should see much more activity in experimental fetal therapy.

### ETHICAL GUIDANCE FOR PRACTITIONERS

There have been efforts to clarify an approach to the central ethical problems that involve practitioners so that the fields of prenatal diagnosis and genetic screening could progress with relative assurance that key values were being respected. In 1976, the Hastings Center's Genetics Research Group organized an interdisciplinary study of the ethics of prenatal diagnosis. This group issued guidelines for practitioners in 1979 that have been widely adopted. The document favored the use of prenatal diagnosis for groups of women who can be well-defined and are known to be at risk, such as the 35 + age group, rather than generalized screening for all pregnancies. On the abortion issue, the emphasis was on the individual choice of the parents, even when the medical practitioner disagrees with their preferred course of action. The document stressed the diversity of views on abortion and the value of respect for the pluralism that exists on the matter. Guidance was offered to practitioners on cases that cause the most disagreement. For example: (1) prenatal diagnosis should not be denied to a woman who has decided from the outset against abortion; (2) parents should be informed about postnatal therapies when these exist; (3) additional findings should not be withheld from parents, even when they are of disputed importance, as in the XYY condition; and (4) practitioners should oppose the use of amniocentesis for sex choice alone, unrelated to a sex-linked disorder.

The approach of the Hastings Center document relies primarily on two ethical principles. The principle of freedom underlies the preference for parental autonomy in choices related to diagnosis and possible abortion.

The principle of fairness supports the evenhanded treatment of parents with different values and disclosure of all the information that prenatal diagnosis will yield. Within the value structure of contemporary institutions, it would be unacceptable to coerce anyone, regardless of the genetic risk, to undergo fetal therapy or to bring the pregnancy to term because a therapeutic option existed at birth. On the side of the practitioner, if he or she disagrees on moral grounds with the request or choice of the parents, there is always the alternative of removing oneself and referring the case to another practitioner.

The historical roots of the principles of freedom and fairness lie in the ideas that form the modern state's approaches to human sexuality, reproduction, and marriage. In the author's view, the injunctions or public policy that bear on pregnancy screening are twofold: "I will respect your freedom of choice to avoid or achieve reproduction with or without technological intervention if you will respect my freedom to do likewise. Further, I will work for a society in which neither of us will suffer harm or punishment because of the differences that exist when freedom is cherished."

### THE CASE OF NEURAL TUBE DEFECTS SCREENING

To screen or not to screen for neural tube defects (NTDs) is a paradigmatic problem that raises ethical issues regarding a whole spectrum of possibilities in prenatal diagnosis and future fetal therapy. Since the prevention of poliomyelitis by vaccine, NTDs are the leading cause of paralysis in children. NTDs are a common abnormality in Ireland, Scotland, and Wales (6 to 8 in 1,000 births). The incidence in the United States is 2 in 1,000 births. Anencephaly and spina bifida are the most frequent forms of NTD. Anencephaly is not compatible with life. Spina bifida lesions can be more or less devastating, depending on the involvement of the spinal cord in the open defect and the location of the lesion.

At this time in the history of the disorder, prenatal diagnosis is accompanied by palliative rather than curative forms of therapy. Surgery closes lesions, shunts drain hydrocephalus, and orthopedic devices ameliorate the effects of paralysis. However, the extent of the damage to the child will have been largely determined in utero. NTDs result from polygenic causes, namely, the effects of several genetic abnormalities interacting with as yet unknown environmental factors. Many researchers are studying these causes and the potential of NTD therapy. A recent report of experimental surgery on monkey fetuses with induced NTDs stated that the results were favorable when the treated group was compared with normal controls after birth. If animal experiments prove beneficial, surgeons will doubtless find parents who are willing to participate in the first trials of human fetal surgery for this defect.

British health authorities widely employ screening for NTDs without significant public reaction. In the United States, a limited amount of screening is done in pilot programs and private practice, but a proposal to regulate conditions under which many more pregnancies could be screened has aroused significant controversy.

Alpha fetoprotein (AFP), a product made only by the fetus and, in rare cases, by cancers in adults, can be detected at elevated levels in maternal blood at 16 weeks of gestation, because more AFP than normal apparently leaks through the placental barrier. This finding has proven to be a suggestive but not a conclusive indication of an NTD in the fetus. The proper medical response to the first positive result is to examine with UL (to rule out other causes) and AM for a more definitive test of elevated AFP in amniotic fluid. Some physicians also employ a second blood test after the first positive finding. Ethically, it is vital that the mother not act on the first positive result to abort the pregnancy on what may be a cause unrelated to NTD, such as twins that may be normal. The follow-up with UL and AM must be timely, well-coordinated, and supplemented by accurate communication with an anxious mother and family.

Fully 9 years after first considering approval of marketing the test kit for a radioimmune assay of maternal serum AFP for laboratory use, the U.S. Food and Drug Administration in 1984 decided to allow its use.

## QUESTIONS FOR DISCUSSION

1. Should every expectant mother be informed at the first obstetrical interview that a blood test is available as a first step to rule out an NTD?
2. Can busy practitioners satisfy the complexities of informed consent for AFP screening?
3. Should the test be given routinely (like a pap smear) without a full explanation unless the result is positive?
4. Can practitioners guarantee that the UL and AM needed to follow up the blood test will be readily provided? Can these services be provided with equity in all parts of the nation?
5. In AFP screening, the rate of false-positive and false-negative results is directly related to the cutoff points established by screening programs. Lower cutoff points for screening normal serum AFP values have a higher detection rate for NTDs but carry a higher false-positive rate. Those that set high cutoff points detect fewer NTDs with a lower false-positive rate. What is the most ethically desirable solution?
6. How should parents be counseled about the potential for treatment of spina bifida?
7. How should parents be counseled about the abortion decision if diagnosis is positive?
8. Who is responsible for the costs of care of a child born with an NTD following errors in laboratory work or in subsequent UL or AM interpretations? Conversely, who is responsible for the loss when a normal fetus is aborted on the basis of erroneous findings?
9. Does abortion for NTDs set a precedent in ethical reasoning for neglect of an infant born with the same degree of handicap? Is there more willingness to do pediatric euthanasia if one is willing to do abortion?

10. In the long run, does large-scale pregnancy screening weaken respect for handicapped persons and commitment to their care?
11. What role, if any, does the federal government play in the regulation of AFP testing? Does any regulation set a precedent that weakens the physician–patient relationship? Are there issues in pregnancy screening that transcend the limits of that relationship and must be addressed by society, as represented by government?
12. Where is pregnancy screening taking us as a society? Will elite groups be able to decide before birth who lives and who dies? What will prevent this outcome?
13. Should research on fetal therapy have a priority as high as or higher than that of research on fetal diagnosis? What reasons support your argument?

## SELECTED BIBLIOGRAPHY

Fletcher, J. C. (1981). Ethical issues in genetic screening and antenatal diagnosis. *Clin. Obstet. Gynecol. 24*:1151–68.

Harrison, M. R., Golbus, M. S., and Filly, R. A. (1981). Management of the fetus with a correctable congenital defect. *J.A.M.A. 246*:774–7.

Herzenberg, L. A., Bianchi, D. W. Schroeder, J., et al. (1979). Fetal cells in the blood of pregnant women: detection and enrichment by fluorescence–activated cell sorting. *Proc. Natl. Acad. Sci. 76*:1453–5.

Hodgen, D. G. (1981). Antenatal diagnosis and treatment of fetal skeletal malformations. *J.A.M.A. 246*:1079–83.

Milunsky, A. (1979). *Genetic Disorders and the Fetus*. New York: Plenum Press.

National Center for Health Care Technology. (1980). *Maternal Serum Alpha-Fetoprotein: Issues in the Prenatal Screening and Diagnosis of Neural Tube Defects*. Conference Proceedings. Washington, D.C.: U.S. Government Printing Office.

National Institute of Child Health and Human Development. (1979). *Antenatal Diagnosis*. Report of a Consensus Development Conference. NIH Publication No. 79-1973. Bethesda, Md.: National Institutes of Health.

National Institutes of Health, Consensus Development Conference. (Feb. 6–8, 1984). The Use of Diagnostic Ultrasound Imaging in Pregnancy.

Powledge, T. M., and Fletcher, J. C. (1979). Guidelines for the ethical, social and legal issues in prenatal diagnosis. Hastings Center Guidelines. *N. Engl. J. Med. 300*:168.

Report of an International Workshop. (1980). Prenatal diagnosis – past, present, and future. *Prenatal Diagn.* (special issue).

Simoni, G., Brambati, B., Danesino, C. et al. (1983). Efficient direct chromosome analyses and enzyme determinations from chorionic villi samples in the first trimester of pregnancy. *Hum. Genet. 63*:349–57.

# COSTS AND BENEFITS OF PREVENTIVE STRATEGIES: CONTAINING HEPATITIS

JEFFREY P. KOPLAN

A general internist in practice in a suburban community of 40,000 is assigned to the hospital infection control committee of a 250-bed community hospital. She is asked to formulate some recommendations for control and prevention of hepatitis B among hospital staff.

After reviewing the pertinent literature and guidelines issued by national bodies, she obtains data and draws some conclusions. Accidental needle-stick exposures are the second most commonly reported injury (after musculoskeletal injury) to the employee health service, and thus result in significant costs to the hospital. In the hospital, the risk of clinical hepatitis B infection following exposure to blood known to contain hepatitis B surface antigen (HBsAg) is approximately 1 in 20. If the blood is of unknown HBsAg status, the risk is much lower, about 1 in 2,000.

Many hospital employees have little or no exposure to blood that would place them at risk for hepatitis B virus infection. Among the remaining employees, there are varying levels of exposure and risk, with the highest risk for laboratory technicians who handle blood specimens.

Similarly, different types of patients are more or less likely to be HBsAg positive (carriers). Thus, blood exposures from certain sources may represent a high risk if the person is a drug abuser, a homosexual, comes from a highly endemic area, and so on.

Diagnostic technologies that are readily available include serological testing for HBsAg and hepatitis B surface antibody (anti-HBs). HBsAg is evidence of current infection, and anti-HBs is evidence of past infection and current immunity. The cost of each test is about $25, but may be lower in a large hospital screening program.

Three therapeutic modalities are available:

1. Immune serum globulin (IG), which has a low titer (1:100) of anti-HBs and which, when given as passive immunization shortly after exposure, may

provide some protection against hepatitis B. IG costs $5 per dose, including administration.

2. Hepatitis B immune globulin (HBIG), which has a high titer (more than 1:100,000) of anti-HBs. Studies have demonstrated an efficacy of up to 75 percent in preventing hepatitis B. HBIG costs $320 for the required two doses.

3. Hepatitis B virus vaccine, which must be given prior to exposure to confer active immunity. It is over 90 percent effective and has few adverse reactions. It must be given in three doses and costs $150.

The average societal cost for a hepatitis case, including direct and indirect costs, is $4,000.

## QUESTIONS FOR DISCUSSION

1. Is it cost effective or practical to screen all patients admitted to a hospital for HBsAg? Describe the factors that contribute to your conclusion.

2. Is it cost effective or practical to screen all staff at the time of employment for HBsAg (as potential hazards) and anti-HBs as an indicator of their immune status? Would you repeat these tests at routine intervals? How would you use the test results in terms of job assignment, any alteration in hospital procedures for patient care, provision of hepatitis B vaccine, and reactions to needle-stick exposures?

3. The persons who incur the different costs used in an analysis may view them differently. For example, although a hepatitis case costs $4,000, this cost is societal. Consider the different perspectives (as well as expenditures and savings) on benefits and costs of hospital administrators, hospital employees, medical insurers, and staff surgeons.

4. Discuss the social, ethical, economic, and legal considerations of serological screening of patients and staff. Should screening be mandatory?

5. To immunize 400 hospital staff persons whose jobs potentially expose them to blood would currently cost $60,000, but would provide long-term immunity and eliminate the need to react to individual exposures. An alternative strategy is reacting to needle-stick exposures with immediate IG administration while testing the source for HBsAg and, if positive, giving HBIG. Several variables are pertinent in choosing between these strategies. Discuss the importance of various components of an analysis, such as patient HBsAg carriage (high-versus low-risk groups), levels of staff immunity, infectivity of exposure, and so on. Might a combination of strategies be necessary? Finally, 90 percent of needle-stick exposures are unrecognized or unreported. How would this influence your choices of strategy?

6. Are cost factors pertinent to hepatitis prevention? Which costs seem most crucial, and how might changing certain ones (lowering them by the use of improved technology or by increased usage and economy of scale, or raising

them because of increasing costs of medical care, equipment, etc.) affect your choice of strategies?

7. Gonorrhea, tuberculosis, genital herpes, leprosy, and syphilis are all infectious diseases with social connotations. Does hepatitis B have similar social stigmata? Why? Discuss the potential for blaming the victim in hepatitis, considering the role of lifestyle/habits in exposure and infectivity, the relative risk to health care workers, and the relationship of the disease to a crucial component of health care, blood products.

8. Would it be useful to establish a registry of HBsAg-positive patients who use the hospital?

## SELECTED BIBLIOGRAPHY

Francis, D. P., and Maynard, J. E. (1979). The transmission and outcome of hepatitis A, B, and non-A, non-B: a review. *Epidemiol. Rev. 1*:17–31.

Koplan, J. P., and Kane, M. A. (1982). Management of needle-stick exposures. *Med. Decision Making 2*:129–31.

Maynard, J. E. (1978). Viral hepatitis as an occupational hazard in the health care profession. In *Viral Hepatitis. A Contemporary Assessment of Epidemiology, Pathogenesis and Prevention* (G. N. Vyas, S. N. Cohen, and R. Schmid, eds.) pp. 321–31. Philadelphia: Franklin Institute Press.

McCormick, R. D., and Makl, D. G. (1981). Epidemiology of needle-stick injuries in hospital personnel. *Am. J. Med. 70*:928–32.

Mulley, A., Silverstein, M., and Dienstay, J. (1982). Indications for the use of hepatitis B vaccine based on cost effectiveness analysis. *N. Engl. J. Med. 307*:644–52.

Pattison, C. P., Maynard, J. E., Berquist, K. R., et al. (1975). Epidemiology of hepatitis B in hospital personnel. *Am. J. Epidemiol. 101*:59–64.

Recommendations of the Immunization Practices Advisory Committee (ACIP). (1981). Immune Globulins for protection against viral hepatitis. *M.M.W.R. 30*:423–8, 433–5.

Reuler, J. B., and Campbell, J. A. (1982). Cost analysis of a needle stick protocol. *Med. Decision Making 2*:133–7.

# TECHNOLOGY AND DIAGNOSTIC EVALUATION

# THE TEST OF THE LABORATORY
# VERSUS THE TEST OF TIME

HAROLD C. SOX, JR.

Most diagnostic tests do not provide definitive information about the true state of the patient. Because nearly all tests are imperfect, test results must be regarded as statements about the probability of disease. Tests sometimes give negative results in patients who have the disease of concern (false-negative results) and sometimes give positive results in patients who are not diseased (false-positive results). The interpretation of a test result depends on these characteristics of the test, and, in addition, on the probability of disease prior to doing the test. The effect of test performance characteristics and the pretest probability of disease on test interpretation is illustrated by a patient with chest pain.

> The patient was first seen in the emergency room one evening with a complaint of severe chest pain that had not been relieved by several nitroglycerin tablets.
>
> The patient described the location of the pain as extending from the middle of the chest across the left breast area. He also said that the pain occurred simultaneously in his left arm. When asked to describe how the pain felt, he used the terms *sharp*, *dull*, and *pressure* at various times in the interview. Although the pain had often been brought on by exertion and relieved by rest in the past, the episode that brought him to the hospital began when he was at rest, and it continued despite the fact that he was lying still. The patient said that the pain appeared to worsen when he took a deep breath. He denied having nausea or sweating with this episode of pain, but did say that he had become somewhat short of breath.

1. Is this man's chest pain due to myocardial ischemia? What do you think?
2. If you answered yes or no, what does this answer mean? Doesn't a yes or no answer mean that you have tried to guess the true physiological state of the patient? Is it wise to guess in this clinical situation if you are prepared to take action based on your guess?

This emergency room visit was the third in several months. On several of the previous visits, the patient had been admitted to the hospital, but there had been no evidence of a myocardial infarction. On this occasion, he was again admitted to the coronary care unit for diagnostic studies to establish the cause of his chest pain.

3. How would you go about establishing the cause of the chest pain? Write down your ideas and refer back to them when you have read through the entire case.

The procedure for diagnosing myocardial infarction is very costly because, according to current practice, the patient must be admitted to a coronary care unit for several days, at a daily charge of at least $500. The main reason for this precaution is to detect potentially fatal cardiac arrhythmias, which often occur in myocardial infarction. During the period of greatest danger, diagnostic tests for myocardial infarction are most likely to be abnormal. These tests are performed one or more times each day that the patient is in the coronary care unit.

Not everyone who is seen in the emergency room because of chest pain is admitted to the coronary care unit. Physicians rely on the patient's history of chest pain to form an initial diagnostic impression. Some patients' histories clearly indicate other causes of pain, and no diagnostic tests for myocardial infarction are required. Other patients' histories clearly indicate that infarction is occurring, and the decision to admit the patient does not depend on diagnostic test results. Often, however, the clinician remains uncertain about the cause of pain. Stated formally, the probability of myocardial infarction, as estimated by the physician, is neither low enough to send the patient home with a clear conscience nor high enough to justify admitting the patient to the hospital. The probability of myocardial infarction below which the physician will send the patient home is the threshold probability for that action. Conversely, there is another, higher threshold probability of myocardial infarction for admitting the patient to the hospital. When the probability of infarction is between these two threshold probabilities, it is difficult to justify either sending the patient home or admitting to the hospital. Sometimes, diagnostic tests can alter the probability of infarction enough that a threshold probability for taking definite action is crossed.

Our patient's history was considered atypical for myocardial infarction because the pain lasted for only about 20 minutes and because the patient had none of the characteristic associated symptoms that usually occur in myocardial infarction. The physical examination revealed normal vital signs; there were no arrhythmias, and there was no evidence of reduced cardiac output. If asked, the emergency room physician might have estimated the probability of infarction to be about 25 percent. About one

Table 1. *Detection of acute myocardial infarction by its classic electrocardio-graphic manifestations*

|  | True-positive rate[a] | False-positive rate[a] |
|---|---|---|
| One ECG in the emergency department | 0.56 | 0.02 |
| Serial ECGs in the coronary care unit | 0.68 | 0 |

[a]Values are weighted means of several studies, in which only new Q waves, ST segment elevation, and deep symmetric T wave inversion were considered classic. The Sox (1982) reference contains citations of the original reports on which the tables in this article are based.

patient in four with this clinical picture might, in the experience of the physician, prove to have an infarction.

4. What information would you use to estimate the probability of myocardial infarction in this patient? Is it important to make an accurate estimate? Why?
5. How would you show that your estimate of the probability of myocardial infarction was correct?

To prove that myocardial infarction has occurred, necrosis of cardiac muscle must be demonstrated, either electrophysiologically or biochemically. In myocardial infarction, the electrocardiogram may show changes that are specific for infarction: new Q waves, ST segment elevation, and symmetric, deep T wave inversion. These classic findings almost never occur except in myocardial infarction (low false-positive rate) (Table 1). Unfortunately, these findings are absent in nearly half of emergency room patients who are later found to have a myocardial infarction. Furthermore, even after daily electrocardiograms in the coronary care unit, one-third of myocardial infarction patients will not have these classic findings (low true-positive rate) (Table 1). Thus, when the classic electrocardiographic evidence of myocardial infarction is present, it is diagnostic; its absence proves nothing.

After several days of diagnostic tests, it is possible to draw definite conclusions about many coronary care unit patients. Patients whose electrocardiograms show the classic findings of infarction are considered to have had a myocardial infarction, because these findings are rarely misleading (Table 1). When the electrocardiogram does not show these findings, the clinician must rely on serum tests for cardiac muscle enzymes. Dead cells release their contents into the circulation. If a particular molecule is found only in cells from one organ, necrosis of that organ may be inferred from finding the molecule in the circulation. This principle is the basis for serum enzyme tests for myocardial infarction. Myocardial muscle cells contain creatine phosphokinase (CPK), an enzyme that is also present in skeletal muscle cells but not to an appreciable degree in any other organs. A small amount of CPK can be detected in the serum of normal individuals. In patients with myocardial infarction, CPK in serum exceeds this

Table 2. *Detection of acute myocardial infarction by elevated serum levels of CPK*

|  | True-positive rate[a] | False-positive rate[a] |
|---|---|---|
| Unfractionated total CPK | 0.94 | 0.10 |
| MB isoenzyme of CPK | 0.97 | 0.003 |

[a]Values are weighted means of several studies.

baseline level about 6 hours after the onset of chest pain, reaches peak levels 24 to 36 hours later, and usually returns to baseline levels by 72 hours after the onset of infarction.

Because minor trauma to skeletal muscle will raise the serum level of CPK above baseline levels, false-positive increases in serum CPK are frequent in patients admitted to the coronary care unit (Table 2). Ideally, it is desirable to measure only CPK from heart muscle. Quirks of the molecular structure of CPK make this feat possible. CPK contains two polypeptides. There are two different forms of these polypeptides: M and B polypeptide. Thus, there are three molecular forms (isoenzymes) of CPK, each corresponding to one combination of the two types of polypeptides: an MM isoenzyme, a BB isoenzyme, and an MB isoenzyme. Each isoenzyme catalyzes the same reaction. The most easily available test for CPK measures the amount of enzyme activity without indicating which of the three isoenzymes is present. The test is inexpensive, and the results are available in about 1 hour. The test characteristics of unfractionated CPK are shown in Table 2. Most patients with myocardial infarction will have an abnormal serum level of CPK (high true-positive rate). The defect of the test is the high frequency of abnormal serum levels of CPK in patients without infarction (high false-positive rate). Nearly all of these false-positive results are due to release of the MM isoenzyme from skeletal muscle. The MB isoenzyme of CPK is present only in heart muscle. As shown in Table 2, the test for the MB isoenzyme has a very low rate of false-positive results and is ideal for detecting infarction. Unfortunately, detecting the MB isoenzyme requires physically separating it from the other isoenzymes or using an immunoassay. The test costs about the same as the unfractionated CPK test but currently takes 24 hours instead of 1 hour to perform. The choice between these two tests may be influenced by the patient's clinical state, in addition to the characteristics of the tests.

When a patient has a history and a physical examination that strongly suggest myocardial infarction, but the electrocardiogram does not show the classic findings of infarction, an abnormal serum level of unfractionated serum CPK raises the probability of myocardial infarction to the point of certainty (Table 3). Normal levels do not eliminate the possibility of an infarction, although the probability is greatly reduced. The test for MB-CPK gives very similar results. Thus, in these patients, unfractionated total serum creatine phosphokinase is an adequate

Table 3. *Interpreting the results of serial electrocardiograms (ECGs) and serum CPK levels*

| Clinical impression from initial history and examination | Probability of infarction based on the history and physical examination[a] | Probability of infarction based on a nondiagnostic ECG[b] | Probability of infarction based on nondiagnostic ECG and CPK results[b] | | | |
|---|---|---|---|---|---|---|
| | | | Total CPK | | MB isoenzyme | |
| | | | Abnormal | Normal | Abnormal | Normal |
| Strong clinical evidence of myocardial infarction | 0.90 | 0.75 | 0.97 | 0.17 | 1.0 | 0.08 |
| Weak clinical evidence of myocardial infarction | 0.25 | 0.10 | 0.51 | 0.007 | 0.97 | 0.003 |

[a] As might be estimated by comparing the patient's findings with those of other patients admitted to the coronary care unit.
[b] Posttest probabilities calculated using Bayes' formula.

test; decisions based on it are unlikely to be changed a day or so later when the results of the MB-CPK test are learned.

The serum test for MB-CPK is of unique value in patients with a relatively weak history of myocardial infarction. These patients have cardiac chest pain that lasts for 15 to 30 minutes, but they lack the typical findings associated with infarction: a history of nausea, sweating, and dyspnea, and physical findings suggestive of reduced cardiac output or arrhythmias. Assuming that the probability of infarction is estimated to be 0.25, the probability of myocardial infarction after a nondiagnostic electrocardiogram and after both types of serum tests for CPK is as shown in Table 3. Patients with the classic electrocardiographic findings of myocardial infarction almost certainly have had an infarction, but the absence of these findings reduces the probability of infarction only slightly. The MB-CPK results either raise the probability of infarction to a very high level or reduce it to a very low level. In either case, the probability of infarction would cross many physicians' threshold values for telling the patient that a myocardial infarction had or had not occurred. Normal serum levels of unfractionated serum CPK reduce the probability of infarction to a very low level, but abnormal serum levels raise the probability of infarction only to 0.5. Clearly, in patients who have an unconvincing history of infarction and lack the classic electrocardiographic findings for infarction, the MB-CPK test is preferable to the unfractionated serum CPK test.

Our patient spent 3 uneventful days in the coronary care unit. Each day, an electrocardiogram was performed, and blood was drawn for the unfractionated CPK and MB-CPK tests. Normal findings were obtained on all of these tests. Since the subjective estimate of infarction had been low before these tests, the normal results excluded the possibility of infarction.

On further review of the entire history, the patient's physicians felt that the history was quite suspicious for an ischemic cause of chest pain. During the previous 6 months, his typical episodes of pain were characterized as follows: restrosternal location with radiation to the left arm; brought on by exertion but also occurring at rest; characterized as sharp, dull, or pressure-like; aggravated by a deep breath; and sometimes but not always relieved within 2 minutes of taking nitroglycerin. He also had a history of hypertension, was a heavy cigarette smoker, and had a family history of coronary artery disease. However, the exertion did not always cause pain, and taking nitroglycerin did not always relieve it. A further atypical feature was aggravation of the pain by a deep breath.

6. Think about the process of interpreting this history. How would you process the information? Are some of the findings more important than others? How does your interpretation take these important findings into account?

7. What is your estimate of the probability that this man's chronic chest pain is due to myocardial ischemia? How did you decide? How might you test the accuracy of your estimate of the probability?

The patient's physicians classified him as having atypical angina. Because the patient was having considerable pain despite the administration of long-acting nitrates and β-adrenergic blocking agents in full doses, he was considered to be a candidate for coronary artery bypass surgery if his pain was caused by coronary artery disease. The next step in management was to ascertain the cause of his chronic chest pain.

One of the principal lessons of this tale is the relationship between test interpretation and what is known about the patient prior to the test. Throughout, we assume that the most useful way to express the meaning of a test result is as a probability of disease. Bayes formula is a simple way to express algebraically the relationship between test performance characteristics (true-positive and false-positive rates) and the probability of disease prior to doing the test (pretest risk) and after the test results are known (posttest risk). This relationship can be expressed as follows:

$$\text{posttest risk (test positive)} = \frac{\text{pretest risk} \times \text{TPR}}{\text{pretest risk} \times \text{TPR} + (1 - \text{pretest risk}) \times \text{FPR}}$$

where TPR = true-positive rate and FPR = false-positive rate

This relationship shows that the pretest risk of disease must be known in order to interpret a test result. Estimating the pretest risk of disease is usually done subjectively, based partly on past experience and partly on intuition. In patients with chronic chest pain, the estimation of the pretest risk is relatively precise, although still somewhat subjective: The more the patient's history fits the description of typical exertional angina pectoris, the higher the probability that the patient has significant coronary artery narrowing. In men who have atypical angina (like this patient), the probability of coronary artery disease is 0.67. In typical exertional angina, it is 0.90.

Because of the patient's history of atypical angina, the physicians caring for him were not sufficiently confident that he had coronary artery disease to proceed directly with coronary arteriography. Instead, they ordered an exercise electrocardiogram.

8. Why not just do a coronary arteriogram at this point? Is an exercise electro-cardiogram a powerful enough test to dissuade you from doing an arteriogram if the exercise test is negative for ischemia?

The principle of the exercise electrocardiogram is that when there is clinically significant coronary artery narrowing, it is possible to increase the workload on the heart to the point where myocardial oxygen requirements exceed that which can be delivered through a narrowed vessel. At this point, energy-dependent cation transport is altered, and there are changes in the membrane potential of myocardial cells. The usual electrocardiographic manifestation of this effect is depression of the ST segment. This ischemic response may be detected by exercising the patient to exhaustion on a treadmill while monitoring the electrocardiogram continuously.

The exercise electrocardiogram is a useful test, but it is often misleading. Patients with significant coronary artery narrowing often do not have ST segment depression (false-negative results). Patients without significant coronary artery narrowing sometimes have ST segment depression when they exercise (false-positive results). The exercise electrocardiogram is unusual in one way: Its true-positive rate increases as the patient's history becomes more characteristic of typical angina pectoris (Table 4). Thus, test performance is not necessarily constant; it can vary systematically with the clinical characteristics of the patient. Table 4 also shows the pretest probability of coronary artery disease in the various chest pain syndromes and the posttest probability corresponding to a positive and a negative test result.

> The patient's history was interpreted as atypical angina, for which the pretest risk in men is 0.67. He exercised on the treadmill for 7 minutes before stopping because of fatigue. His pulse reached and maintained a rate that assured an adequate stress on the heart, yet there was no ST segment depression. Therefore, he had a negative exercise electrocardiogram.

9. Is the term *negative test* useful? What do you think the term means? Does it mean that the patient does not have ischemic heart disease? Ask yourself the same questions about a *positive test*.

Although the physicians caring for this patient were surprised at the negative exercise electrocardiogram, they correctly maintained their suspicion that he had coronary artery disease, presumably because they knew that the exercise electrocardiogram is often normal in patients with this disease. Still, they were unwilling to subject the patient to coronary arteriography without more convincing evidence that he had coronary artery disease. They therefore ordered a radionuclide myocardial scan during exercise.

10. Do you think it makes sense to withhold a test because you think that the chances that it will be positive are too low? Give some reasons supporting this reasoning.

The radionuclide scan of the myocardium images the distribution of myocardial blood flow. The principle of the test is that thallium-201, a radioactive isotope, behaves like potassium, which is the major intracellular cation. When thallium-201 is injected into a vein, it is rapidly extracted from the circulation by myocardial cells. An area of myocardium that has a poor blood supply will contain little thallium-201 and will appear as a dark spot within the white background that represents normal myocardial uptake of thallium-201. The scan during ex-

Table 4. *Test performance and interpretation of the exercise electrocardiogram (ECG) in men*

| Cardiologist's clinical diagnosis | Test performance[a] | | Prevalence of CAD prior to test[a] | Test interpretation | |
|---|---|---|---|---|---|
| | True-positive rate of exercise ECG | False-positive rate of exercise ECG | | Probability of CAD when the test is positive[b] | Probability of CAD when the test is negative[b] |
| Nonanginal chest pain | 0.46 | 0.21 | 0.22 | 0.38 | 0.16 |
| Atypical angina | 0.72 | 0.20 | 0.67 | 0.88 | 0.42 |
| Typical angina | 0.84 | 0.29 | 0.88 | 0.96 | 0.62 |

[a] As shown in a multi-institutional study involving several thousand patients: Weiner, D. A., et al. (1979). Exercise stress testing: correlations between history of angina, ST segment response, and prevalence of coronary-artery disease in the Coronary Artery Surgery Study (CASS). *N. Engl. J. Med.* 301:230–51.

[b] Posttest probability of coronary artery disease (CAD) calculated using Bayes' formula.

ercise is particularly able to identify partial coronary artery narrowing. Blood flow through normal vessels increases fivefold during exercise, but blood flow through narrowed vessels increases relatively little. Therefore, exercise enhances the contrast between thallium-201 uptake by normally perfused myocardium and thallium-201 uptake by myocardium whose blood supply is partially obstructed. The results of the radionuclide myocardial scan during exercise have been compared with those of coronary arteriography in many clinical studies. Overall, about 77 percent of patients with coronary artery disease had an area of reduced thallium-201 uptake that appeared or enlarged during exercise (true-positive rate). Only 7 percent of patients without coronary artery disease had these findings (false-positive rate).

Interpreting the radionuclide scan requires knowing the pretest risk for patients with atypical angina who have had a normal exercise electrocardiogram. The pretest risk for such patients is 0.42 (Table 4). The posttest risk for a patient with an abnormal radionuclide scan is 0.89; the posttest risk for one with a normal scan is 0.15.

11. What would the posttest risk for a radionuclide scan be if the pretest risk (after the normal exercise electrocardiogram) had been 0.20? Would you have done such a scan under these circumstances? If not, what would you have done?

12. Suppose you had misinterpreted the patient's history, and the pretest risk of ischemic heart disease was really only 5 percent. Would this information have changed your decision to do an exercise electrocardiogram? Would it change your thinking about doing a radionuclide scan now that the exercise electrocardiogram has been shown to be negative? You may want to use Bayes' formula and the information in Table 4 to help answer this question.

This outpatient's radionuclide scan during exercise revealed defects in the apex and intraventricular septum that appeared at his maximum exercise level. This result was considered to be strong evidence of coronary artery disease, and the patient underwent coronary arteriography. The arteriogram revealed that the luminal diameter of the left anterior descending coronary artery was 80 percent occluded.

13. Does an 80 percent narrowing of one coronary artery prove that the patient's chest pain was ischemic? If not, what evidence would you require to make this conclusion?

Intracoronary injection of the vasoconstrictor ergonovine caused typical chest pain, ST segment elevation, T wave inversion, and disappearance of a branch of the left anterior descending coronary artery. The coronary spasm was promptly reversed by an intracoronary injection of nitroglycerin. The findings were taken as proof that the patient's pain was due to myocardial ischemia. The coronary spasm was thought to explain the inconsistent relationship between exercise and chest pain, because it was assumed that coronary spasm caused the episodes of chest pain at rest.

The patient underwent percutaneous balloon angioplasty of the fixed left anterior descending coronary artery stenosis. A coronary arteriogram done at the time of the procedure showed a reduction in luminal stenosis from 80 to 30 percent. The residual stenosis was considered to be too little to cause myocardial ischemia.

Up to this point, there was every reason to believe that the diagnostic tests had provided accurate information about the cause of the patient's pain. This depends on the assumption that the coronary arteriogram is an absolutely reliable indicator of coronary artery disease. There are two problems with this assumption. First, the measurement of luminal narrowing is subject to error. The arteries are quite small, and it may be difficult to measure reduction in luminal diameter accurately, especially in branches of the main coronary arteries. In addition, reduction in luminal diameter does not necessarily reflect cross-sectional narrowing, which determines blood flow. A more important problem is that significant coronary narrowing does not always cause chest pain. Half of the patients with myocardial infarction do not have cardiac pain in the months prior to infarction. Furthermore, 11 percent of asymptomatic males over age 50 have significant coronary stenosis. Therefore, when a patient has nonspecific chest pain and significant coronary narrowing, rigorously proving that the chest pain is due to coronary artery disease can be very difficult. When a perfect test for proving that chest pain is caused by myocardial ischemia is invented, we will probably find that the coronary arteriogram is not a reliable test for explaining chest pain.

The patient's chest pain was virtually unchanged by the angioplasty procedure, which had reduced the stenosis to 30 percent. After a year of disabling pain, the patient was reevaluated. At that time, an exercise electrocardiogram and a radionuclide myocardial scan were both negative. A repeat coronary arteriogram showed the same 30 percent fixed stenosis; intracoronary injection of the vasoconstrictor ergonovine did not cause coronary spasm. With this new information, several aspects of the patient's past history took on new significance. Several months prior to the onset of his chest pain, his wife had undergone coronary artery bypass surgery. Shortly thereafter, the patient requested a retirement pension on the grounds of medical disability. Following his second coronary arteriogram, the discharge diagnosis was probable psychogenic chest pain.

This cautionary tale helps us to understand that it may sometimes be very difficult to understand the truth about a patient. Despite the most sophisticated diagnostic tests, no one knew if the patient's pain was caused by myocardial ischemia, but there was no way to be sure without an imaginary perfect test for the ischemia. Because most tests are not perfect, we usually cannot interpret test results as revealing the true state of the patient. A much more realistic view is that test results alter the probability that the patient is diseased. This view is not only realistic, it also provides a framework for relating diagnostic test results to action: The decision to order a test can be based on whether the posttest probability of disease will cross a threshold for taking action.

This case history is an extreme example of how tests can mislead. The physicians caring for this patient interpreted the test results sensibly, and only the test of time revealed their apparent error. Errors in test interpretation tend to occur when the test result comes as a surprise: A positive test in a low-risk patient is likely to be a false-positive result, and a negative result in a high-risk patient is likely to be a false-negative result. Experienced diagnosticians are skeptical about surprises.

## SELECTED BIBLIOGRAPHY

Diamond, G. A., and Forrester, J. S. (1979). Analysis of probability as an aid in the clinical diagnosis of coronary-artery disease. *N. Engl. J. Med. 300*:1350–8. This article uses existing data to estimate the pretest probability of coronary artery disease and shows that the exercise electrocardiogram is most useful in certain subsets of patients with chest pain.

Goldman, L., Caldera, D. L., Nussbaum, S. R., et al. (1977). Multifactorial index of cardiac risk in non-cardiac surgical procedures. *N. Engl. J. Med. 297*:845–50. A clear description of an empirical method for estimating the pretest probability of an event.

Pauker, S. G., and Kassirer, J. (1980). A threshold approach to clinical decision making. *N. Engl. J. Med. 392*:1009–17. This article shows how the concept of a threshold probability for taking specific action can be used in clinical medicine.

Rifkin, R. D., and Hood, W. B. (1976). Bayesian analysis of electrocardiographic exercise stress testing. *N. Engl. J. Med. 297*:681–6. The authors explain clearly how to use Bayes' formula to aid in test interpretation.

Sox, H. C. (1982). The emergency department evaluation of chest pain. In *Emergency Medicine Annual* (B. Wolcott and D. Rund, eds.), pp. 43–60. Norwalk, Conn.: Appleton-Century-Crofts. This article has an extensive bibliography of articles that document the performance of cardiovascular diagnostic tests.

# THE PENALTIES OF EXCESSIVE INQUISITIVENESS

MICHAEL ANBAR

You are an intern in surgery in a big city university hospital. The time is 3:15 A.M., and you are taking a nap on the cot in the emergency room (ER) when the nurse wakes you up to take a call from another hospital. This is a small hospital in a village 50 miles away, stating that they have transferred to you a patient whom they cannot handle. A head-on collision had occurred at 11:30 P.M. on a nearby highway. One driver was killed and the other, who is now on his way to your hospital, suffered a head injury, and additional traumas. His vital signs are relatively normal: The heart rate is 85, the blood pressure 120/80, and the breathing rate somewhat high – about 18/minute. The patient, however, is confused, and in view of the head injury it has been decided to send him to your hospital, which has a computed tomography (CT) scan and a good neurosurgery group.

About 40 minutes later, the ambulance arrives and the patient is brought in. He is a male in his mid-50s, with a smashed face and a bleeding forehead. There is bleeding from the nose and evidence of blood in the left ear. There are also substantial hematomas on the left shoulder and left chest, and although the chest movements suggest multiple rib fractures on the left side, the patient breathes voluntarily but somewhat rapidly (about 20 inhalations per minute). The heart sounds are normal, no rub sounds are heard, and the electrocardiogram (ECG) is normal. Auscultation of the lungs does not indicate any asymmetry in spite of the rapid breathing rate. You take the blood pressure, which is 115/76. The patient is evidently confused and not cooperative, but he is definitely not comatose; his reflexes and pupil responses are normal. Because jthe ER's portable x-ray machine broke down 2 hours ago, you send the patient to the Radiology Department to (1) ascertain the absence of any spine fractures in the upper vertebrae, (2) find out whether there are any apparent skull fractures, and (3) determine the extent of the chest injury.

Ten minutes later, the nursing aide comes back in panic. The patient stopped breathing while she was waiting for the x-ray technician, and the immediate attempts of both her and the technician to resuscitate him by cardiopulmonary resuscitation (CPR) have failed. The patient is being worked on by the x-ray technician. You rush to the Radiology Department while telling the nurse to call the attending physician. By the time the attending physician arrives 15 minutes later, the patient, who was returned meanwhile to the ER, is dead.

The Pathology Department reports that the patient died of respiratory failure following pneumothorax, caused most probably by the chest injury.

In retrospect, what went wrong? Why did this patient die? Could this tragic outcome have been prevented? The attending physician tells you angrily that if instead of sending the patient to the Radiology Department you had intubated the chest and put him on a respirator, he could have left the hospital in 2 weeks. Is this true? After all, the purpose of sending the patient for x-ray was to assess the extent of the injury so as to know what to do next. How could you have anticipated that this patient, who seemed to be in stable condition 3 hours after the accident, would suddenly die while you were trying to find out the nature and extent of his injury?

Try to answer these questions before reading the discussion.

### DISCUSSION

A number of mistakes in judgment were made in this case. We will discuss two of them.

### *Overreliance on "objective" quantitative information*

We do not know whether this patient was in shock and therefore in partial respiratory failure when he arrived at the hospital. The "normal" blood pressure is meaningless since we do not know what this patient's *regular* blood pressure is. This is a classic mistake in judgment brought about by medical technology – where the availability of a quantitative measurement that fortuitously fits normality may bias the reasoning of the clinician. If the patient had a blood pressure of 90/60, the physician would have been much more worried about him, but this might also have been his regular blood pressure. There are false-positive and false-negative results even in a simple quantitative measurement such as blood pressure.

### *Inappropriate use of diagnostic medical technology*

There is only one justification for the use of diagnostic medical technology: The result should potentially change the course of remedial action. This, however, is a *necessary* but not a *sufficient* condition: The latter condition is that the benefit of the diagnostic technology should exceed its cost (or risks).

In the case under discussion, the only justified x-ray examination at the time was that of the spine. This was necessary to ensure that moving the patient's head would not result in paralysis. Skull x-rays were not called for, because the partial consciousness and normal reflexes of the patient did not indicate an emergency head injury. Even if there was a broken skull, it would be detected by regular x-rays in less than 50 percent of the cases; furthermore, even if it was detected, the extent of the internal head injuries could not be determined without CT. Thus, in view of the patient's neurological responses, neurosurgical intervention should not be have been undertaken before morning.

Chest x-rays could have detected the pneumothorax, but this was not the purpose of the examination. If there was a reasonable probability of pneumothorax, the indication would have been *immediate* treatment of the chest (insertion of a chest tube).

The argument that the physician must obtain maximal information about the state of the patient for general medical and legal reasons does not hold in a life-threatening, emergency situation.

The use of health care technology often involves delegation of the patient's care to personnel who are not sufficiently knowledgeable and appropriately equipped to handle acute situations. Moreover, technology specialists are generally not informed about the clinical condition of the patient to be examined. In many cases, they are not informed even about the particular problem for which the examination in question has been requested. These factors must be added to the overall cost (in terms of risk) of the examination. The series of x-rays requested in this case did not involve financial costs and radiation exposure risks alone. The *time* spent in the Radiology Department became extremely expensive for this patient. Without adequate supervision, it had cost him his life.

There is little doubt that the technology was inappropriately used in this case. It should be noted that stories about patients dying while undergoing x-ray examinations or CT scans are familiar to ER personnel.


CONCLUSION

Following this discussion, did you change your position regarding the actions of the hypothetical intern? In what respect?


SELECTED BIBLIOGRAPHY

Hall, F. M. (1976). Over-utilization of radiologic examinations. *Radiology 120*:443–8.

Patrick, J. D., Doris, P. E., Mills, M. L., et al. (1983). Lumbar spine x-rays: a multi-hospital study. *Ann. Emergency Med. 12*:84–7.

Streitwieser, D. R., Knopp, R., Wales, L. R., et al. (1983). Accuracy of standard radiographic views in detecting cervical spine fractures. *Ann. Emergency Med. 12*:538–42.

Zuiderma, G. D., Rutherford, R. B., and Ballinger, W. F. (1979). *The Management of Trauma*. Philadelphia: W. B. Saunders.

CASE 11

# REIMBURSEMENT INCENTIVES AND
# CLINICAL STRATEGIES

STEVEN A. SCHROEDER and BERNARD LO

## THE PHYSICIAN

Dr. R is a 31-year-old internist who is in her first year of private practice in a large metropolitan community. She recently completed her residency training in internal medicine and a subspecialty fellowship in gastroenterology at a nearby university medical center. Dr. R elected to practice in this area because of family considerations, even though she is aware that its physician/population ratio is one of the highest in the country and that competition for patients is intense. She is married to a young lawyer, and they would like to have children soon. However, she still owes $22,000 for debts incurred in medical school, in addition to a recent loan to set up her practice. She and her husband would like to defer having children until their financial circumstances are more secure.

Dr. R has started her practice by joining a six-person multispecialty group that practices fee-for-service medicine. She is accepting cases in either general internal medicine or gastroenterology, but hopes to build a practice that is about 75 percent gastroenterology. The group members share expenses equally, but their net income is determined by the fees generated by each physician. Dr. R felt fortunate to be invited to join the practice for several reasons: it enjoys a good reputation; such opportunities are relatively infrequent in this area; and it minimizes the amount of overhead and equipment for which she is responsible. Nevertheless, she had to negotiate a loan of $25,000 (at 18 percent interest) in order to purchase appropriate equipment, including an upper gastrointestinal endoscope, and a table.

## THE REFERRAL

Dr. R has been referred a patient by Dr. S, a middle-aged general practitioner, who has been in the area for 25 years and has a very busy practice. Dr. R is

283

aware that Dr. S could be an important source of patients for her practice, and is pleased at her first referral from him. Dr. S's patient is a 37-year-old insurance company executive who has had episodic abdominal pain for the past 6 months. He asks that the patient be evaluated and considered for upper gastrointestinal endoscopy.

The patient arrives at Dr. R's office, and at registration is found to have a high-option Blue Cross/Blue Shield health insurance plan that covers all hospital care and most ambulatory tests and procedures, but not simple office visits.

Dr. R takes the patient's history and performs a physical examination. Pertinent historical findings include moderate use of alcohol, coffee, and cigarettes, and occasional salicylate ingestion. The patient has occasionally used antacids, but never regularly; he has never taken cimetidine. Dr. R is impressed that the patient's pain seems to be exacerbated by personal stress, both at home and at work.

On physical examination, the only pertinent finding is moderate epigastric tenderness. The stool guaiac test is negative.


## THE MANAGEMENT

At this point, Dr. R has made a presumptive diagnosis of either peptic ulcer disease or gastritis. She now faces a number of decisions in the subsequent management of this patient. To begin with, should she order more tests?

The tests that Dr. R is considering (and their costs) include complete blood count (CBC), $10.40; screening panel (SMA-12), $28.80; upper gastrointestinal (UGI) series, $144.00; and upper gastrointestinal endoscopy, $300. The fee for the endoscopy would go toward Dr. R's costs and income; the fee for the UGI would go to the radiologist. Endoscopy can establish some diagnoses that cannot be detected on a UGI. In this case, endoscopy might show gastritis in addition to ulcer disease. Although endoscopy may establish the diagnosis more accurately than UGI, it is not clear that a more accurate diagnosis provides therapeutic benefits to the patient. The treatment for both ulcer disease and gastritis is the same: the initiation of antacids or cimetidine, and the discontinuation of gastric irritants such as alcohol or aspirin. Indeed, a negative result on either test would probably not alter the diagnosis or the therapy, given the test characteristics (sensitivity and specificity) of both procedures. In this case, the clinical diagnosis is so strongly established that a negative result on either test is likely to be a false negative. Should Dr. R start an empirical therapeutic trial of antacids or cimetidine, and recommend UGI or endoscopy only if the therapeutic regime is unsuccessful?

Some patients find endoscopy uncomfortable or are frightened by its rare complications. Other patients are concerned about long-term radiation risks from x-rays. Still others may expect sophisticated testing to be done, because they equate advanced technology with high-quality medical care. Under the doctrine of informed consent, the physician should inform the patient of the proposed tests or treatments, their risks and benefits, and the likely outcomes and alternatives. Once so informed, the competent patient must consent to the plans. Dr. R is also concerned that Dr. S expects endoscopy to be performed. If she does not perform the procedure, he might refer the patient (and other patients) to gastroenterologists who are more willing to do endoscopies.

What roles should the wishes of the patient and the referring physician (Dr. S) play in Dr. R's decisions? What are the malpractice implications of the various actions she might take? Consider her long-range objectives in establishing her practice when responding to these questions.

In chronic diseases such as peptic ulcer disease, an important part of the care is educating the patient and discussing how lifestyle, stress, diet, cigarettes, and alcohol affect the disease. Yet the physician reimbursement schedule offers disincentives for such education and discussion. If Dr. R spends 25 minutes performing endoscopy, she charges $300, a fee that will be totally reimbursed by the patient's insurance. However, if she spends 45 minutes in education and counseling, she charges $60, which may not be covered by the patient's insurance. How might the reimbursement implications for Dr. R influence the various diagnostic and therapeutic strategies she might undertake for this patient? To what extent does third-party payment influence clinical decisions? Consider both the services covered and the extent to which the covered services are valued in answering these questions.

How could an oversupply of physicians influence the way medicine is practiced, as illustrated by this case?

### SELECTED BIBLIOGRAPHY

Almy, T. P. (1981). The role of the primary physician in the health care industry. *N. Engl. J. Med. 304*:225–8.

Marton, K. E., Sox, H. C., Wasson, J. H., et al. (1980). The clinical value of the upper gastrointestinal tract roentgenogram series. *Arch. Intern. Med. 140*:191–5.

Roe, B. (1981). The UCR boondoggle. *N. Engl. J. Med. 305*:41–5.

Schroeder, S. A. (1980). Editorial. The complications of coronary arteriography: a problem that won't go away. *Am. Heart J. 99*(2):139–41.

Schroeder, S. A., and Showstack, J. A. (1978). Financial incentives to perform medical procedures and laboratory tests: illustrative models of office practice. *Medical Care 16*:289–98.

Showstack, J. A., Schroeder, S. A., and Steinberg, H. R. (1981). Evaluating the costs and benefits of a diagnostic technology: the case of upper gastrointestinal endoscopy. *Med. Care 198*:498–509.

# THE COST OF THE ROUTINE ORDER

PHILIP GREENLAND and PAUL F. GRINER

### CASE HISTORY

A 78-year-old widowed woman comes to the emergency room of the university hospital with a chief complaint of abdominal pain of 2 weeks' duration. The patient has a number of serious chronic illnesses including high blood pressure, asthma, cerebral and cardiac atherosclerotic vascular disease, a chronic cardiac muscle disorder (idiopathic hypertrophic subaortic stenosis), and a recent history of recurrent rectal bleeding considered to be due to diverticular disease of the colon. She is followed at the university hospital in the general medicine and cardiology clinics. She has been admitted to the hospital three times in the past year for other problems.

The patient describes her pain as constant and severe, located deep in the epigastrium (mid-upper abdomen) and left upper quadrant. She denies knowledge of any exacerbating or alleviating factors including meals. Her bowel movements and urinary habits have been normal. There has been no fever. Her appetite was normal until 2 days prior to admission, when near constant nausea began. She has been able to drink liquids but has vomited on several occasions. This pain syndrome is unlike anything she has experienced in the past.

The patient is taking numerous potentially toxic medications including prednisone (a steroidal antiinflammatory agent), verapamil (a newly developed drug for her heart condition), and several others for high blood pressure and asthma.

An additional factor is the known presence of calcified gallstones, detected incidentally during an earlier hospitalization. She has, however, had no definite attacks of cholecystitis (inflammatory disease of the gallbladder due almost exclusively to gallstones) in the past.

The patient is widowed and lives with one of four devoted daughters; the others live nearby. She is well educated and articulate. The family, as always, is quite concerned over the patient's new problem, especially in light of her many previous ones.

Examination reveals an uncomfortable, obese woman. She has no fever, and other vital signs are consistent with her known baseline values. The only new findings are tenderness to palpation in both the right upper abdominal quadrant and the left lower quadrant. The remainder of the abdominal and general examinations are unrevealing. The stool examination reveals no blood, and the rectal examination is normal.

## HOSPITAL COURSE

*Day 1.* The patient is seen by her primary internist (a third-year medical resident) and several other medical and surgical residents in the emergency room. All of them agree that the history and findings on examination are not characteristic of any disease process, and a long list of diagnostic possibilities is given including cholecystitis, diverticulitis, peptic ulcer disease (possibly due to the prednisone therapy), and vascular disease of the abdominal vessels. An attending physician sees the patient later that day and agrees that the patient's illness represents a puzzling diagnostic problem, although cholecystitis appears to be most likely.

Because of the many diagnostic possibilities, a number of tests are planned, including an acute abdominal x-ray series, an ultrasound study of the abdomen, an upper gastrointestinal (GI) x-ray series, barium enema, and sigmoidoscopy. The acute abdominal series is completed on day 1 and reveals only the calcified gallstones, a normal abdominal gas pattern, stool present in the colon, and no free abdominal air or abnormal masses.

*Day 2.* The patient is started on intravenous fluids and given nothing to eat or drink by mouth. Her symptoms persist. An SMA-6, SMA-12, and complete blood count are ordered. Only a slightly increased alkaline phosphatase level is discovered.

*Day 3.* Symptoms persist. The abdominal ultrasound test is done. The gallstones are again detected, but dilatation of the bile ducts or thickening of the gallbladder are absent. The diagnosis remains uncertain.

*Days 4 and 5 (Saturday and Sunday).* Symptoms persist, and the patient remains on intravenous fluids. An SMA-6 and SMA-12 are ordered daily and show no changes.

*Day 6.* A barium enema is performed and demonstrates diverticulae of the colon, which was previously known. No masses are detected. The pain seems to worsen after this test. As yet, there is no definitive diagnosis.

*Day 7.* The pain improves slightly. The patient is prepared for an upper GI series with cathartics. She is now able to tolerate liquids by mouth.

*Day 8.* The upper GI series is canceled due to retained barium from previous x-ray tests. Right upper quadrant pain persists. The attending physician and the residents feel that cholecystitis is the most likely diagnosis, but cannot say this definitively because the test results are nonspecific, as is the clinical condition. The family and patient question the doctors extensively about the diagnosis and the workup.

*Day 9.* The patient's symptoms improve, and she can drink liquids. Her preparation for the upper GI series continues.

*Day 10.* The patient's symptoms are nearly gone. The upper GI series is again postponed due to persistent retention of barium. The physicians disagree about the need to complete this test. The absence of a definitive diagnosis and concern over drug-induced ulcer disease finally convince them to obtain upper GI x-rays after all.

*Days 11 and 12 (Saturday and Sunday).* The patient's symptoms improve. She is now off intravenous fluids. No blood work or x-rays are done.

*Day 13.* The patient is now asymptomatic and back to her normal self. She has the upper GI series, which she describes as ''awful.'' The x-ray shows no ulcer or other abnormality. The patient is discharged home with a diagnosis of probable acute cholecystitis. No surgery is planned for the near future due to the patient's chronic state of debility.

### SUMMARY OF TESTS

During the hospitalization, the patient underwent 5 radiological procedures, 15 hematology tests, 16 clinical chemistry tests, and several other routine tests including an electrocardiogram.

### SUMMARY OF CHARGES

The total hospital bill is $3,503.35. Approximately one-quarter of the charges are for the laboratory tests. The patient's attending internist, who saw her daily in the hospital and spoke at length with several family members, bills for the usual and customary Blue Shield charges, which amount to less than $250 for the entire 13-day hospitalization. The radiology department bills for its five procedures; this amount, also covered by Blue Shield, is over $400. Therefore, the total charges for this hospitalization exceed $4,000.

### QUESTIONS FOR DISCUSSION

1. What is the effect of doing multiple ''inexpensive'' tests on the overall care of hospitalized patients?
2. Who are the high-cost users of medical care?

3. What is the additive value of any given test?
4. What are the risks of iatrogenic illness induced in the course of diagnostic evaluation?
5. How many physicians were involved in this patient's care? Was this beneficial, harmful, or neutral?
6. How many of this patient's tests do you think were performed as a part of hospital routine?
7. What role, if any, did the educational system in a university hospital play in determining the number of tests this patient had?
8. How much of a role did the patient and her family play in determining the number of tests ordered?
9. Direct laboratory charges were about one-quarter of the total hospital bill. How much of the bill was indirectly related to laboratory tests? What was the total impact of laboratory tests on the cost of this patient's care?
10. What is your opinion of the distribution of charges rendered by the hospital, the radiologist, and the internist?
11. Did lack of knowledge of the tests or their characteristics appear to be important in this patient's evaluation?
12. Were many of this patient's laboratory tests redundant, that is, was more than one test performed to rule in or rule out any given condition?
13. Could this patient's evaluation have been completed more expeditiously?

### SELECTED BIBLIOGRAPHY

Altman, S. H., and Blendon, R., eds. (1977). *Medical Technology: The Culprit Behind Health Care Costs?* Proceedings of the 1977 Sun Valley Forum on National Health. DHEW Publication No. 79-3216. Washington, D.C.: U.S. Department of Health, Education, and Welfare.

Delbanco, T. L., Meyers, K. C., and Segal, E. A. (1979). Paying the physician's fee. Blue Shield and the reasonable charge. *N. Engl. J. Med. 301*:1314–20.

Greenland, P., Mushlin, A. I., and Griner, P. F. (1979). Discrepancies between knowledge and use of diagnostic studies in asymptomatic patients. *J. Med. Educ. 54*:863–9.

Griner, P. F. and the medical house staff, Strong Memorial Hospital. (1979). Use of laboratory tests in a teaching hospital: long-term trends. *Ann. Intern. Med. 90*:243–8.

Moloney, T. W., and Rogers, D. W. (1979). Medical technology – a different view of the contentious debate over costs. *N. Engl. J. Med. 301*:1413–19.

Schroeder, S. A. (1981). Medical technology and academic medicine: the doctor-producers' dilemma. *J. Med. Educ. 56*:634–9.

Schroeder, S. A., and Martin, A. R. (1981). Editorial: will changing how physicians order tests reduce medical costs? *Ann. Intern. Med. 94*:534–6.

Schroeder, S. A., and O'Leary, D. S. (1977). Differences in laboratory use and length of stay between university and community hospitals. *J. Med. Educ. 52*:418–20.

Wertman, B. G., Sostrin, S. V., Pavlova, Z., et al. (1980). Why do physicians order laboratory tests? A study of laboratory test request and use patterns. *J.A.M.A. 243*:2080–2.

Zook, C. J., and Moore, F. D. (1980). High-cost users of medical care. *N. Engl. J. Med. 302*:996–1002.

CASE 13

# PROSPECTS AND DILEMMAS
# OF THE CONSULTANT:
# THE MEDICAL IMAGING SPECIALIST

A. EVERETTE JAMES, JR., ALAN C. WINFIELD, JEREMY J. KAYE,
FRANK A. SLOAN, RONALD R. PRICE, C. LEON PARTAIN,
W. HOYT STEPHENS, RALEIGH J. HAMILTON, and
HENRY P. PENDERGRASS

The rapidity with which technical advances in medical imaging have developed in the recent past has been quite remarkable, and there is a promise of continuing escalation of progress in the immediate future. Today's diagnostic imaging techniques bear little resemblance to the primitive radiographic procedures of the pioneers of radiology at the turn of the century, following the discovery of the x-ray by Wilhelm Conrad Roentgen in 1895. The new technology is also modifying traditional relationships of referring physicians with medical imaging specialists. In this case, we will explore the development of this technology and the difficulties of seeking its appropriate use.

### DIGITAL RADIOGRAPHY

Medical imaging is primarily concerned with data accumulation, analysis, and transfer. Beginning in the 1960s, biomedical engineering techniques developed in physics, engineering, and computer sciences, and have since been used to develop new radiological techniques. Digital radiography is notable among them. It replaces the traditional x-ray image on silver halide film with an electronic sensor controlled by a computer (Erickson et al. 1981). The term *digital* refers to the conversion of information currently available as an analog x-ray image into a mathematical form that permits its integration by a computer.

The most common type of digital radiography is the image intensifier video fluoroscopic system. The procedure most frequently performed using this system is referred to as digital subtraction angiography (DSA). Of all the digital techniques, DSA has received the most attention, because it has provided physicians with the ability to image arterial vascular structures by the injection of relatively small amounts of contrast material into the venous system. Therefore, the patient can now have a study as an outpatient that would previously have required a hospital admission. Direct digitization of the radiographic images from the image intensifier also has the advantage over traditional film subtraction techniques of increased contrast sensitivity.

The digital subtraction technique requires the capturing of an image in the computer's memory immediately prior to the appearance of the contrast material in the arterial system. The basic image, or mask, will later be used to subtract the density of soft tissue and osseous structures overlying and otherwise obscuring the vascular structures of interest. Subsequent images of the opacified arteries (containing contrast medium, or dye) are then digitized and stored in the computer's memory. The computer is used to carry out a subtraction by the difference of the mask and postcontrast images. The result is a relatively good diagnostic image of the arterial system.

Thus, the physician now faced with a clinical problem suggesting a vascular insufficiency (such as a transient ischemic attack) or stenosis (such as an arteriosclerotic change) can consult the imaging physician about a noninvasive digital angiogram.

## ULTRASOUND TECHNIQUES

No less exciting in the clinical setting of today's practice is ultrasound technology, particularly real-time imaging. Diagnostic sonography had its origin in techniques that had been previously applied to submarine navigation and to the testing of industrial materials. Its use in clinical diagnostic medicine is several years old. However, it came into its own in 1974 with the production of improved diagnostic devices that showed the internal nature of organs and vessels, and has become an area of medical imaging much in clinical demand (Fleischer and James 1983). It finds particular use in obstetrics because it obviates the need to expose the patient and the fetus to potentially harmful ionizing radiation. With pulsed Doppler modifications that measure and quantitate blood flow, its role in the diagnosis of occlusive vascular disease is significant, all the more so when its noninvasive capabilities are realized. Because of the minimal biological hazard when employed at diagnostic levels, the relatively low cost of the equipment, and the ease of the study, ultrasound will be increasingly utilized in the future. The physician having a patient with right upper quadrant pain can order a real-time ultrasound study of the pancreas, liver, and gallbladder. This requires no patient preparation and little cooperation, is noninvasive, and can be performed in minutes. Gallbladder wall thickening, calculi, or dilatation of the biliary tract can be shown in a matter of minutes, and the diagnosis established with certainty.

Real-time ultrasound also can be effectively utilized to examine carotid artery insufficiency and stenosis of peripheral vessels, and to diagnose obstetrical problems of all types.

## DEVELOPMENTS IN NUCLEAR MEDICINE

Nuclear medicine has progressed dramatically over the last 20 years, and has demonstrated a surprising flexibility in modifying, in a noninvasive, low-radiation exposure format, areas of study that have not been as well handled by other means. In particular, cardiac nuclear medicine is a subject of present intense interest and growth, because of its ability to yield functional data on the cardiovascular system. Incorporation of physiological observation using radionuclide tracers permits recognition of areas of myocardial ischemia and abnormal cardiac function. These observations find ready clinical application in the area of ischemic heart disease and are assuming increasing importance in its management. With the improvement of radiopharmaceuticals that localize to the myocardial muscle and those that are confined to the blood pool, physicians can now image the area of ischemia in order to "size" infarcts and to quantify the loss of function and the response to treatment or recovery. We are also presently witnessing the emergence of positron emission tomography (PET), a highly specialized, rapidly advancing technique whose potential and capabilities are only now beginning to be explored. Short half-lived metabolic tracers such as compounds labeled with $^{11}$C, $^{15}$O, and $^{13}$N will provide data regarding fundamental metabolic processes (Patton 1981). These will not be in routine clinical use, but will assist in exploring the data available from nuclear medicine studies that can be obtained in most hospitals and private physicians' offices. The previously mentioned modalities have demonstrated enhanced utility and flexibility because of numerous advances in biomedical engineering technology. The utilization of computer techniques in the field of medical imaging has been revolutionary and is found in many areas (Price et al. 1982). One capability of interest to the primary physician is the capture of data from an imaging study at a remote site such as a private office, outpatient clinic, or another hospital.

### NUCLEAR MAGNETIC RESONANCE TECHNOLOGY

Another similarly exciting imaging technique involving computer reconstruction is being rapidly developed. Nuclear magnetic resonance (NMR) is a technique that provides high-quality images in numerous projections without utilizing ionizing radiation and without, at least so far as can be determined today, any significant adverse biological effects. Magnetic fields and radiofrequency waves are employed to produce signals that reflect the atomic composition of the body in health and disease. Further, like nuclear radiology, NMR imaging has the potential ability to evaluate pathophysiological measurements and may possess the specificity to differentiate disease processes into categories (such as neoplasia) on the basis of abnormal function rather than abnormal anatomy. The devices are currently being evaluated vis-à-vis other alternative imaging methods in several dozen centers, and by 1984 will be installed in over 100 institutions.

### IMAGING DEPARTMENTS OF THE FUTURE

It is important for physicians to attempt to understand the role of these evolving imaging techniques as they might relate to and partially displace some of the more conventional radiographic examinations better known to those now involved in patient care. Virtually all the new techniques just described are computer related, and therefore will, of necessity, require conversion of information to a digital state. It is not difficult to see that most future medical imaging will be converted to digital data, computer manipulated, transferred and stored electronically, and ultimately reviewed or interpreted remotely, with no need for conventional film exposure or storage. Imaging departments functioning in a filmless setting are easily conceived (Capp 1981). Steps are underway to develop such departments. The technology now exists to create areas of imaging with computer storage, analysis, and reconstruction, with final conversion from digital to analog visual form. Gray scale may be replaced by color. Color will allow a much wider portrayal of signals from the diagnostic methods employed. However, the traditional gray-scale format will remain the one most commonly used for the next decade. The prospects for image acquisition, manipulation, and transfer are exciting and include such advances as on-line remote consultations, instantaneous transfer of data from area to area within a hospital or medical delivery system, computer comparison of images, and so on.

## NEW PROSPECTS AND PROBLEMS FOR IMAGING SPECIALISTS

These developments promise to change the relationship between the referring clinician and the consultant radiologist or medical imaging specialist. It is no longer adequate for the medical imager to act solely as an interpreter of findings depicted on radiographs, fluoroscopic screens, cathode ray tubes, or tape recorders. The complexity and expense of the technology, the numerous options available in determining a pattern of diagnostic study, and the variation in expense, safety, and efficacy of the various modalities at our disposal require medical imaging physicians to play a more active role than they do at present in planning the diagnostic examination of the patient. Attending clinicians, unsettled about which of the myriad possible diagnostic studies will be the most practical, prompt, and cost effective in achieving therapeutic goals, will increasingly need help. If radiologists are to provide it adequately, they must become involved more directly in the care of the patient, and increasingly leave the imaging suite for the bedside, at least to the extent that the goals of diagnosis and therapy are understood and agreed upon by both the clinician and the radiologist. To do less than this is to allow the referring physician to navigate without adequate guidance through a complicated maze of diagnostic imaging studies, hoping to sift from a sometimes overabundant mass of data answers to the questions posed by the patient's problem. To facilitate this, some departments have named a radiologist of the day (ROD) to be immediately available for this purpose.

However, the medical imaging specialist (radiologist or other) may not personally possess all of the physics and basic science skills necessary to interact effectively with this new technology; therefore, a symbiotic relationship must be established with those scientists who have the capabilities and interest to develop and modify the technology at the physician's disposal. The technologists, basic scientists, and other investigators, individually and collectively, must also understand the needs of the clinician. Radiologists, as middlemen, must supply the stimulus and interest, and must participate in the financial support of these groups to ensure that the developing technology continues in an atmosphere of unencumbered and creative research, with guidance on its possible clinical utilization. If the practicing radiologist can effectively serve as the catalyst between these groups, this will ensure that the technology of medical imaging will continue to achieve the exciting gains for improved patient care it has shown over the past several decades.

## CASE STUDY

To examine the issues raised by the technological complexity of imaging techniques, and the changing role of the medical imaging specialist as consultant to the referring physician, we present the following case:

You are a radiologist in a large hospital, and receive a request from a physician on the staff for a diagnostic examination of his patient. The referring doctor supplies the following information: This is a 15-year-old boy who was brought to the hospital with left flank trauma. On admission he was found to have hematuria. Follow-up observation demonstrates a dropping hematocrit. The doctor requests the radiologist to do an intravenous pyelogram (IVP). He wants to take the boy to the operating room following the procedure.

As the consultant radiologist, you do not believe that the imaging examination requested is the best procedure to yield the information sought by the referring doctor. Increasingly interested in assuming a more active role in helping clinicians apply imaging technologies appropriately, you ask for both a meeting with the clinician and the opportunity to visit the patient's bedside with him.

## SCENARIO 1

The referring doctor responds that he is too busy to meet with you; further, he does not see how your bedside visit would help clarify matters. He asks you simply to perform the imaging procedures he requested; he will then bring the patient to the operating room to deal with his injuries. Taking account of clinical and ethical considerations, how should you act in this situation?

## SCENARIO 2

The referring doctor agrees to your request. You visit the patient, and after reviewing the case recommend a set of imaging tests different from those originally requested. You, as the radiologist, urge the physician to forego the IVP because the injury and symptoms make you suspect the existence of vascular injury to the left kidney. In that case, the diagnostic examination of choice is angiography of the kidney and its vicinity, which may lead to embolization of the artery, stop the bleeding, and avoid the need for immediate operation. The referring doctor, somewhat uneasy over these developments, agrees to your suggestions, but indicates that he holds you responsible for any untoward outcome. Should you, the consultant radiologist, assume such a responsibility?

### QUESTIONS FOR DISCUSSION (BOTH SCENARIOS)

1. In general, what are the clinical and ethical problems of the consultant in medicine?
2. Specifically, what are the benefits and dangers for patients, referring doctors, and medical imaging specialists when the last group ask for a more direct role in diagnostic decision making and patient care?
3. What, ideally, should be the role of the medical imaging specialist?

### SELECTED BIBLIOGRAPHY

Capp, M. P. (1981). Radiological imaging – 2000 A.D. *Radiology 138*:541–50.
Coulam, C. M., Erickson, J. J., Rollo, F. D., et al., eds. (1981). *The Physical Basis of Medical Imaging*. New York: Appleton-Century-Crofts.
Erickson, J. J., Price, R. R., Rollo, F. D., et al. (1981). A digital radiographic analysis system. *RadioGraphics 1*(2):49–60.
Fleischer, A. C., and James, A. E., Jr. (1983). *Real Time Ultrasound*. New York: Appleton-Century-Crofts.
Patton, J. A. (1981). Emission tomography. In *The Physical Basis of Medical Imaging* (C. M. Coulam, J. J. Erickson, F. D. Rollo, et al., eds.), pp. 253–63. New York: Appleton-Century-Crofts.
Price, R. R., James, A. E., Jr., Monahan, W. G., et al. (1982). *Digital Radiography*. Philadelphia: Grune & Stratton.

# THE PATIENT'S PERCEPTION OF RISK

KEITH I. MARTON

This case illustrates some of the psychological aspects of technology use, particularly those that concern the perception of risks and probabilities. By psychological aspects, we refer to intrinsic rules that people use to perceive and process information, which are not always intuitively obvious. In fact, such rules sometimes result in systematic distortions of information.

Because these common perceptual rules may distort the information we receive, it is important to understand them. Consider, then, the following scene in a medical office.

The patient, a 28-year-old man, has sought consultation because of abdominal discomfort of several weeks' duration. He is accompanied by his wife. There is a discussion of the physician's plans for evaluating the patient's symptoms after the initial history and physical examination have been completed. The physician indicates some uncertainty about the cause of the symptoms, but suggests that the best course is a trial of antacids to see if they will be relieved. But the patient is concerned that the doctor is not sure about what is wrong, and asks if any tests could be done to learn with more certainty the nature of his complaint. The doctor says that an upper gastrointestinal (GI) x-ray could help clarify the situation, and the patient accepts the suggestion. The patient's wife, having read newspaper accounts of the dangers of x-rays, expresses anxiety about her husband's being exposed to them unnecessarily. The patient becomes anxious too, and asks about the risks of x-ray-induced cancer. He notes that recently a friend with abdominal complaints had died of cancer. The doctor indicates that although there are some risks, they are minimal. He makes plans for the x-ray, prescribes the antacids, and asks to see the patient in 2 weeks.

When the patient returns, he reports that the pain stopped the day after the x-ray was done. The doctor tells him that the test was negative. The patient is relieved, and says that if the pain returns he would like a second radiological examination. The doctor, puzzled, asks whether this normal x-ray has reassured him. "This time, sure," replies the patient. "But I'd want to make sure there wasn't something serious next time too."

QUESTIONS FOR DISCUSSION

The preceding interchange illustrates a number of issues that influence people's view of sophisticated technology. In thinking about the following questions, consider that our perception of technology is likely to be colored by our need for certainty, how we view risks, and what we perceive our own situation to be (e.g., do we see ourselves as standing to gain or lose from an intervention?).

1. We see, in this case, an example of a test that did little to change the physician's diagnostic thinking and had no effect on the choice of therapy. Nonetheless, the patient appeared to be reassured by the test. Can you think of other situations in which both physicians and patients seem to place a high value on small increases in certainty?

2. The patient's wife was quite concerned about the harmful effects of radiation. Do you think her fears were excessive? Why or why not? What factors may be important in determining our concerns about the dangers of radiation?

3. Note that the patient was concerned about the possibility of cancer, an extremely unlikely event in a healthy young man. Do you think the patient really understood how low the probability of cancer was? How good are people at conceptualizing low probabilities? What factors other than probability are likely to color our views about whether or not to worry about an unpredictable event? (Hint: Think about how bad the event might be.)

4. The patient seemed to be more reassured by the x-ray than by the physician's judgment after taking a history and doing a physical examination. Is this common? Why might this be the case? What do you think would have happened had the physician more vigorously resisted the patient's request for an x-ray? Could the physician have been more effective in reassuring the patient?

5. The patient seemed to improve as soon as the upper GI was done. Do you think tests might have placebo effects? If so, would this be a legitimate reason for ordering a test?

6. In this situation, the patient seemed to be temporarily reassured by the test but indicated that he would want the same sort of reassurance again in the future. Do you think this attitude is common? What do you think this indicates about what the patient learned from the experience?

7. The patient illustrated his fear of malignancy by referring to a friend with similar symptoms and cancer. How do you think this form of reasoning affected the accuracy of his estimate of the likelihood of cancer? Can you think of other ways in which we may bias our estimates about uncertain events? (Hint: The article by Tversky and Kahneman cited in the selected bibliography is very helpful.)

SELECTED BIBLIOGRAPHY

Child, A. W., and Hunter, E. D. (1972). Non-medical factors influencing use of diagnostic x-rays by physicians. *Med. Care 10*:323–35.

Sinclair, W. K. (1981). Effects of low-level radiation and comparative risk. *Radiology 138*:1–9.

Slovic, P., Fischhoff, B. and Lichtenstein, S. (1980). Facts and fears: understanding perceived risk. In *Societal Risk Assessment: How Safe Is Safe Enough?* (R. C. Schwing and W. A. Albers, Jr., eds.), pp. 181–214. New York: Plenum.

Sox, H. C., Jr, Margulies, I., and Sox, C. (1981). Psychologically mediated effects of diagnostic tests. *Ann. Intern. Med. 95*:680–5.

Tversky, A., and Kahneman, D. (1974). Judgement under uncertainty: heuristics and biases. *Science 185*:1124–31.

Tversky, A., and Kahneman, D. (1981). The framing of decisions and the psychology of choice. *Science 211*:453–8.

# TECHNOLOGY AND SPECIALIZED HEALTH CARE

CASE 15

# BIRTH:
# ELECTRONIC FETAL MONITORING

MIRIAM D. ORLEANS and ALBERT D. HAVERKAMP

### WHAT DOES EFM DO

Electronic fetal monitoring (EFM) is a means of continuously recording the fetal heart rate and uterine contractions. This can be achieved through external monitoring, in which a Doppler belt with an ultrasonic flow rate meter is strapped over the mother's abdomen. The internal method requires rupture of the membranes in order to place an electrode directly upon the fetal scalp. The electrode is passed through the cervix and twisted to embed it in the fetal scalp. The use of this technique requires that the patient be in labor; otherwise, induction must occur. EFM records both the infant's heart rate and the mother's uterine contractions on a graph.

Historically, fetal heart rate was followed (and today still can be followed) by auscultation, which involves listening to the fetal heart rate with a stethoscope placed against the mother's abdomen. A similar, more recent method is the use of a hand-held Doppler ultrasonic flow rate meter that magnifies the fetal heart tones so that they are easily heard. Both auscultation and the use of the hand-held Doppler meter require personal attendance to the patient, because the tones must be counted by an observer. These earlier techniques do not provide continuous information, as does EFM. EFM is a more accurate diagnostic technology than either the Doppler method or auscultation.

There is a long-held belief among obstetricians that a number of perinatal outcomes can be improved by improving intrapartum management. The three outcomes that have been principal targets are (1) the reduction of intrapartum deaths or stillbirths, (2) the reduction of mental retardation, and (3) the reduction of cerebral palsy. Research evidence shows that most fetal deaths do not occur intrapartum. In the United States Collaborative Perinatal Study, the total incidence of intrapartum fetal deaths was found to be 4.4 per 1,000 live births.

303

Among infants weighing more than 2,500 g, the incidence of intrapartum fetal death was only 1.5 per 1,000. Low birth weight infants, then, account for the larger fraction of the incidence of intrapartum deaths. However, low birth weight infants constitute 8.2 percent of all births. The implication is that in a small number of cases, the monitor might be useful if it revealed information that made it possible to reverse a morbid condition or save low birth weight infants from death.

In the mid-1970s, it was suggested by some writers that 50 percent of the cases of mental retardation might be averted by the use of EFM. However, actual studies of the severely mentally retarded show that there are only 3 to 4 per 1,000 children with intelligence quotients below 50 who have suffered a bio-logical insult to the brain. Among those children only 10 percent are damaged by events at the time of birth – including labor itself.

Cerebral palsy tends to occur among 2.5 per 1,000 school-age children; this incidence is found in most Western countries. It has been estimated that 20 to 40 percent of cerebral palsy cases are the result of intrapartum hypoxia, which means that most cerebral palsy occurs for other than intrapartum reasons. Al-though there are some intrapartum events with deleterious effects that can be identified by EFM, in terms of their low incidence one must ask whether they are sufficient to warrant the current almost universal monitoring of low-risk mothers with good health and pregnancy histories.

Using EFM, excellent infant outcomes are obtained. However, in all of the five randomized prospective trials of EFM, the use of monitoring was accom-panied by an increased rate of intervention, particularly cesarean section.

In their roles as fetal advocates, obstetricians have employed increasingly complicated technologies such as EFM, amniocentesis, and ultrasound, along with an increased use of cesarean section as part of their effort to reduce intra-partum death and neurological damage.

The use of EFM to record fetal heart tones has greatly increased in the past decade. This trend has not been without controversy. EFM, which is available in almost every delivery room in the United States, is often routinely used. This has caused concern and reevaluation among members of the health professions and by the public. Questions concerning the efficacy of EFM, the extent of its benefit, the significance of the loss of "naturalness" of the delivery, and the need to monitor in order to protect professionals against malpractice suits are all being discussed in professional journals. To probe these issues, we present two cases.

## CASE 1

A 27-year-old woman with a second pregnancy has just arrived at the community hospital at term and in good labor. Her first delivery had been uncomplicated, and she had given birth to a healthy 7 1/2 lb boy. She asks not to be given intravenous fluids, does not want continuous EFM, and wants to walk around in labor. The nurses state that hospital policy requires electronic monitoring of everyone in labor. The patient responds that she did not need such monitoring before, and that her first pregnancy and delivery had gone very well. She was hoping for the same experience again. She appeals to the resident doctor in charge, who requests time to talk over the matter with other staff.

The house staff debates the issues. One doctor argues that the hospital policy is intended to maximize the safety of infants and thus is wise. Further, the evidence provided by EFM helps protect staff from accusations that the best care was not provided in the event of a bad outcome connected with the birth. Another doctor, who opposes the procedure, points out that the risks for the fetus without monitoring are extremely small with respect to either fetal distress or intrapartum death. Without monitoring in 1965, the intrapartum death rate was only 1.5 per 1,000 among all labors and among infants who weighed 5 1/2 lb or more. The mother's risk status is altered, however. The chances of delivering her baby by cesarean section appear to be increased. The doctor indicates that a careful British study of low-risk patients revealed a doubling of the rate of cesarean section from 4.4 to 9 percent when EFM was used. If this woman is allowed to labor with reasonable surveillance of her infant, and if the obstetric unit has the capability to resuscitate the infant if an unexpected event occurs, she argues, the risks are indeed very low for mother and infant. What would you do, taking account of the desires of the mother, the health of the baby, the costs of care, the malpractice issue, and the experiences of obstetric house staff?

### CASE 2

A 27-year-old woman carrying her second child has had her pregnancy complicated by diabetes that started when she was 10 years old. She also has hypertension and renal disease. She is now 37 weeks pregnant. In her last pregnancy, she had a stillborn infant from an abruptio placenta at 38 weeks. Now she has developed preeclampsia along with her diabetes. An amniocentesis showed that the fetus has mature lungs. Her cervix is dilated to 2 to 3 cm, a pitocin drip is begun to induce labor, the membranes are ruptured, and it is learned that meconium is present. The resident recommends that a direct scalp electrode be placed on the fetus.

The woman is reluctant to have the EFM. The resident in charge tells his staff that given the presence of severe maternal disease and major risks for the infant, EFM is warranted. Before EFM, he explains, a preemptive cesarean section would have occurred, as the risks for the infant were seen as too great. With EFM, one can follow a labor involving a woman with severe medical and obstetrical problems, but if the fetal heart rate pattern is reassuring, the infant is well. In this case, EFM would help the doctor in deciding to allow a vaginal delivery and avoid a cesarean section, which would be complicated in a diabetes patient with preeclampsia. But another staff member urges that given the situation, one shouldn't "fool around" with EFM, but instead go immediately to cesarean section. What would you do in this situation (1) if you were the patient's doctor and had these facts? (2) if you were the patient and were told these facts?

## SELECTED BIBLIOGRAPHY

Banta, H. D., and Thacker, S. B. (1979). Assessing the costs and benefits of electronic fetal monitoring. *Ob/Gyn. Surv. 35*:627–42.

Goodlin, R. C., and Haesslein, H. C. (1977). When is it fetal distress? *Am. J. Obstet. Gynecol. 128*:440–7.

Haverkamp, A. D., Orleans, M., Langendoerer, S., et al. (1979). A controlled trial of the differential effects of intrapartum fetal monitoring. *Am. J. Obstet. Gynecol. 134*:399.

Kelso, A. M., Parson. R. J., Lawrence, G. T., et al. (1978). An assessment of continuous fetal heart rate monitoring in labor. *Am. J. Obstet. Gynecol. 131*:526–32.

Neutra, R., Fienberg, S. E., Greenland, S., (1978). The effect of fetal monitoring on neonatal death rates. *N. Engl. J. Med. 299*:324–6.

Quilligan, E. J., and Paul, R. H. (1975). Fetal monitoring, is it worth it? *Obstet. Gynecol. 45*:96–100.

Renou, R., Chang, A., Anderson, I., et al. (1976). Controlled trial of fetal intensive care. *Am. J. Obstet. Gynecol. 126*:470–6.

# THE PREMATURE INFANT:
# PROGNOSTIC DILEMMAS FOR
# PARENTS AND PRACTITIONERS

I. DAVID TODRES

T is a 5-hour-old, premature infant, weighing 900 g (2 lb), who is experiencing severe breathing difficulties in a New England community hospital. He is the first child born to an 18-year-old mother. The infant is blue because of inadequate oxygenation, and has started to have seizures because of lack of oxygen to his brain.

The condition he is suffering from is known as *hyaline membrane disease*. It is a life-threatening condition, and sophisticated medical technology is required to monitor his disease and provide lifesaving therapy. This requires transporting the infant to a medical center (neonatal intensive care unit) where the special technology exists and skilled personnel are available to apply it.

The pediatrician taking care of the infant is administering oxygen to sustain his life. The pediatrician informs the parents that the infant is critically ill and may not survive. The best solution is to provide him with further intensive care in a special unit at a nearby medical center. Should the infant survive, there is a strong possibility that he may be permanently handicapped mentally and physically as a result of a period of oxygen deprivation to his brain. The parents are uncertain about pursuing vigorous therapy, afraid of the possibility of having a "bad baby." They feel overwhelmed by the situation and passively accept the recommendation of the physician and nurses to transport the infant to the major medical center for further care. Dr. J, the pediatrician who has just met Mrs. J for the first time, reassures her that all will be well.

An emergency transport team is summoned from the neonatal intensive care unit. Doctors and nurses are dispatched in an ambulance with a special incubator designed to take the infant from the community hospital safely back to the neonatal center. This incubator will maintain the infant's body temperature within a normal range. In addition, special cardiac and respiratory monitoring devices are attached to detect any critical changes. An infusion pump designed to administer very small, precise volumes of fluid to the infant is available. Special emergency equipment is taken along.

At the community hospital, the team assesses the infant's condition. Increasing respiratory difficulty now necessitates the insertion of an endotracheal tube, which passes into the windpipe. A blood sample is sent to the laboratory and confirms the clinical impression of deteriorating lung function, as evidenced by decreasing oxygen tension and increasing carbon dioxide tension. Because of the infant's failure to breathe adequately on his own, a device is attached to the endotracheal tube and the infant is ventilated to compensate for his inadequate breathing. With the breathing problem under control, a special catheter is placed through the umbilical stump into the umbilical artery and threaded up into the aorta. The catheter is taped in position, and dextrose water is infused through it. An x-ray is taken of the chest to determine the nature of the respiratory difficulty and to verify the position of the endotracheal tube. In addition, an x-ray of the abdomen confirms the correct position of the umbilical artery catheter.

The umbilical catheter is connected to the infusion pump. The infant is placed in the transport incubator. A mechanical respirator now replaces the manual breathing device used in the emergency situation. The infant is transported safely to the newborn intensive care unit.

Radio communication from the ambulance has alerted personnel to the expected arrival of the infant and his special needs.

Once in the newborn intensive care unit, the infant is placed on a special table with an overhead infrared heating device to maintain his body temperature constant via a skin sensor probe.

Artificial ventilation is continued through a mechanical respirator, and a paramagnetic oxygen analyzer intermittently checks the appropriate amount of oxygen delivered to the infant. A transcutaneous oxygen electrode (a heated skin electrode, which measures oxygen diffusing from the bloodstream through the skin) continuously monitors oxygen levels in the blood. Heart rate, respiration, and blood pressure are constantly monitored through pressure transducers on an oscilloscope.

Intermittently, catheters are passed through the endotracheal tube, and suctioning of secretions is carried out. This is vital, as buildup of secretions may block the tube and endanger the child's life. A dedicated team of physicians and nurses is involved in the infant's care. In addition, a large support system attends to the special needs of the infant and family. Radiologists are consulted daily, as x-ray examinations of the infant's chest are vital in the assessment of any developing complications. Multiple blood tests are performed by technologists, who analyze these micro-samples in an adjacent laboratory. In addition, a team of specially trained respiratory therapists closely monitors the effects of the mechanical respirator and adjusts the device according to the infant's clinical needs. The social service department is actively involved in helping the parents to keep in touch with their sick infant. The social service worker has analyzed the Js' ability to cope emotionally and financially with the future care of their infant. Mr. J is 20 years old and unemployed. To the social worker, the parents appear to be incapable of appreciating the responsibility for future care, especially with a strong possibility of brain damage. She wonders whether efforts to save the life of this infant are "appropriate."

For 3 days, T has made excellent progress. He still requires the mechanical ventilator, but his own spontaneous breathing efforts are improving, and it is expected that he will be weaned from the ventilator on the fifth or sixth day of life.

Suddenly, on the fourth day of life, T's condition takes a turn for the worse. His symptoms suggest that he has suffered an intracranial hemorrhage, which sometimes occurs in very ill, low birth weight infants and is responsible for much morbidity and death.

To verify the diagnosis, special tests are carried out. A lumbar puncture is performed with a needle, and a sample of cerebrospinal fluid is taken. Analysis of the fluid shows it to be blood-stained.

An ultrasound device is now passed over the infant's head and demonstrates the presence of an intraventricular bleed. Further confirmation of this condition is obtained by performing a computerized axial tomography (CAT) scan.

The parents are informed of this, and told that this bleed may seriously affect their infant's neurological status. With potentially serious damage already present, additional damage must be considered. The physician and nursing team begin to raise questions about the wisdom of continuing to support the infant. The medical student member of the team begins to challenge his colleagues, stating, "You appear to be more interested in making machines work and keeping organs functioning better than doing what's best for the baby." There is a sense of uncertainty among the physicians and nurses. How much damage has already taken place? How much more has been added?

The neurology consulting team has been involved. At this stage in the development of the case, and with a limited understanding of the human brain, it is very difficult to prognosticate with reasonable certainty. Left with this uncertainty, the physicians and nurses feel obligated to continue to support the infant, owing it to the child to give him the benefit of the doubt. The parents do not appear to comprehend the gravity of the situation.

One of the residents on the physician's team feels that a decision should be made not to pursue further vigorous therapy. She believes that this decision should be made by the health care team and that the parents are too young and inexperienced to do so. In addition, she states: "They would feel awfully guilty doing this for the rest of their lives."

QUESTIONS FOR DISCUSSION

1. Without the application of special technology, the infant would certainly die. What causes us to use machines because we are able to operate them, rather than selecting special situations in which the machine is appropriately applied? Given T's initial story and his family situation, was the use of technology appropriate (a) at the start and (b) following the brain hemorrhage?
2. Who should decide to begin to apply this lifesaving technology? What is the role of the pediatrician, nurse, and family in this situation? Should the director

of the neonatal intensive care unit triage the admission? If the unit is filled to capacity and a more viable infant requires admission, should treatment for T continue, and who should make that decision?

3. Should technology be utilized to its ultimate conclusion, or is there a point at which we must decide that the technology is not fulfilling its therapeutic purpose? How do we know when we have reached this point? Having raised these issues, who decides whether to continue to pursue heroic therapy, or withdraw it and apply comfort and care measures to the patient? Should experimental devices and drugs be employed when all acceptable medical therapy has failed?

4. T's condition is precarious. Further intracranial hemorrhage may lead to cardiac arrest. The issue of resuscitation is discussed among the medical and nursing personnel and with T's parents. His parents are concerned that resuscitating him would only bring back a hopelessly damaged child. The physicians and nurses express uncertainty. There is no technology available that can predict the outcome with certainty, although advances in technology continue to resolve some of the present uncertainties. Where does one draw the line on further resuscitation procedures? At what point is an infant considered to be hopelessly damaged? Can this judgment be scientifically quantified?

5. From an ethical standpoint, how should the parents' youth, and their social and financial status, enter into an evaluation of whether to strive to keep the infant alive? From the viewpoint of ethics, should the ability of the technology to sustain this baby's life, independent of its likely quality, be the principal criterion in the clinical decision? If not, what should be?

### SELECTED BIBLIOGRAPHY

Duff, R. S. (1981). Counseling families and deciding care of severely defective children: a way of coping with "medical Vietnam." *Pediatrics 67*:315–20.

Duff, R. S., and Campbell, A. G. M. (1973). Moral and ethical dilemmas in the special nursery. *N. Engl. J. Med. 289*:890–4.

Jonsen, A. R., Phibbs, R. H., Tooley, W. H., et al. (1975). Critical issues in newborn intensive care: a conference report and policy proposal. *Pediatrics 55*:756–68.

Ramsey, P. (1979). *Ethics at the Edges of Life.* New Haven: Yale University Press.

Shaw, A. (1973). Dilemmas of "informed consent in children." *N. Engl. J. Med. 289*:885–90.

Todres, I. D., Krane, D., Howell, M. C., et al. (1977). Pediatric attitudes affecting decision-making in defective newborns. *Pediatrics 60*:197–201.

*Editor's note*: For a discussion of U.S. government guidelines published in 1984, concerning the treatment of infants with severe disabilities, see "Procedures relating to health care for handicapped infants." *Federal Register*, vol. 49, pp. 651–4, January 12, 1984.

# NEUROLOGICAL DISORDERS: DECISION ANALYSIS AND THE PATIENT'S WORKUP

ARTHUR S. ELSTEIN, JOHN I. BALLA, MARILYN L. ROTHERT, and DAVID R. ROVNER

The objectives of this case are:

1. To introduce decision trees and the method of averaging out and folding back to choose a clinical strategy. The choice between skull x-rays and computed tomography (CT) scan in cases of traumatic head injury serves as an example of a more general evaluation logic.
2. To demonstrate that laboratory tests and diagnostic procedures can be rationally selected, and that not every available procedure needs to be ordered to evaluate a problem accurately and efficiently.
3. To introduce some of the issues in technology assessment and the proliferation of expensive technology.
4. To introduce public health and economic perspectives by considering the social and economic costs of illness.
5. To provide opportunities for discussion and exploration of thoughts and opinions regarding the provision of medical services to patients whose lifestyles may be distasteful or who are viewed as self-destructive, and to explore related ethical issues.
6. To examine our prevalent system of reimbursing more generously for medical procedures than for histories and physical examinations, and to offer opportunities for reflecting on the possible effects of this policy on the utilization of technology.

## THE CASE: MR. B

It is Saturday evening, January 9, 1984. You are a first-year resident in internal medicine who is called to the emergency room of a 300-bed county hospital at about 10 P.M. to see Mr. B. He is a 58-year-old man who is well known to the emergency room staff and the local police because he is frequently brought in drunk. The police state that they "picked him up off the street" and want him "checked over" before they take him to jail to "sleep off his binge."

He is disheveled, loud, and abusive, reeking of alcohol, the front of his shirt stained with vomitus. He is placed in a room, shouting obscenities, thrashing about and kicking, accompanied and restrained by two police officers.

You arrive at 10:30 P.M. By this time, Mr. B appears to be sleeping and is difficult to rouse. The vital signs are as follows: temperature 100 F, pulse 98 and regular, respiration 16, and blood pressure 120/76. Meanwhile, a nurse has obtained three older emergency room records for the past 2 months on Mr. B; he was brought in twice by "good samaritans" while severely intoxicated, once for examination after being "rolled" by youngsters. She related that he frequently comes to the emergency room inebriated and disoriented, but tonight he seems more hostile than usual. An orderly who usually gets along with him is unable to calm him down tonight. The police remain with the patient.

1. What immediate steps should be taken to prevent potential brain injury?
2. What significant information from the history and physical examination can be rapidly obtained that help you manage this patient?

You find Mr. B's blood pressure and pulse to be unchanged. His breathing appears to be regular, with snoring respirations, so you insert an oral airway and administer oxygen via a nasal cannula at a rate of 2 liters/minute. You draw blood for laboratory studies, start an intravenous (IV) line, and administer 50 ml of 50 percent dextrose IV. There is no response, but his condition appears to be stable. You approach the police in an effort to obtain information that might be helpful to you.

The police state that they found Mr. B at 9:30 P.M. propped against a mailbox on a street near his hotel room. He was loud and obscene, so one of the local tenants had called the police to remove him. He has been known to the police for about 15 years, is often brought to jail for vagrancy while intoxicated, and usually stays there until he sobers up and goes to court. The police have noticed him becoming more confused and forgetful over the past 2 to 3 months, and these officers feel that his behavior tonight is not characteristic of him. Mr. B has no known family, is sometimes employed as a day laborer, lives in a local hotel room, and receives general assistance. The police are unaware of any serious medical problems and/or medications, although one officer thinks he may have "sugar." They have no knowledge of any recent trauma.

3. What are the most likely causes of this patient's altered state of consciousness? Estimate the probability of each. Keeping these in mind, on what specific factors should the physical examination be focused?

### Physical examination

*General.* The patient is a 58-year-old, thin, unshaven, unwashed man who appears to be older than his stated age. There is a strong odor of alcohol from the patient, and he appears to be sleeping. He responds to being shaken and having his name called loudly by groaning.

*Respiration*. His respiration rate is 16, and appears to be regular, with occasional deep sighs.

*Eyes*. The pupils are small–dilated 2 mm, round, equal, and react to light. The patient does not cooperate in the test for pupillary accommodation. Doll's eye movements are present. Funduscopic examination reveals questionable blurring of the right disc margin, but is otherwise normal.

*Motor responses*. There is spontaneous movement of all limbs but the left arm. Pressure on the supraorbital ridge results in movement of all limbs. Passive resistance to limb movement is present bilaterally.

*Reflexes*. Deep tendon reflexes are 2+ on the right and 3+ on the left (on a scale of 0 to 4+). The Babinski sign is absent on the right side but present on the left.

*Head*. No trauma is noted.

*Neck*. The neck is supple. Carotid bruits are not heard.

*Chest*. The lungs are clear to auscultation.

*Heart*. The rate is 90, with a regular rhythm. No murmurs, S-3, or S-4 sounds are heard.

*Abdomen*. The abdomen is soft, without masses. Active bowel sounds are heard. The liver is firm and palpable 4 cm below the right costal margin.

4. How do these physical findings change the probabilities for each problem on the list?
5. Should a skull x-ray be done *at this time*? Under what circumstances do skull x-rays provide useful information? (What is the usual cost of a skull x-ray?) Suppose a skull fracture is demonstrated in this patient. How would the treatment and management change as a result of this information?

You call the attending physician to let her know what is going on, as well as a neurosurgeon for consultation.

By 1 A.M., you have arranged for Mr. B's admission to the intensive care unit and are awaiting the arrival of the neurosurgeon. The nurse alerts you that the patient's clinical status is deteriorating. You examine Mr. B and find a blood pressure of 160/100, pulse 68, and respirations rapid and deep. He does not respond to his name, and is responsive only to deep noxious stimuli, with decorticate posturing on the left side of the body. The right pupil is dilated 10 mm and fixed, unresponsive to light. The left pupil is dilated 4 mm and responds to light. Funduscopic examination shows a blurred right disc margin. The right eye is deviated outward and is unresponsive to head turning. The left eye is normal.

6. Of what significance are these findings?

You administer 50 g mannitol by IV push. A Foley catheter is inserted. Decadron, 6 mg, is then given IV. A rapid diuresis occurs over the next 30 minutes.

At 1:30 A.M., reexamination shows Mr. B to have regular respiration. The right pupil is dilated 4 mm and responsive to light. The left pupil is dilated 2 mm and responsive to light. Doll's eye movements are absent. Caloric stimulation causes the patient to groan and exhibit avoidance movement.

7. What is the significance of this reexamination?

The neurosurgeon and radiologist arrive. You explain the situation thus far. Several tests might be done, but time is pressing and the situation is reasonably urgent. They ask you for your views about the advisability of several procedures.

8. Consider the following diagnostic procedures: cerebroarteriogram, CT scan, radionuclide scan, pneumoencephalogram, lumbar puncture and spinal fluid examination (cell count, glucose, protein, and gram stain only; cultures would add to the cost), electroencephalogram, skull x-rays, and electrocardiogram. Develop a rationale for ordering or omitting each. Consider the costs of the tests, their invasiveness, and their contribution to a treatment decision.

A CT scan is ordered, and the radiologist on duty interprets it at 6 A.M. It shows a large right subdural hematoma. Mr. B is taken to the operating room immediately. Emergency burr holes are placed in the biparietal areas, yielding a large right subdural hematoma. Within minutes of evacuation of the hematoma, Mr. B becomes alert. Your subsequent neurological evaluation reveals no deficit. The rest of his stay in the hospital (7 days) is uneventful.

9. Suppose you are a physician on a committee responsible for developing a protocol for managing traumatic head injuries in your community hospital. The committee is considering three strategies:
   a. Operate on everyone with a history of head trauma.
   b. Do a neurological examination on all patients with a history of head trauma; then do a CT scan only on patients with abnormal neurological findings. Operate only on patients with abnormal CT scans.
   c. Do skull x-rays on all patients with a history of head trauma; then do a CT scan on patients with fractures. Operate only on patients with abnormal CT scans.

Which of these strategies has the lowest expected mortality and highest expected survival? Which has the highest dollar cost? Which strategy would have the

Table 1. *Summary of charges for Mr. B's illness that will be paid by Medicaid*

| Procedure | Charges ($) |
|---|---|
| Test costs (write in your own) | ___ |
| CT scan (with report) | 290 |
| Operating room charges | 350 |
| Intensive care unit charges (2 days at $426 per day) | 852 |
| Regular hospital day charges (5 days at $180 per day) | 900 |
| Other hospital charges (per day for a surgical patient) | 72 |
| Emergency room charge | 45 |
| Emergency room physician's charges | 36 |
| Neurosurgeon's charges (consultation and surgery) | 1,500 |
| Radiologist's charges | 70 |
| Attending physician's charges | 170 |
| Pharmacy charges (IVs, anesthetic, mannitol) | 125 |
| Anesthesiologist's charges | 350 |
| Total charges | ___ |

greatest impact on other patients who might need neurosurgical services for other problems? What principles would you use in developing a protocol in your hospital?

Answer the first question by considering the decision trees in Figures 1, 2, and 3, and by averaging out and folding back.

10. With rising criticism that hospitals are acquiring too much high-cost technology, what community and social factors need to be considered in the purchase of expensive medical technology such as a CT scanner?

11. Suppose a CT scanner had not been available at this county hospital. How would you, as a physician, provide for your patient's care if a CT scan was

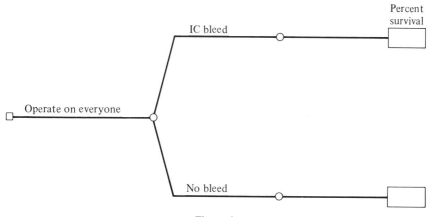

Figure 1

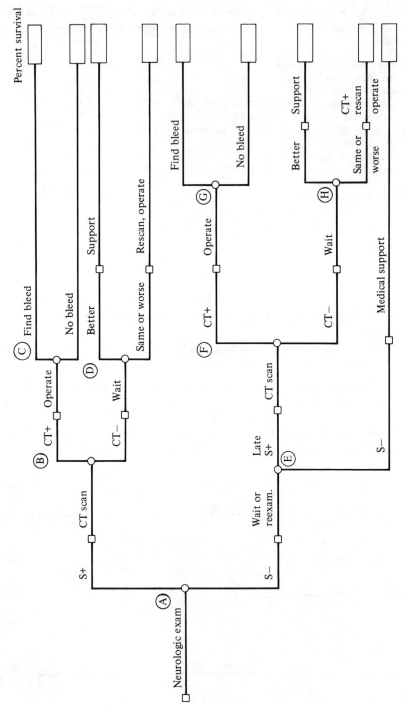

Figure 2

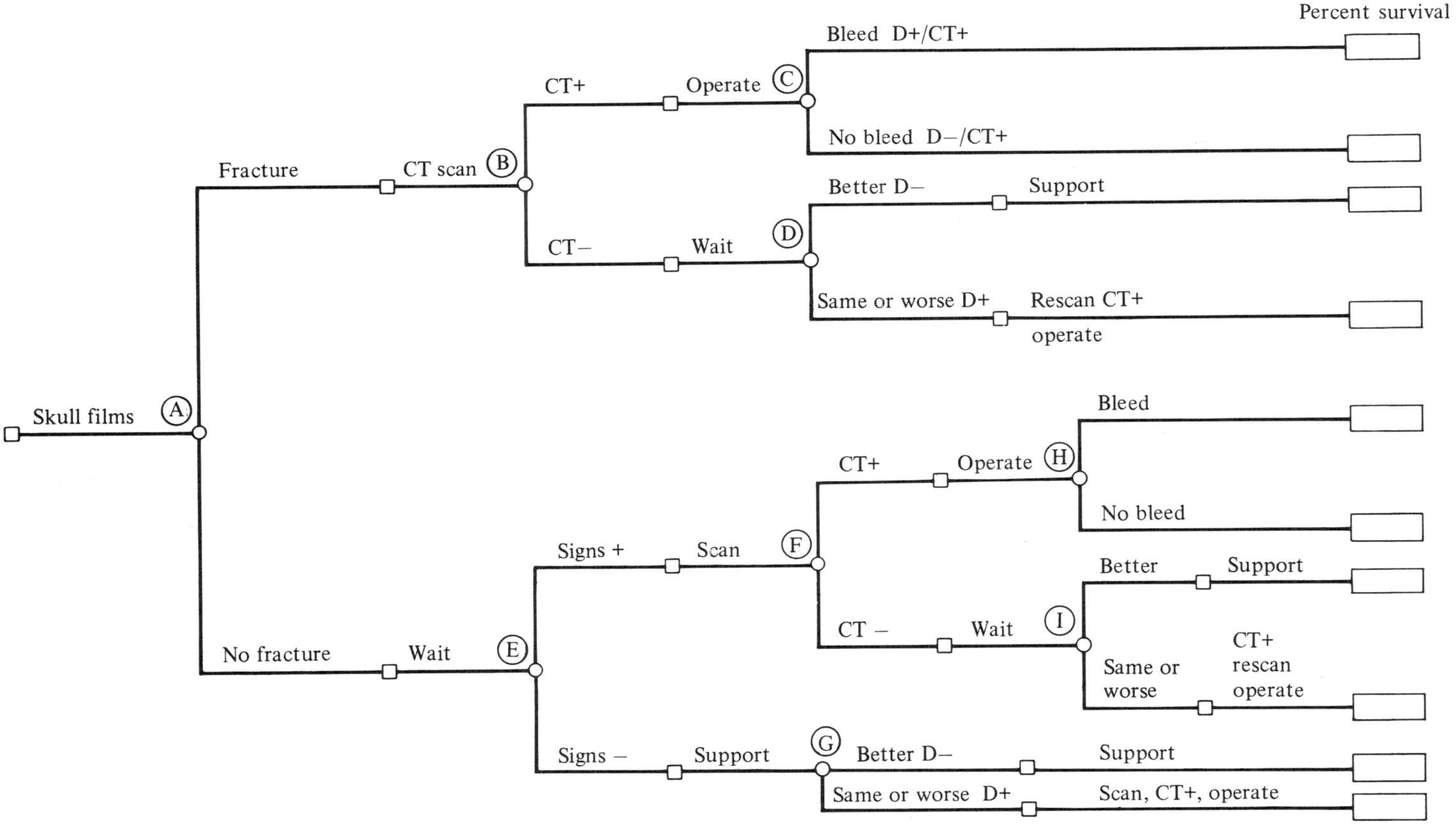

Figure 3

needed? What could hospital administrators do to make scanners more accessible?

12. Discuss the economic impact and costs of chronic alcoholism to society and the current approaches to the reduction of alcoholism.

13. Is there any need for, or way of providing, follow-up health care for Mr. B? Regular medical care? Alcohol treatment? Financing of his health care? What are the obligations of physicians, and of society in general, to provide health care services to patients such as this one? Do self-destructive patients have a right to health care?

14. Suppose that, instead of being an alcoholic, Mr. B is a busy physician who requires hospitalization for control of back pain that he has failed to treat conservatively at home because he is "too busy." Should his hospitalization insurance pay for this hospitalization when he has refused adequate home care?

15. a. Why is the neurosurgeon compensated at an hourly rate nearly 10 times that of the attending physician for his involvement in Mr. B's case?

    b. Some critics of the health care system have suggested that primary care physicians may be utilizing an increased number of unnecessary technological procedures (electrocardiograms, laboratory tests, x-rays, etc.) because such procedures are reimbursed at higher rates per hour of work than history taking, physical examinations, and patient education. Discuss this proposition.

### INTRODUCING UTILITY THEORY

In considering this case from a decision analytic standpoint, survival and death are treated as the dichotomous outcomes of any possible clinical strategy, and the value of any strategy is calculated in terms of the expected rate of survival. Of course, with head injury as with many other problems, matters are not always that simple, and the clinician may have to reckon with the possibility of survival in any one of a number of intermediate states of dysfunction. This case also introduces utility theory as a means of evaluating preferences for these intermediate states and states of function between total cure and death, and incorporating these evaluations into decision making. The case is expanded by considering five possible outcomes instead of the two used initially: cure with no significant residual disability, survival with moderate physical disability, survival with severe mental disability, persistent vegetative state, and perioperative death. Readers are asked to order these alternatives and then evaluate intermediate outcomes by the classic method of choices between gambles. The resulting utilities are incorporated into the decision trees of Figures 1, 2, and 3, and averaging out and folding back with utilities is introduced.

The case also introduces a discussion of the possibility that there are dysfunctional states that some people would evaluate as worse than death. In almost any group of 12 or more medical students, there is usually at least one who is prepared to rank a persistent vegetative state as the worst outcome, whereas others assert that as long as there is some hope of recovery, that state is preferable to death. Our case thus links the technical decision analytic considerations to discussions of ethical principles.

## CONCLUSION

As this brief discussion shows, the topics touched on span a wide range: emergency room treatment of head injury; CT scanning and the use and misuse of skull x-rays; introducing technology assessment; the use of decision analysis to evaluate clinical strategies; averaging out and folding back; the basics of utility assessment; and a brief glance at one of the more troubling ethical issues of our time – the possibility of survival in an extremely dysfunctional state that some might regard as worse than death. Our aim was to present these diverse topics in the context of a clinical case and thereby to demonstrate that decision analysis, technology assessment, and ethical problems are not simply topics for academic analysis but also touch ineluctably upon the clinical practice and social organization of health care.

### SELECTED BIBLIOGRAPHY

Balla, J. I., and Elstein, A. S.. Skull x-ray assessment of head injuries: a decision analytic approach. Submitted for publication.

Beck, J. R., (1982). Quantitative logic and new diagnostic tests. *Arch. Intern. Med.* *142*:681–2.

Bryden, J. F., and Jeannette, B. (1983). Neurosurgical resources and transfer policies for head injuries. *Bri. Med. J.* *286*:1791–3.

Galen, R. S., and Gambino, S. L. (1975). *Beyond Normality*. New York: Wiley.

Weinstein, M. C., and Fineberg, H. V. (1980). *Clinical Decision Analysis*. Philadelphia: W. B. Saunders.

# RESPIRATORY FAILURE: TECHNOLOGICAL CARE IN THE HOME AND HOSPITAL

KATHLEEN A. McCORMICK and FAYE G. ABDELLAH

### CASE REPORT

Mrs. J was a 45-year-old housewife with a husband on disability due to diagnosed coronary artery disease, a 16-year-old son with a delinquent record, and a 5-year-old mentally retarded daughter with inoperable congenital heart disease. Mrs. J was admitted to the hospital in severe respiratory distress. She had noticed shortness of breath with strenuous exercise 8 years prior to admission, which increased in severity over the next several years. She neglected her own medical needs because she was caring for her disabled husband and daughter. Two months prior to admission her symptoms worsened, and by the time of admission she was no longer able to perform her household duties, slept kneeling in a chair, and drank only fluids for nourishment.

On physical examination she was breathing rapidly. The patient was told by the doctor that it was necessary to insert a nasotracheal tube and control her ventilation with a volume-cycled ventilator, to begin intensive respiratory therapy, and to transfer her to the intensive care unit. The patient pleaded: "Please let me go home. We have no money to pay you. I have to go home to take care of my daughter and husband." The physician considered her behavior inappropriate, the result of a mental state created by the low oxygen and high carbon dioxide levels indicated by laboratory tests. He telephoned her husband, who agreed that his severely ill wife should be treated and signed all the consent documents.

Ventilatory support to the patient was complicated by several episodes of pneumonia. On the 19th hospital day, the patient's pulmonary impairment was incapacitating. It became apparent to the physician that unless an operation was performed to correct large bullae in both upper lung fields, the patient would have no improvement in gas exchange and would be unable to care for her family and home. Yet the outcome and rationale for the surgical procedure were uncertain (Brown et al. 1973).

The patient underwent surgery, and the operation was successful. Ventilation was assisted with a volume-cycled ventilator for 10 postoperative days. During this period, a dispute arose between the respiratory therapist and the physician concerning the appropriate time and manner of weaning the patient from the ventilator. In arguing their positions, each asserted a technical knowledge and a moral responsibility to the patient. They finally reached a mutually satisfactory decision. But the rancor troubled the staff, and the patient was aware of the dispute.

The patient's recovery was gradual, and she was ready for discharge to her home after 90 hospital days. She required supplemental oxygen, suction equipment, and ventilation assistance four times daily. For these needs, equipment was placed in her home and professional help provided to maintain her there. A visiting nurse called on the family weekly.

The total hospital bill was $250,798. The husband signed the house mortgage and his life insurance policy over to the hospital. The family would live on welfare and Medicaid assistance. The average monthly bill for oxygen in the home alone was $275.

Nine months after the patient's discharge from the hospital, her husband died from a heart attack. Her son, who needed money to support the family, was arrested for armed robbery 1 month later. The daughter died six months after the father. One year after the operation, the respiratory crippled woman was able to pursue her activities of daily living. However, 4 years after the surgery, Mrs. J finally succumbed to the complications of her illness. The cause of death was respiratory failure.

ISSUES

"Life-prolonging," "lifesaving," "life-supporting," and "life-controlling" are the phrases describing the history and equipment specifications of ventilators. Prolonged, controlled ventilation outside the operating room began during the Scandinavian poliomyelitis epidemics in the 1950s. By the 1970s the applications had greatly expanded, and the ventilator became an important tool in the treatment of a variety of disorders. The use of ventilators involves a number of difficult issues: (1) who has the right to refuse a ventilator; (2) how to manage patients on ventilators; (3) economics; and (4) home care and nursing home treatment. Each of these issues is commented on briefly, followed by questions for discussion.

### Refusal to put a patient on a ventilator

Such a refusal, when long-standing disease is present, or in an emergency situation when a respiratory arrest occurs, has been described in the legal and ethical writings related to *no-code orders*. Legislative concern arising from dilemmas involving ventilator technology have resulted in "right to die or natural death acts," which permit individuals considered competent to outline in living wills the circumstances under which they would allow life to be prolonged with life-sustaining equipment, and which discuss the rights of a person who has a terminal condition in relation to life-sustaining measures that would prolong the process of dying. When a patient is not competent, is unconscious, or is a minor, the family or guardian may need a court order for a no-code or no-treatment order (Memel and Lemkin 1978; Cushing 1981). How would you have treated Mrs. J's request not to be put on the ventilator? Knowing the outcome of the case, would you say that the decision to treat was a good one from the patient's, the family's, and society's perspectives?

## Managing patients by the team approach

In this approach, which has been described in the literature since 1971, the role of the doctor is the diagnosis and management of the disease (Petty 1971). The continuum of care rests with the nurse (Bushess 1973; McCormick and Birnbaum 1974; Nett 1974). The physical therapist teaches patterns of breathing while weaning patients off the ventilator, and performs chest physiotherapy for patients on the ventilator. The respiratory therapist provides clean, adjusted, and technically safe equipment at the patient's bedside and monitors the volume, pressure, and time of respiration.

Patients on mechanical ventilators require extensive monitoring. The elements monitored and the persons often accountable for the measurements are listed in Table 1. But the functions of team members in the intensive care unit often overlap. This group must understand the importance of hospital procedures, accuracy in the communication of doctors' orders, monitoring of patients, and delivery of treatments.

Analogous to the issue of patient care management is role clarification for team members and knowledge of the specialized care required for patients who need ventilator technology. For over 20 years ventilators have been used to treat severely ill hospitalized patients; yet, articles in the literature still appear that ask "Does the MA-1 Respirator Make You Nervous?" (Moses and Steinberg 1979). Hospital surveys show that inservice programs to train nurses in intensive care techniques increased 379 percent between 1973 and 1976 (Kralovec 1978). In this case, on what grounds could the respiratory therapist justify pressing her position against that of the doctor? Discuss the general problems of assigning technical and moral responsibility for patient care when it is fragmented among such a diverse group of personnel.

## The cost for respiratory care services

One study estimates such costs account for as much as 20 to 30 percent of the expenses of all hospitalized patients (American Association of Respiratory Ther-

Table 1. *Management of patients on ventilators: team responsibilities in monitoring*

| Element monitored | Responsible person(s) | | | |
|---|---|---|---|---|
| | Physician | Nurse | Respiratory therapist | Physical therapist |
| Tidal and minute volumes | X | X | X | |
| Airway pressures | X | X | X | |
| Skin color | X | X | | |
| Level of consciousness | X | X | | |
| Vital signs | X | X | X | |
| Oxygenation | X | X | X | |
| Carbon dioxide | X | X | X | |
| Humidification | X | X | X | |
| Airway patency | X | X | X | |
| Congestion | X | X | | |
| Infection | X | X | | |
| Fluids | X | X | | |
| Posture | X | X | | X |
| Adequate nutrition | X | X | | |
| Medication administration | X | X | | |
| Physiotherapy | X | X | | X |
| Elimination/catheters | X | X | | |
| Cardiac output | X | X | X | |
| Alveolar-arterial $O_2$ difference | X | X | X | |
| Psychosocial milieu | X | X | | |
| Electrocardiogram | X | X | | |
| Blood withdrawal | X | X | X | |
| Weaning | X | X | X | X |
| Auscultation/percussion | X | X | | |
| Weight | X | X | | |
| Compliance (lung and chest wall) | X | X | X | |
| Oxygen consumption | X | X | X | |
| Dead space ventilation | X | X | X | |
| Functional residual capacity | X | X | X | |
| Diffusion capacity | X | X | X | |
| Cardiopulmonary resuscitation | X | X | X | |
| Equipment safety | X | X | X | |

apy 1981). To train new graduate nurses to function in a technological intensive care environment costs about $9,500 compared to about $5,700 for recruiting, hiring, orienting, and inservice training for a new nurse in a nonintensive care environment (Wagner 1980). Discuss from the perspective of the patient and family in this case, and from the viewpoint of society, the $250,000 medical care bill for Mrs. J's illness: Was it fair to require the family to sign over the home's mortgage and the husband's life insurance to the hospital? Examine the economic and ethical issues of seeking to reduce medical costs in general.

## Home and nursing home facilities

Health care teams provide services to patients in need of ventilator support in the home, skilled nursing homes, intermediate care facilities, and hospices. The patients in these settings require personnel with skills to maintain safe respiratory equipment and assess its adequacy, and to provide simple and minimally expensive therapy. Out-of-hospital types of equipment include humidification devices, nebulizers, ventilators, suction apparatus, mechanical vibrators and percussors, and in special situations, rocking beds, phrenic nerve stimulators, and apnea alarms (George 1977; American Lung Association 1978). A recent survey of Medicare-funded health care costs revealed that durable medical equipment (which includes oxygen and ventilators) accounted for 50 percent or $100,000,000 of the home health care costs it paid (Janssen and Saffran 1981).

According to the 1977 National Nursing Home Survey, 15 percent of nursing home residents have chronic respiratory disease, and 50 percent of nursing home patients require intensive nursing care including oxygen administration (Van Nostrand 1979). This survey did not include data concerning the use of ventilators in these populations. For patients with chronic lung disease who need ventilatory and oxygen therapy at home, the costs ranged from $250 to $450 per month in 1978 (Gessner 1978). In this case, what might have been done through home services to improve the outcome for this family? What are the general social and medical implications of transferring technological care from the hospital to the home?

In the future, new ventilators will provide servo-control by sampling the patient's end-expired carbon dioxide in order to adjust the minute volume, and a microcomputer attached to them will give staff quick access to review the patient's profile and calculate pulmonary physiological variables (Mushin et al. 1980). However, these new technologies, like the older ones, will continue to present health professionals with complex ethical, legal, economic, educational, and management problems resulting from their use.

### SELECTED BIBLIOGRAPHY

A committee report of the American Association of Respiratory Therapy. (1981). Approaches to the review of respiratory therapy services: Technical assistance document. *Resp. Care 26*: 460–78.

American Lung Association. (1978). Respiration care services in skilled nursing facilities and intermediate care facilities. A report. New York, unpublished paper.

Braun, S. R., do Pico, G. A., Birnbaum, M. L. et al. (1973). Bullae and severe generalized disease: successful treatment with bullectomy. *J. Thorac. Cardiovasc. Surg. 65*:926–9.

Bushness, S. S. (1973). *Respiratory Intensive Care Nursing*. Boston: Little, Brown.

Cushing, M. (1981). "No code" orders: current developments and the nurse director's role. *J. Nurs. Admin. 11*:22–9.

George, R. B. (chairperson, ATS Respiratory Therapy Committee). (1977). Home use of equipment for patients with respiratory disease. *Am. Rev. Respir. Dis. 115*:893–5.

Gessner, D. M. (1978). New developments in oxygen-therapy equipment for home use. *Respir. Ther. 8*:2951, 58.

Janssen, R. J., and Saffran, G. T. (1981). Reimbursement for durable medical equipment. *Health Care Financ. Rev. 2*:85–96.

Kralovec, P. (1978). Survey shows increase in hospital training programs. *Hosp., J.A.H.A. 52*:173–80.

McCormick, K. A., and Birnbaum, M. L. (1974). Acute ventilatory failure following thoracic trauma. *Nurs. Clin. North Am. 9*:181–94.

Memel, S. L., and Lemkin, J. W. (1978). The legal status of "no code orders." *Hosp. Med. Staff 7*:1–8.

Moses, R. M., and Steinberg, S. (1979). Does the MA-1 respirator make you nervous? *R.N. 42*:34–44.

Mushin, W. W., Rendell-Baker, L., Thompson, P. W., et al. (1980). *Automatic Ventilation of the Lungs*, 3rd ed. London: Blackwell Scientific Publications.

Nett, L. (1974). The use of mechanical ventilators. *Nurs. Clin. North Am. 9*:123–36.

Petty, T. L. (1971). *Intensive and Rehabilitative Respiratory Care*. Philadelphia: Lea & Febiger.

Van Nostrand, J. F., Zappola, A., Hing, E., et al.: (1979). *The National Nursing Home Survey: 1977 Summary for the United States*. Series 13-No. 43, DHHS No. (PHS) 79-1974. Hyattsville, Md.: National Center for Health Statistics.

Wagner, D. L. (1980). Nursing administrators' assessment of nursing education. *Nurs. Outlook 28*:557–61.

# HEART DISEASE:
# THE ETHICAL QUANDARIES OF
# TREATING THE AGED

ERIC J. CASSELL

Mr. W was 84 years old. His wife was alive, and he was enjoying the material advantages of a productive life and the personal satisfaction of having raised a family of loving and successful children. Two years earlier, the diagnosis of polymyalgia rheumatica had been made, and he remained on very low-dose steroids. Mild hypertension was being controlled with a thiazide diuretic. Despite these two problems, he considered his health excellent until a Sunday in May, when, while eating breakfast, he lost consciousness. He regained consciousness and was alert again within a few moments. Everyone attributed the spell to exertion on the previous day. One week later, while going to the bathroom, he fell to the floor unconscious; again he recovered within moments and felt "like new."

He went to see his internist accompanied by his son. Detailed questioning failed to reveal a similar history, any clear-cut precipitating episode, or any neurological symptoms. On auscultation of his heart, as in past examinations, a moderately loud decrescendo systolic murmur was heard. Otherwise his physical examination revealed only a healthy man who appeared to be younger than his years. The doctor said that he was not sure what the trouble was; such events were not uncommon as one aged. "Why not wait a little bit, and see what happens before we do any tests, or anything."

Within the next 3 weeks, the patient suffered three more episodes of syncope, one of which occurred in a supermarket. In separate telephone conversations with the patient and his son, the physician suggested that the time had come for further tests, and both of them quickly agreed. Arrangements were made for an echocardiogram and a 24-hour electrocardiogram (Holter monitor) to be done by a cardiologist.

The echocardiogram showed moderate calcific aortic stenosis. The 24-hour electrocardiogram did not provide an explanation for the syncope. The cardiologist who did the studies told the patient that there was "something the matter with a heart valve, but it's not very important; some medication ought to take care of things.'' The patient told his son about the conversation, asking whether the son knew what that meant.

After the tests, the son called to ask about the results. The physician explained that the stenosis of the aortic valve might be the source of Mr. W's syncope. If that was the case, the doctor continued, eventually one of the episodes would probably be fatal (there was a 1-year mortality of about 50 percent). The only treatment of known effectiveness was surgery to replace the tight valve. However, before surgery could be considered, a cardiac catheterization would be required to provide further information about the disease and the possibility of operation. However, both the doctor and the patient's son were loath to broach the subject of surgery to the patient, and they elected to do another Holter monitor study in the hope that an abnormality of heart rhythm would be found that might have escaped detection on the first occasion. They agreed that the test would give them more time to think about the decision. ''Besides, W will know we're doing something.''

At this point, we will present two different scenarios of what followed.

### SCENARIO 1

The second Holter study was also negative. The son, after thinking about the matter, refused to let the physician discuss the possibility of surgery with his father. The son had heard all about heart operations (indeed, his father-in-law had died during cardiac surgery in 1963), and he wanted nothing to do with them. The doctor offered to discuss the various probabilities in detail. He planned to show the son how greatly things had changed since 1963 and to use modern decision analysis to help in making things clear.

The son finally agreed to have his father participate in the discussions, and Mr. W took the same position: He refused to consider cardiac surgery or catheterization. Mr. W said that he understood the risks and was not afraid of dying. Within 2 months, he was admitted to the hospital because of chest pain. The entire history was known to the house staff, including his continued refusal of cardiac catheterization. While there, he suffered a cardiac arrest. He was resuscitated, but did not regain consciousness. He was maintained on a respirator and intravenous fluids for 72 hours before he suffered an arrest again and died.

### SCENARIO 2

Mr. W agreed to enter the hospital for cardiac catheterization, but said that he did not think he would ever permit surgery. The cardiologist believed that it was unlikely that the patient's syncope was due to the aortic stenosis, because of the presence of hypertension. He felt that a demonstration of hemodynamically *unimportant* valvular disease would allow refocusing on an arrhythmia as the cause. Cardiac catheterization had an extremely low mortality at his hospital, and he thus felt justified in using this approach, which might speed up the diagnosis. Further, the cardiologist thought that he could interest the cardiac electrophysiologist in the case, so that after the catheterization, sophisticated studies of cardiac conduction could be done that might reveal the difficulty.

At the time Mr. W was hospitalized, a study was in progress comparing cardiac catheterization with radionuclide cineangiography. Mr. W was asked to participate, and after carefully reading the consent form, he agreed. The radionuclide cineangiogram appeared to confirm the cardiologist's opinion that aortic valvular stenosis was not the problem, but the staff went ahead with plans for the cardiac catheterization. Others argued that the finding on the radionuclide cineangiogram obviated the need for catheterization.

The cardiologist's opinion prevailed, and to everyone's surprise, the cardiac catheterization demonstrated a tightly stenotic aortic valve. Once again, the patient was approached on the question of surgery. By now, Mr. W was so intrigued and impressed by all the interesting things that he had experienced in the hospital that he had changed his mind about being operated on. The chances of his dying or being disabled by the operation were presented in detail. It did not occur to his physicians to discuss with him the long period of convalescence usually experienced by patients of his age. One of the reasons that Mr. W was willing to take the risks of surgery was his fear that he would otherwise be forced to give up the active life he cherished.

Mr. W underwent surgery, and his aortic value was successfully replaced. He gradually resumed his activities but was never quite as vigorous as he had been preoperatively, in part because his family was so protective of him. Two years later, a pacemaker was implanted by the same surgeon because of recurrent bradyarrhythmia. The following year he began to show signs of organic mental syndrome, and because his family was unable to care for him, he was admitted to an extended-care facility. He died in the nursing home at age 88.

QUESTIONS FOR DISCUSSION

## General questions

1. Why did the physician deal with the patient's son (a common occurrence when the patient is aged) as well as with the patient? Did this imply that aging itself changes one's autonomy and competence? Was the fact that the son was paying a portion of his father's bills a consideration? Should it have been?

2. Should the cardiologist who performed the electrocardiogram and echocardiogram have told the patient about the findings? Does the information "belong" to the patient, to the person performing the tests, or to the patient's physician?

*Questions referring to Scenario 1*

3. The physician planned to use a systematic decision analysis method in evaluating the appropriateness of surgery. Should such a method be seen as a procedure or a technology insofar as it influences therapy and patient care? When physicians use decision analysis or make statistical inferences, are they obliged to seek consent, as if for a new operation, test, or drug?
4. a.  In Scenario 1, should resuscitation attempts have been made in view of the patient's previous refusal of definitive therapy?
   b.  Since cardiac arrest might have been expected, given the patient's history, should the issue of resuscitation have been discussed with the patient, his family, or both?

*Questions referring to Scenario 2*

5. If the cardiologist believed that the catheterization would yield negative results, was he justified in exposing the patient to the small risk involved?
6. If catheterization was being done in order to offer the electrophysiologist a more attractive case, should the patient have been informed of this reason?
7. The result of the radionuclide cineangiogram was treated by some as reliable. How thoroughly must the sensitivity and specificity of a new test be established before it enters clinical practice? Should the results of a new test be revealed to a patient when the meaning of those results remains in doubt?
8. What is the obligation of those who are conversant with technology in regard to "selling" its capabilities? Is the physician obliged to protect the patient from decisions based on the patient's enthusiasm for the technology, or from the doctor's own enthusiasm for a procedure?
9. Should the long convalescence period have been included in the physician's discussion of the risks of cardiac surgery?
10. Were all of these technological interventions worthwhile?

### SELECTED BIBLIOGRAPHY

Cantor, N. L. (1977). A patient's decision to decline lifesaving medical treatment. In *Ethics in Medicine: Historical Perspectives and Contemporary Concerns* (S. J. Reiser, A. S. Dyck, and W. J. Curran, eds.), pp. 152–72. Cambridge, Mass.: MIT Press.
Cassell, E. J. (1976). Permission to die. In *Dilemmas of Euthanasia* (J. A. Behnke and S. Bok, eds.), pp. 121–31. New York: Anchor Press.
Cassell, E. J. (1976). *The Healer's Art*. New York: J. B. Lippincott, pp. 164–82.
Edmund-Davies, L. (1977). The patient's right to know the truth. In *Ethics in Medicine:*

*Historical Perspectives and Contemporary Concerns* (S. J. Reiser, A. S. Dyck, and W. J. Curran, eds.), pp. 235–38. Cambridge, Mass.: MIT Press.

Mayerson, E. W. (1976). *Putting the Ill at Ease*. New York: Harper & Row, pp. 97–126, 249–69.

McCormick, R. A. (1976). To save or let die. In *Bioethics* (T. A. Shannon, ed.), pp. 123–34. New York: Paulist Press.

Meyers, D. W. (1975). The legal aspects of voluntary medical euthanasia. In *Dilemmas of Euthanasia* (J. A. Behnke and S. Bok, eds.), pp. 51–67. New York: Anchor Press.

Reiser, S. J. (1978). *Medicine and the Reign of Technology*, New York: Cambridge University Press, pp. 174–95.

Saunders, C. M. S. (1977). Telling patients. In *Ethics in Medicine: Historical Perspectives and Contemporary Concerns* (S. J. Reiser, A. S. Dyck, and W. J. Curran, eds.), pp. 238–40. Cambridge, Mass.: MIT Press.

# REHABILITATION:
# THE DECISION TO REPLACE
# A HUMAN FUNCTION WITH A MACHINE

RUTH B. PURTILO

## THE PATIENT

Mr. C, a 56-year-old motel owner and manager in a small town, suffered a stroke. Initially, he was comatose. Six months later, he is still paralyzed on the left side, and is unable to walk because of spasms in his left arm and leg. He has some perceptual difficulty that is manifested when he attempts to guide his wheelchair. He is right-handed, so that he can feed and almost completely dress himself. He needs assistance in getting on and off the toilet.

During the 6-month rehabilitation course as an inpatient, he has shown gradual improvement in functioning. However, during the last 2 weeks his condition has plateaued, and a decision has been made to discharge him. He will return home to be cared for by his wife, a healthy, vivacious woman in her early 50s. They will hire a part-time nurse to assist her in the morning and evening, and he will continue to be seen as an outpatient. Mr. C states that he intends to return to his position in the motel. His wife maintains that she will take over the business and that he will have to stay at home, because he cannot possibly manage it in his present condition.

The medical rehabilitation team is meeting to discuss his discharge. A question has arisen as to whether or not Mr. C should be given an electric wheelchair. The team is split in its judgment. Some believe that it will increase his motivation to continue his rehabilitation efforts; the others maintain that it will reduce his continuing efforts to achieve independent ambulation. They also fear that he will develop decubitus ulcers (bed sores) or a renal infection, because there will be less motivation for him to change positions often. Not only are bed sores and kidney infections extremely expensive to heal, in some instances they are life-threatening to an already vulnerable individual such as Mr. C. Mrs. C worries that the electric wheelchair will be a sign to her husband that he must give up his hope of ever walking again: "He'll take it as a signal that he's been written off." She is completely opposed to the idea. He says, "All I know is that I have to get back to work or I'll ... " and he makes a gesture of slitting his throat.

The reader enters the story at the moment when a group of well-meaning and discerning health professionals are trying to make a sound clinical judgment about what is best for Mr. C. On the surface, the discussion focuses on a practical consideration: the effect of a technological device on the continued progress of a patient. But beneath the surface rhetoric is a matrix of deep-seated assumptions and projections about the effect of this technological aid on the quality of life of a man whose very identity seems to be at stake. In this relatively simple case example, the reader catches a glimpse of how the effect of medical technology spreads from physical questions into the realm of human values, and how technology affects a patient who has a condition such as stroke requiring long-term rehabilitation services. Not only does stroke rank near the top of disabling conditions (Sahs et al. 1976a), but an estimated 2,750,000 persons in the United States today have suffered a stroke some time in the past; of these, 1,110,000 have required long-term services (Sahs et al. 1976b).

## IMMEDIATE AND BROADER FUNCTIONS OF TECHNOLOGICAL INTERVENTION

The rehabilitation team responsible for planning Mr. C's discharge is committed to ensuring that he not lose the gains he has made during his rehabilitation. In medical circles, the term used to describe the loss of recovered function is *deconditioning*. It occurs when the body, already in a debilitated state because of conditions such as stroke, again starts to break down. Failure to take strict precautions leads to such a relapse in rehabilitated patients, with the reappearance of acute symptoms and, in extreme cases, death. Health professionals must provide appropriate instruction, encouragement, medications, follow-up visits, and technological devices to ensure that this discharged stroke patient can continue to enjoy the fruits of his efforts and to improve his functioning.

### Lifesaving versus quality of life-enhancing intervention

Members of Mr. C's rehabilitation team express different opinions on whether an electric wheelchair is indicated. One group views the wheelchair as a mechanical mood elevator and a source of motivation to improve. The other group, supported by Mrs. C, views it as an impediment – a mechanical sedative leading to lethargy at best, and possibly to severe deconditioning in the form of contractures or bed sores. Some technologies are interventions that enhance the quality of life, whereas others are lifesaving. The group in favor of using the wheelchair argue that the device has no direct bearing on Mr. C's mortality, but will enable him to live a fuller life. However, it is viewed by the second group as posing a threat to life, and is rejected by them on these grounds.

### Technology and the rehabilitation setting

Traditionally, the term *lifesaving* has been reserved for dramatic interventions such as a heart-lung machine or a defibrillator. Presuming that the second group's perception of the wheelchair's power to affect life and death is correct, their position demonstrates that mundane interventions such as a wheelchair may sometimes have such implications. Devices that affect deconditioning should be treated as seriously as the more dramatic technologies. To do less is to underestimate technology's power.

#### TECHNOLOGY AND THE INDIVIDUAL

Considering the immediate and long-term effects of a technology helps health professionals to decide why they strongly support or oppose a given intervention, and whether other technologies can better deal with the patient's hopes, dreams, skills, illusions, and fears. In the example of Mr. C, the following types of information may be relevant as means of individualizing his treatment:

1. The relationship between Mr. and Mrs. C: how the decision will affect their interaction at home
2. Mr. C's idea of what it means to be in a wheelchair
3. How Mr. C spent his leisure time before the stroke
4. Mr. C's activities at work
5. The C's home: architectural and other barriers to his movement with or without an electric wheelchair

#### QUESTIONS FOR DISCUSSION

1. In health care, lifesaving technology is often defined in the narrow sense of being high-cost interventions for acute conditions. How could the terms and concepts surrounding a health professional's understanding of lifesaving technology be expanded or modified to include less dramatic applications of technology?
2. In what ways does our present language about technology influence our attitudes toward different types of patients? That is, do you think that a patient whose life could be "saved" by applying an expensive lifesaving technology is more valued than one whose signs and symptoms require less dramatic measures?
3. Do you believe Mr. C ought to have an electric wheelchair? Which of the following factors do you think would significantly influence your judgment if you were a member of the rehabilitation team?

    a. Mr. C's age

    b. Mr. C's residual physical impairment

    c. Mr. C's ability to pay for the wheelchair

    d. Mrs. C's judgment about what she thinks is best for her husband

    e. Your own experience with a wheelchair

4. What other factors would significantly influence your judgment? Give reasons why each of the factors you would consider legitimate ought to be accepted by the others involved in this decision.

## SELECTED BIBLIOGRAPHY

Anderson, T. P., and Kottke, F. J. (1978). Stroke rehabilitation: a reconsideration of some common attitudes. *Arch. Phys. Med. Rehabil.* *59*:175–80.

Burke, T. R. (1975). A survey and critical evaluation of long-term care reimbursement policies under medicaid. *J. Long-Term Care 3*:1-15.

Chaudhuri, G. (1980). Rehabilitation of the stroke patient. *Geriatrics 35*(10):45–54.

Childress, J. F. (1977). Priorities in the allocation of health care resources. In *No Rush to Judgement.* (David H. Smith, ed.), pp. 129–48. Indianapolis: Poynter Center.

Dahlberg, C. C. and Jaffe, J. (1977). *Stroke: A Doctor's Personal Story of His Recovery.* New York: Norton.

Granger, C. V., and Green, D. S. (1975). Measurement of outcome of care for stroke patients. *Stroke 6*:4–9.

Haber, L. D. (1966). Identifying disability: concepts and methods in measurement of disability. *Report No. 1. Social Security Survey of the Disabled.* Washington, D.C.: U.S. Government Printing Office.

Hyman, M. (1971). The stigma of stroke: Its effect on performance during and after rehabilitation. *Geriatrics 26*:132–41.

Hyman, M. (1972). Social-psychological determinants of patient's performance in stroke rehabilitation. *Arch. Phys. Med. Rehabil. 53*:217–26.

Knowles, J. H. (1977). Introduction. In *Doing Better and Feeling Worse: Health in the United States.* (John H. Knowles, ed.), pp. 1–8. New York: Norton.

Labi, M. L., Phillips, T. S., and Greshman, G. E. (1980). Psychosocial disability in physically restored long-term stroke survivors. *Arch. Phys. Med. Rehabil. 61*(12):561–5.

McCall, S. (1976). Human needs and the quality of life. In *Values and the Quality of Life* (J. K. Farlow and W. R. Shea, eds.), pp. 6–24. New York: Science History Publications.

Purtilo, R. B. (1976). Similarities in patient response to chronic and terminal illness. *Phys. Ther. 56*:279–84.

Purtilo, R. B. (1979). A just medical care delivery and the "permanent patient": The severe stroke patient as a test case. Ph.D. dissertation, Harvard University Graduate School of Arts and Sciences, Cambridge, Massachusetts.

Robbins, S. (1976). Stroke in the geriatric patient. *Hosp. Pract. 11*:293–7.

Sahs, A. L., Hartman, E. C., and Aronson, S. M. eds. (1976a). *Guidelines for Stroke Care.* Washington, D.C.: U.S. Government Printing Office, p. 18.

Sahs, A. L., Hartman, E. C., and Aronson, S. M., eds. (1976b). *Report of the U.S. Joint Committee for Stroke Facilities.* Washington, D.C.: U.S. Government Printing Office, p. 358.

# CASE 21

# MULTIPLE INJURY:
# BURNS AND HEROIC MEASURES

## JANET A. MARVIN

A 28-year-old highway patrolman involved in a high-speed chase rolled his vehicle and was trapped in the burning car. Firefighters and paramedical personnel arriving at the scene had to extinguish the fire before medical care could begin and the patrolman be extracted. While rescue personnel were working to release him, paramedics secured his airway by intubation and started intravenous fluid therapy. The extraction procedure took approximately 15 minutes after the fire was extinguished.

When the patient arrived at the hospital, he had a stable blood pressure, was breathing spontaneously with an orotracheal airway tube in place, and was noted to have sustained a 47 percent total body surface area (TBSA) burn, almost all of which was a full-thickness injury. The burn involved his face, ears, scalp, hands, and lower extremities. The patient had also sustained an open fracture of the left knee and concussion to the head, lacerations of the lips with loss of two teeth, and laceration of the gingiva. Should the patient, with an injury that will lead to severe disfigurement and disability and a high likelihood of mortality, be vigorously resuscitated? Who should be involved in the decision?

After additional stabilization procedures in the emergency department, the patient was taken to surgery for debridement and closure of the left knee injury by the orthopedic surgeons, repair of the lip and gingival lacerations by the maxillofacial surgeons, and escharotomies of the right and left arms and hands by the burn/plastic surgeons. During these procedures, the patient received 2 units of blood, the first of approximately 50 units he was to receive over the next 2.5 months.

Upon completion of the surgical procedures, the patient was admitted to the burn intensive care unit. The care in this specially designed unit was aimed at: (1) control of infection by strict isolation techniques; (2) resuscitation of the patient with large volumes of intravenous fluids; (3) monitoring of the patient's hemodynamic status with continuous measurements of cardiac electrical function, cardiac output, and pulmonary artery pressure monitoring; and (4) management of the patient's deteriorating pulmonary status due to the effect of smoke inhalation with mechanical ventilation.

In addition, the patient's nutritional needs were estimated to be 4,000 to 4,500 kcal per day, including 165 to 180g of protein per day. To meet these needs in a patient who could not eat at first and who would not eat later in his course of treatment, intravenous alimentation and tube feeding were required. Without adequate caloric and protein intake, poor wound healing and infection become major complicating factors.

Wound care for this patient included twice daily hydrotherapy treatments, with painful debridement and exercise therapy. In addition, special splints were made to maintain his hands in the best position for eventual rehabilitation and function. This patient probably had the worst hand and face burns of any patient admitted to the burn center in 3 to 4 years (in a unit that admits about 350 patients per year). Therefore, wound care was more difficult for the staff than usual, because of the perceived problems with long-term disfigurement and disability.

On the fourth day after injury, the patient was taken to the operating room for the first of a series of excision and grafting procedures. The burns on the patient's legs and right arm were excised, and autografts were taken from all available donor sites. This yielded about 3,000 cm$^2$ of autograft. In addition, approximately 1,000 cm$^2$ of homograft (cadaver skin) were used to complete the grafting of the excised areas. At this time, wires were inserted in the distal part of each digit on both hands to allow the hands to be positioned in a metal basket-type apparatus know as a *hay rake*, which allows for maintenance of proper hand position for optimal function. Continued problems with exercise and position for maintenance of function challenged the ingenuity of the physical and occupational therapist.

By the eighth postburn day, the patient seemed to be much improved and no longer needed the aid of the endotracheal tube. Dressing changes on that day showed that about 75 percent of the skin grafts had survived. Although this was encouraging to the staff, the patient continued to require heavy sedation for pain, and began to show signs of depression and frequent periods of disorientation. Although wound cultures remained negative, infection and sepsis were always a concern. Intravenous catheters were changed every 3 days to prevent sepsis, even though this was time-consuming for the staff and often painful for the patient. Strict adherence to isolation techniques increased the time required to care for the patient.

By the 11th day after injury, it was noted that as the dead tissue from the patient's head began to separate, large areas of the bony skull were exposed. On the 15th day after injury, the patient was beginning to ask questions about the future, and about how his face would look and how his hands would heal. Although there was much support from family members and friends, as well as the staff, family members suffering from the stress began to argue among themselves. The patient began to express concerns about whether he really wanted to survive. At this stage, how would you treat a request by the patient to discontinue therapy, if you were a member of the hospital staff?

A psychologist began working with the patient and staff to prepare them for the upcoming surgical procedures for his face. Progress notes from the psychologist warned that ''attempts to show the patient pictures of other burn patients or the use of mirrors so that he can see his own face would be ill advised at present. Too much information, too soon, and an inadequate opportunity to process this information could easily overwhelm the patient and/or increase suidical ideations.'' What would you recommend if the patient now insisted on seeing how he looked?

The social worker continued to work with the family to resolve the interpersonal problems and help them understand their responses to the stress. Efforts were made to have only certain members of the health care team interact with the family in order to eliminate confusion and misinformation. Family conferences were planned frequently with the primary attending physician, primary nurse, social worker, and psychologist to provide the necessary information about the patient's progress and answer their questions.

On the 17th postburn day, the patient was taken back to the operating room for excision and homografting of the face, including both eyelids, nose, cheeks, forehead, and upper and lower lips. At this time, a halo (metal frame) was attached to the patient's skull to prevent pressure on its posterior aspects. Two days later, the patient was again taken to the operating room for autografting of the face and application of a specially fabricated face mask. The mask was used initially to immobilize the face grafts, and later to apply pressure to reduce scar formation and maintain the normal commissures of the face.

On the 25th postburn day, the patient became septic, with a pseudomonas infection in the ungrafted wounds. He was treated with large doses of antibiotics, excision of the remaining infected eschar, and temporary closure of these areas with homograft. The patient began to improve slightly about the 30th postburn day. Over the next week, he improved to the point where he was again lucid and began to eat small amounts while continuing to be fed intravenously and with tube feeding. The patient's family was encouraged by his progress, but tension among family members continued.

On the 50th postburn day, the patient had another episode of sepsis, at which time he aspirated his tube feedings and required reintubation and management on the ventilator, as well as antibiotic therapy for several days. After this episode, the patient continued to improve. On the 65th postburn day, the patient returned for more debridement of his scalp and debridement and grafting of areas on his chest and hands. On the 75th postburn day, the patient had more debridement and grafting of his hands. At this time, the bony tips of several digits on each hand required amputation. This was one of the more traumatic surgical procedures for the patient and his family, who finally had to face the fact that he would have limited use of his hands and would not be able to return to his original occupation as a highway patrolman.

Over the next 6 weeks, the patient had two additional operative procedures for grafting of small open areas on his hands. In addition, he developed a bone infection at the site of the original fracture, which required two operative procedures. After almost 4 months in the hospital, the patient was transferred to the rehabilitation unit, where he began to regain his independence and be trained so that he could accomplish the activities of daily living. In addition, psychological counseling continued to be provided, and with the help and assistance of his employer, he was retrained for a job in communications for the State Patrol.

After almost 7 months in the hospital, the patient returned home to resume life with his wife. For 5 to 6 months the patient continued to require outpatient physical therapy, splinting to maintain function, and appliances to adapt to his home and work environment. He and his wife continued to require psychological counseling. Although he was eventually able to return to work, the physical and emotional scars remain. One year after his accident, he has hands with which he can grasp, but no fine movements because he has lost all the digits except two on one hand and all the digits except his thumb on the other hand. The grafted areas of his face healed with an acceptable cosmetic result, but his entire scalp was eventually grafted, so that he has no hair. His ears were also severely burned and are now gone. He has had a hairpiece made that looks very similar to his original hair, as well as artificial ears that make his facial appearance more acceptable. In fact, his facial appearance is more acceptable than his nurses, physician, and therapist ever dreamed possible during the first 2 months of his care.

Consider the cost of the care of such a patient in monetary terms (the original hospital bill was in excess of $120,000 in 1981 dollars), in personal time and stress, and in the utilization of precious resources such as blood, homograft, and other items in short supply, and the outcome for the patient. Was the decision to begin and continue this therapy wise in this case?

## SELECTED BIBLIOGRAPHY

Bernstein, N. R. (1976). *Emotional Care of the Facially Burned and Disfigured*. Boston: Little, Brown.

Childress, J. F. (1979). Bioethics: the burn victim and medical paternalism. *New Physician 28*(8):37–8.

Imbus, S. H., and Zawacki, B. E. (1977). Autonomy for burned patients when survival is unprecedented. *N. Engl. J. Med. 297*(6):308–11.

# GASTROINTESTINAL ILLNESS:
# THE HUNGER FOR CERTAINTY

HOWARD M. SPIRO

A 55-year-old man, previously always vigorous, over the past 2 months noticed pain in the middle of his abdomen, in the epigastrium. At first, he ignored it. As it became more insistent, he found that it was present at night, worse when he lay flat on his back but less when he sat up, and less still when he leaned forward. At times the pain seemed to be worse after he ate, and upon reflection, he noted that his appetite was not as keen as it had been. Weighing himself one day, he found that he was 10 pounds lighter than he had ever been over the previous 10 years. Otherwise, he felt fit. He worried about the pain but hoped it would go away. After about 2 months, when he could no longer deny that the pain was becoming more pervasive and even radiated to his upper back, he called upon his physician.

The physician examined him after considering the possibilities that the story raised. There seemed little doubt to the clinician that the story was classic for a pancreatic tumor; the nature of the pain, its persistence, and the conditions that relieved or worsened it made a retroperitoneal lesion seem most likely. Little else could simulate a disorder in that location, aside from two other not uncommon possibilities – chronic pancreatitis or a retroperitoneal tumor, a lymphoma. Because the patient was not an alcoholic, chronic pancreatitis did not seem to be a reasonable consideration, for this condition occurs almost exclusively in alcohol abusers. The possibility of a retroperitoneal lymphoma also seemed unlikely after the physical examination; apart from some tenderness in the midepigastrium, the physician found nothing amiss. He could feel no palpable nodes, and the liver and spleen were not enlarged. Indeed, the physical examination added nothing to the physician's considerations. He could not feel the gallbladder in the right upper quadrant as a globular mass, a finding that would have indicated that carcinoma of the pancreas had already obstructed the common bile duct, causing the gallbladder to swell.

The likely diagnosis, pancreatic tumor, seems obvious from the history and physical examination. It remains for the physician to prove by diagnostic techniques what the history has suggested. Ten years ago, in such circumstances, the physician would have been likely to admit the patient to the hospital for rapid assessment, knowing that the most expeditious way of confirming the diagnosis and relieving the patient as rapidly as possible was to act on each test ordered sequentially with a logical plan. As the result of each study was obtained, the physician had immediate access to it, and could review it, explain the next step to the patient, and then choose the next study most likely to give help.

In contrast, practitioners today order a barrage of tests all at once, the so-called data base, because the cost of each hospital day is so enormous. The other major change in the diagnostic approach has been the remarkable increase in the number and variety of diagnostic images the physician can now obtain to help predict what an operation will disclose and to see on film what the patient has already reported. The rapid development of technological diagnostic aids in the past decade, the imaging revolution, has prevented too rigid an approach; changes have occurred so quickly that no one has had a chance to assimilate them. In the flush of enthusiasm and with a wish to be up-to-date and to assess all the new images, physicians have tended to adopt a somewhat uncritical attitude and striven to obtain all of them, with little regard for cost.

The next diagnostic step in a case such as this is to obtain laboratory data, usually a routine SMA-12 or SMA-24. With a specific diagnosis in mind, fewer tests could be ordered, and few indeed are necessary, but they are all available and can be obtained automatically by checking off one box on a form. The more tests that are easily available, the more are carried out. Liver function studies offer a particularly good example of excess information given and received because it is "cheap." In the 1980s, in the jaundiced patient at least, most liver function studies have become less useful than they once were, having been supplanted largely by the imaging studies to be discussed. However, because the full range of liver function studies, and many others besides, are obtainable by checking one box, all of them are ordered. This happens despite the fact that the partition of serum bilirubin into conjugated and unconjugated fractions is of help in very few clinical situations, and that the lactate dehydrogenase (LDH) universally found in every SMA-12 test, has almost no value to the clinician interested in the liver – or, for that matter, the heart. Yet these tests are ordered, dutifully reported, and ignored, and tradition carries on.

In the laboratory assessment, the physician looks for indirect evidence that the pancreatic tumor has begun to obstruct the bile duct, at least slightly. A rise in the alkaline phosphatase level or even the bilirubin level will give such a clue. The presence of such obstruction will support the probability of a pancreatic tumor, but its absence will not change the diagnostic approach, at least in the mid-1980s. The clinician will also look for a rise in the amylase or lipase level as evidence that the pancreatic duct is obstructed. In the patient under discussion, other chemical tests are also available, but the only one of diagnostic significance is the blood sugar level. Any evidence of diabetes would further incriminate the pancreas, and in the patient under discussion would make the diagnosis of a pancreatic tumor almost inevitable.

Let us suppose that the laboratory tests show that the patient is not anemic, that his alkaline phosphatase level is elevated to about twice normal, and that his amylase and lipase levels are slightly high. Basically, the clinician's diagnosis has now been confirmed by numbers, because the chemical test results fit the clinical setting. Ten years ago, the physician next would have ordered a barium study of the stomach and duodenum to try to see, however vaguely, the outlines of a swollen pancreas. Almost no other diagnostic studies would have been available, requiring a serious consideration of exploratory laparotomy to confirm the diagnosis and to decide on a course of action. Today, however, the physician tends to follow each diagnostic clue separately and sometimes exhaustively. I consider this to be the partial result of the so-called problem-oriented approach, which divides up the clinical complaints so that each one can be analyzed separately, without any synthesis. However, I also believe that this is done because the physician is taught in medical school to abhor uncertainty and follow everything down to the last diagnostic test, and because synthesis of the diagnostic process is no longer emphasized. What seems logical, indeed irrefutable, must be depicted visually if it is to be believed, and if the physician is to be satisfied and considered up-to-date.

Of physicians tempted, at this stage of the diagnostic process, to operate on the patient under discussion, it would be said that time has passed them by, that they have not kept up with the latest technology. Impressing one's peers is an important reason for the multiplication of studies. Therefore, it is likely that the practitioner will fractionate the alkaline phosphatase to be sure that it is not arising from bone, as it well might be in an older person, instead of from the bile ducts, and ignoring the fact that its elevation fits in beautifully with the other formulations.

It is likely that while these laboratory tests have been ordered, the patient will have been sent for an ultrasound examination of the pancreas and bile ducts. This study may show dilated intrahepatic bile ducts, conceivably some dilatation of the common bile duct itself, and possibly evidence of tumor spread to the liver. Depending upon the technical resources available and the visual acuity of the person reading the images, the head of the pancreas may or may not seem enlarged. If the ultrasonographer reports only the "crow's-foot" enlargement of the intrahepatic bile ducts, and indicates that he or she cannot see the entire extent of the common duct or any evidence of tumor in the liver, and cannot rule out a mass in the pancreas, the clinician then has the choice of several different diagnostic approaches.

In terms of time, the most economical study is endoscopic retrograde cholangiopancreatography (ERCP), the passage of an endoscope into the duodenum, and a catheter into the common bile duct and the pancreatic duct, to depict the sites of obstruction and, by implication, to prove the presence of a tumor, and possibly even to take a biopsy of the tumor. Indeed, such an examination is doubly indicated in this patient to exclude the possibility, which is reasonable so far, that the supposed pancreatic tumor is actually a tumor of the ampulla arising at the duodenal exit of the pancreatic duct. This tumor is worth detecting because it is more amenable to long-term surgical care than is the usual pancreatic tumor.

The tests more likely to be chosen, however, because they are noninvasive (even if less specific), and therefore usually justified in a clinical setting where cost is not yet a serious consideration, and where the clinician delights in being up-to-date, are computed tomography and possibly a disofenin scan. This latter radionuclide study gives a functional view of the liver and biliary tree, and can show evidence of obstruction, although at this writing it does not depict the cause of the obstruction. Computed tomography will probably prove to be more useful than ultrasonography in delineating lesions of the pancreas, but hospital cost commissions have, mistakenly I believe, restricted the widespread use of this instrument because of its high cost. Currently, at least in Connecticut, where I practice, computed tomography is not as freely available as it ought to be.

At this writing, there is much debate about the specificity of images and the preferable technique, with results depending – as has already been suggested – upon the kinds of patients studied and the techniques most favored at various institutions. At any rate, ERCP will ordinarily be deferred because it is invasive and unpleasant, until the physician has scrutinized the results of the easier but less reliable noninvasive images.

Let us assume that the disofenin scan shows partial obstruction of the common bile duct and that computed tomography suggests a tumor in the head of the pancreas, confirming the presence of dilated bile ducts. Now that the physician has undeniable evidence that his clinical assessment is correct, several paths are available along the diagnostic route. These will depend upon the physician's convictions, the aggressiveness of the surgeon who has by now been called in to follow the patient along with the physician and – let us hope – the patient's preferences.

If the physician believes, contrary to all published evidence, that some pancreatic carcinomas are curable by operation, then he or she may choose to send the patient for exploratory surgery to determine whether this can be done, a procedure to which the surgeon will usually agree. Most surgeons will try to resect a pancreatic tumor unless there is extensive spread, but that choice does not concern us here. Let us assume, instead, that the physician is of a more scholarly bent and proceeds along the slower imaging diagnostic path in order to be certain of the patient's condition. At this juncture, the physician can now choose between transhepatic cholangiography – the passage of a needle through the skin and liver into the bile ducts to depict more clearly the nature of the obstruction at the distal end of the bile duct, although not its cellular characteristics – or the aforementioned ERCP. Some surgeons claim that seeing the upper border of the tumor at transhepatic cholangiography is more important to planning an operation than any histology that may be found by ERCP, but internists and gastroenterologists generally prefer using the ERCP route to learn the histology if possible.

Let us assume that the patient has undergone ERCP, that it proves obstruction of the bile duct and the pancreatic duct at sites classic for carcinoma of the pancreas, but that biopsies prove to be impossible or at least unhelpful. Once again, several choices can be made, always assuming that the physician has kept the patient well informed.

At this point, the physician can elect to find out whether the radiologist can pass a needle directly through the body wall into the tumor detected at computed tomography or ultrasonography, in order to confirm the diagnosis histologically before considering operation, or can choose surgery. Increasingly, physicians and surgeons want as much certainty as possible before laparotomy, adding each diagnostic study for its minimal increment to their certainty and justifying it with the argument that "you would want your mother to have all these studies before she underwent an operation." So it is likely that the patient will undergo a preoperative percutaneous biopsy in an attempt to prove the nature of the tumor and to plan the surgical attack. From 6 to 15 needle passes may be made in an attempt to retrieve tumor cells, but the results of such cytologic biopsy studies depend upon the skill of the pathologist and his or her ability to make cytologic diagnoses on the basis of small bits of tissue. The major justification for such percutaneous biopsies is avoidance of operation.

Yet, regardless of whether the biopsies are positive or negative, most of the time the physician is likely to proceed to operation, partly because something should be done about the obstruction of the various ducts and partly because, despite all the available data, physicians continue to believe that extirpation of a pancreatic carcinoma gives a better 5-year survival for groups of patients than treating it without debulking the tumor. At such an operation, the surgeon will resect either the tumor or the entire pancreas, or at the least will bypass the obstruction in the common bile duct and carry out an anastomosis between the jejunum and the stomach in order to prevent potential obstruction in the duodenum.

Postoperatively, physician and patient face a host of therapeutic options, which are to some extent conditioned by technology. They can choose a passive course, relying on pain-killing drugs and awaiting the inevitable end, accepting the fact that most patients with carcinoma of the pancreas live only 3 to 6 months after diagnosis, or they can choose more aggressive therapy, usually radiation therapy of 5,000 to 6,000 rads, often in combination with chemotherapeutic drugs. As the number of oncologists increases, and as federal government agencies sponsor ever-increasing activity in cancer research, I believe that about one-third of patients in university hospitals today have cancer and are receiving some form of active cancer therapy. Some types of therapy for cancer of the pancreas lengthen life by 3 to 6 months, but studies so far have not convincingly suggested that such prolonged life is pleasant or even tolerable. It is not appropriate to discuss the various forms of therapy here, but simply to emphasize that their availability justifies their use. Physicians often suggest that such aggressive therapy at least tells patients that they are not being abandoned. Curiously, however, internists and gastroenterologists today generally turn such patients over to oncologists rather than caring for them personally.

Having opted for aggressive therapy, the clinician must decide whether to add the latest technological triumph, intravenous hyperalimentation, a form of parenteral feeding that maintains the nutrition of the cancer patient. On the supposition that a well-nourished patient is better able to withstand chemotherapy than a malnourished one, and on the ill-justified assumption that feeding the patient may not also feed the tumor, physicians are increasingly recommending that patients receiving such aggressive therapy also be given hyperalimentation, which can involve long periods in the hospital. We do not know, however, whether such intensive therapy provides enough palliation. Let us leave the patient now receiving radiation and chemotherapy, and securely tied to the hospital by parenteral hyperalimentation, with a life expectancy of 3 to 6 months.

In the preceding discussion, I have tried to show how many diagnostic studies can be carried out in the patient with a complaint of what even a third-year medical student would recognize as carcinoma of the pancreas. I have stressed that the hunger for certainty has led to the abandonment of diagnostic laparotomy and replaced what used to be a short diagnostic sequence – from physical examination and history to operation – with a tortuous and highly expensive series of diagnostic procedures, all of which are justified because they are noninvasive. Many physicians tend to forget that the important aspect, for the patient at least, is the outcome, and in dealing with carcinoma of the pancreas, at least, there is little that can now be done.

### QUESTIONS FOR DISCUSSION

1. How should physicians structure the diagnostic process in such a case? Should the patient's present comfort or risk of future complications be weighed for or against a diagnostic procedure? In these circumstances, should the physician save the patient 10 days of worry and a host of uncertain test results by operating as soon as he or she thinks that cancer of the pancreas is present? Should the doctor choose first the most definitive study, even though it is unpleasant? What should a physician do when he or she is certain of the diagnosis, considers it possible, or wants to rule it out? Are there psychological as well as medical advantages or justifications to proceeding from one indirect test to another? Should the physician think about the cost of noninvasive tests and discard them because they will add only a minimal amount of information? How much information justifies a noninvasive and nondefinitive test? How certain should the diagnosis be before the physician advises operation? How would you feel if you were the patient?

2. Assuming that pathologic study proves that a cancer of the pancreas is present before operation, what are the odds of cure that justify advising an operation – 1 in 10, 1 in 100? How heavily should the pain and suffering of an operation

be weighed against the chance of providing help? How much should the patient be involved in making that decision? If the physician in this case called in a surgeon who recommended an extensive operation to remove the tumor, but the physician disagreed, should that disagreement be discussed with the patient? Will the worry engendered by disagreement and uncertainty be important, or should decisions be made and presented as a unanimous conclusion by the physicians? What does "5-year survival" mean for the individual patient? How are such survival statistics calculated, and what meaning do they have?

3. When does a new diagnostic study become routine? When is it still considered experimental? Should a physician tell a patient that the latest study is unproven in value but may help? If a new unproven study is painless but expensive, who should pay for it? The physician who is learning from the study? The patient? Should patients be charged more as the physician learns more and more from the study? How can we ensure that a study or technique that has proven useful in the research center where it was first developed will be interpreted correctly the first few times it is used in a community hospital? Should the insurance companies pay for such studies? What does "quality assurance" mean in these circumstances? If a study is no longer useful because it has been superseded by a more definitive one, should third-party payors or outside agencies decide that such a study should not be carried out or at least should not be paid for?

### SELECTED BIBLIOGRAPHY

Feinstein, A. R. (1967). *Clinical Judgment*. Baltimore: Williams & Wilkins.
Reiser, S. J. (1978). *Medicine and the Reign of Technology*. New York: Cambridge University Press.
Spiro, H. M., Burrell, M. I., and Zeman, R. K. (1982). Clinical-radiologic perspectives on radiology of the gallbladder and biliary ducts. In *Diagnostic and Interventional Radiology of the Gallbladder and Bile Ducts* (E. R. N. Berk, F. J. T. Ferrucci, and G. R. Leopold, eds.), Philadelphia: W. B. Saunders.
Spiro, H. M. (1980). The physician and the ikon. *Pharos 43*:2–5.
Spiro, H. M. (1981). Images, isaurians, and internists. *Am. J. Roentgenol. 136*:667–72.
Spiro, H. M. (1980). Diagnostic technology and the times. *J. Clin. Gastroenterol.* 2:5–6.

# KIDNEY DISEASE:
# THE DIALYSIS–TRANSPLANTATION
# DILEMMA

PATRICIA L. SCHAFFER, J. MICHAEL LAZARUS, and
STANLEY JOEL REISER

A 38-year-old lawyer, A, suffered slow progressive renal failure due to polycystic kidney disease present since the age of 19. With the aid of drugs and dietary therapy, he nevertheless managed to combine a successful career with a happy family life. His wife, L, owned and operated a plant nursery on property adjacent to their home in a suburb of Cincinnati. They have two children, C, aged 15, and H, 10.

Recently, A felt unusually fatigued, especially during his 45-minute commute from his law office in Cincinnati. He consulted his physician, Dr. T, who informed him that he had developed end-stage renal failure. In a family conference, Dr. T outlined the alternatives before him: a kidney transplant that required either a related or a cadaver donor, continuous ambulatory or cyclic peritoneal dialysis, or hemodialysis either in the home or at the Cincinnati Dialysis Unit, an out-of-hospital facility associated with the hospital. Of these alternatives, Dr. T recommended transplantation from a willing related donor, because a successful transplant gave the most promise of a return to a normal life. Organs donated from relatives tend to be more histologically compatible and therefore less likely to be rejected. Dr. T urged A to explain the circumstances to his family and to bring them to his office for a discussion of the alternatives. Meanwhile, until A found a suitable donor, Dr. T would initiate hemodialysis in the hospital unit and then transfer A to the out-of-hospital dialysis unit after he stabilized.

Although L was frightened upon hearing the news, she tried to cheer her husband by reminding him that he was fortunate to live in an age of expanding medical technology, which offered hope and life to patients once considered terminal. She reminded him that his father, himself a victim of kidney disease, had no such opportunities and choices to make.

Potential kidney donors included his mother and his two brothers, N and S. The children were not candidates because they were too young and might be threatened with the development of polycystic kidney disease in the future. Although A knew that his mother would be willing to donate a kidney, Dr. T felt that she could not bear the stress of an operation due to hypertension and heart disease. When A asked his brother S to consider undergoing histocompatibility testing, he confessed that a serious operation might prove to be a burden on his wife and children, as well as threaten his blooming career. Nevertheless, S promised his brother that he would think seriously about it. A hesitated to call his other brother, N, since the two had never gotten along well. Moreover, N was a professional athlete, and an operation might jeopardize his promising future. But he finally decided to try. As A expected, N expressed his regrets that because of his career, he could not donate a kidney.

Bitter and depressed, A began hemodialysis in the hospital and soon transferred to the out-of-hospital unit to begin a three-times-weekly, 4-hour dialysis regimen. He tried to schedule his dialysis at 6 P.M. after his working hours, but was told that this time was the most popular one and that he would have to be on a waiting list. He could, however, select any slot from 10 P.M. to 2 P.M. Although these periods were inconvenient to his work schedule and family life, he chose the 6 A.M. shift and thus, could arrive at work at 10:30. After dialysis, however, he often went to work feeling fatigued and depressed that he had to schedule his life around a machine. The long commute to and from work now began to be quite exhausting. A became disgruntled with the regimentation of the dialysis unit and the high turnover of staff. He dreaded seeing a new nurse assigned to him, but understood the necessity for the new nursing staff to learn fistula cannulation on patients. As was the usual practice, he was encouraged to learn about his condition, and was taught to monitor all aspects of his own dialysis and eventually to place his own needles. One of the more communicative nurses, D, was particularly helpful in getting A involved in his own therapy. He also discovered a community of support in fellow patients, each following the progress of the other.

As A became more comfortable with the intimidating machine that had become his umbilical cord to life, Dr. T and the staff encouraged him to switch to home hemodialysis. The costs of both center and home dialysis were covered by the federal government, but home dialysis would allow him to spend more time with his family and free him from the rigid center schedule. After he discussed the idea with his wife, she agreed to train with him for home hemodialysis. During their training at the hospital, L felt very uneasy working with the needles, the blood, and the complex machinery. Even after 6 weeks of training and several months at home, she expressed anxiety that something would go wrong. The stress of raising a family, helping her husband, and running her own business became apparent to her friends. Yet A was so pleased with the increased freedom that home dialysis offered that he failed to notice the burden on his wife.

After A's son C overheard two neighbors saying that he might have inherited his father's disease, he began to shower his mother with questions about whether he was going to have his blood cleaned by a machine like his father. His daughter

H was also affected by the therapy. After she saw her father's blood percolating through a series of tubes during the first home dialysis, she refused to go into the room while he was on the machine.

After 8 months had passed, A's brother S contacted him saying that he was now willing to donate a kidney. Although they were not completely histocompatible, Dr. T was encouraging and the operation was performed. During the postoperative period, both A and S recovered quickly. Although the immunosuppressive medication used to prevent rejection of the kidney caused A to become mildly obese and moon-faced in appearance, he was overjoyed to have control over his body again.

Four months later, he slowly rejected the transplant and had to return to dialysis. Devastated and bitter, he felt that Dr. T had expressed false optimism and failed to prepare him for the psychologically sinking experience of transplant rejection. Seeing his independence slip away from him again, and thinking himself a burden to his family, he contemplated refusing treatment. After all, he had been a proud, successful man. Now he felt reduced to an infantile, impotent creature living on borrowed time. He was also guilt-ridden for having lost the kidney that his brother had so generously given. He became furious with the physicians, psychiatrists, and social workers who tried to convince him that life was worth living when they had never experienced his suffering.

With his family's support, his depression slowly faded. Reviewing his immediate options with Dr. T, he could chose peritoneal dialysis, home hemodialysis, or center hemodialysis. Ideally, A wanted that procedure that gave him greatest freedom. Although continuous ambulatory or cyclic dialysis would free him physically from an inflexible schedule at the dialysis unit and remove the stress of home hemodialysis from his family, A felt it would bind him psychologically – an annoying, ever-present reminder of his condition. He would constantly have to change the fluid in his abdomen four to five times a day, 7 days a week. Night-time cyclic peritoneal dialysis was objectionable to both him and L. His wife begged him not to choose home hemodialysis or peritoneal dialysis, because neither she nor the children could continue to cope well with the stresses involved.

A reflected that if he had to return to the dialysis unit, perhaps the family should move into Cincinnati so that he would not have to face the tiresome commute. Yet, if the family moved, L would have to sell her business and the children would have to change schools and leave their old friends. A now recognized that his chronic disease had become a chronic family disease.

Because he did not want to disrupt his family's life further, he decided to continue to commute to the dialysis unit. Fortunately, on this occasion he was able to obtain a 6 P.M. shift. He was relieved that D still worked there, although he was surprised to find that two of his old friends were gone. When he asked D what had become of them, he learned that one had had a successful transplant and the other had died. When A commented on the pathos of the situation, D recalled the early days of ethical dilemmas when the technology first became available, and physicians and committees literally chose who would live and who would die when allocating the limited and expensive therapy. Even now, she told A, physicians often elected not to dialyze patients they viewed as hopeless – that is, whose quality of life would be made worse by dialysis.

When A returned the following week, he noticed that D was not there. When he inquired about her, he was told that she had quit because she was "burned out," tired of dealing with demanding dialysis patients who felt that they knew more than she did. Although A now inserted his own needles, he watched the other patients with sympathy as they waited for a nurse-in-training to attempt her first fistula cannulation. He noticed that ironically it was often the patients themselves who were responsible for the high turnover of nurses.

A year passed, and with the availability of a new immunosupressive drug, cyclosporine, and improved results with cadaver transplantation, the staff recommended to A that he try another transplant operation. The potential freedom was alluring, but to face the emotionally draining experience of rejection left him on the brink of indecision.

### QUESTIONS FOR DISCUSSION

1. Discuss the problems for A in evaluating the following therapeutic choices:
   a. Hemodialysis versus peritoneal dialysis versus transplantation in the hospital.
   b. Home dialysis, considering the effect of disease and therapeutic options on the marriage and on children or other family members. Think about the patient's chronic disease becoming the family's chronic disease.
   c. In the selection process, consider the following issues:
      i. Freedom from machines, schedules, doctors, and nurses (i.e., patient independence).
      ii. Increased or decreased mortality and/or morbidity (long- and short-term) with each form of therapy.
      iii. Cost to the patient and society.
   d. If you were A, what would you do?
2. Discuss the problems for the staff associated with informed consent or advice given for treatment, considering:
   a. The thoroughness of the explanation given to the patient by the staff, and how much to disclose.
   b. The conflict of interest of physicians and surgeons in advising patients.
3. Examine problems of long-term care for the patient, considering how the frequent contact with doctors and nurses raises questions of:
   a. The patient's familarization with personnel.
   b. Overtreatment by physicians.
   c. The patient's conflict with staff over treatment, that is, the informed consumer disagreeing with the provider's decisions.

4. Explore problems for health providers regarding:
   a. Scheduling in dialysis units so that all patients will have the benefit of treatment.
   b. The need for nurses, technicians, renal fellows, and other personnel to learn by treating patients.
   c. Modification of treatment for cost conservation.
5. Examine staff problems in dealing with this disease such as:
   a. Anger, rage, or lack of attention to patients in response to noncompliance or disagreements.
   b. Emotional attachment and subsequent loss.
   c. Anxiety and guilt over treatment errors.
   d. Constant recipients of patients' anger, frustration, and depression, which lead to ''burn-out'' in nurses, technicians, and physicians.
6. Evaluate the problems of a medical staff in selecting patients for end-stage renal disease treatment considering:
   a. The quality of life for the patient.
   b. The economic costs.
   c. Other social issues in prolonging life.
7. When new drugs and technology become available in scant quantities, who should determine which patients can benefit from them? Would you give priority to certain types of patients?
8. Even when the technology is available, physicians may elect not to use it if they view a case as hopeless. Should physicians have this right?
9. Should the federal government be involved, as it is, in subsidizing most of the expense of kidney dialysis and transplantation, medical technology that benefits only a small percentage of the population?
10. What right does a patient have to refuse treatment? Would you define refusal to dialyze as suicide? Consider how advanced medical technology may change our definition of suicide.

## SELECTED BIBLIOGRAPHY

Cestero, R. V. M., Jacobs, M. O., and Freeman, R. B. (1980). A regional end-stage renal disease program: twelve years experience. *Ann. Intern. Med. 93*:494–8.

Hollenberg, N. K., and Tilney, N. L. (1981). Renal transplantation: donor selection and surgical aspects. In *The Kidney* (B. M. Brenner and F. C. Rector, eds.), p. 2599. Philadelphia: W. B. Saunders.

Lazarus, J. M. (1981). Hemodialysis in chronic renal failure. In *Contemporary Issues of Nephrology*, vol. 7 (B. M. Brenner and J. H. Stein, eds.), p. 153. London: Churchill-Livingstone.

Lazarus, J. M., and Kjellstrand, C. M. (1981). Dialysis – medical aspects. In *The Kidney* (B. M. Brenner and F.C. Rector, eds.), p. 2490. Philadelphia: W. B. Saunders.

Lowrie, E. G., Lazarus, J. M., Mocelin, A. J., et al. (1973). Survival of patients undergoing chronic hemodialysis and renal transplantation. *N. Engl. J. Med. 288*:863–7.

Marshall, J. R., Rice, D. G., O'Mera, M., et al. (1975). Characteristics of couples with poor outcome in dialysis home training. *J. Chronic Dis. 28*:375–81.

Mock, L. A., and Kopel, K. (1977). Psychological aspects of home and incenter dialysis. *Dialysis Transplant.* 6:36–42.

Nolph, K. D. (1981). Continuous ambulatory peritoneal dialysis. *Amer. J. Nephrol. 1*:1–10.

Nolph, K. D. and Sorkin, M. I. (1981). Continuous ambulatory peritoneal dialysis. In *Contemporary Issues of Nephrology*, vol. 7 (B. M. Brenner and J. H. Stein, eds.), p. 193. London: Churchill-Livingstone.

Rajapaksa, T. (1979). Maintenance hemodialysis: how to help patients cope. *Residents Staff Physician J. 6*:72–80.

Roberts, J. L. (1976). Analysis and outcome of 1063 patients trained for home hemo-dialysis. *Kidney Int. 9*:363–74.

Shambaugh, P. W., Hampers, C. L., Bailey, G. L., et al. (1967). Hemodialysis in the home: Emotional impact on the spouse. *Trans. Am. Soc. Artif. Intern. Organs 13*:41–5.

Strom, T. B., Tilney, N. L., and Merrill, J. P. (1981). Renal transplantation: clinical management of the transplant recipient. In *The Kidney* (B. M. Brenner and F. C. Rector, eds.), p. 2618. Philadelphia: W. B. Saunders.

Tsaltas, M. O. (1976). Children of home dialysis patients. *J.A.M.A. 236*:2764–6.

# INDEX

Abel, John J., 50–1
abortion, 255, 257
acid–base balance, 111
action potential of neurons, 39
acute care hospitals, 78
acute respiratory illness, 169
acute rheumatic fever (ARF), 143, 145, 146,
    147, 148
administrators, hospital, 78
adoption of technology, 75–7
    factors influencing, 77–81
air compressors, 248
algorithms
    branching logic of, 164, 167, 173
    decision trees vs., 168
    defined, 167–8
    design of, 173–4
    evaluation of, 172
    limitations of, 172–4
    multivariate analysis vs., 172
    partitioning, 165
    reasons for, 168–72
al-Khowarizmi, 167
allergic reactions, 146, 147
allied health personnel, 9
Allwall, N., 51
alpha fetoprotein (AFP), 259
ambulances, 106
ambulatory patients, 202
American College of Surgeons, 10
American Medical Association, 106
American Rheumatology Association's Medi-
    cal Information System (ARAMIS), 163
amniocentesis (AM), 255, 256, 304, 305
    in alpha fetoprotein testing, 259
anaphylaxis, 147
anencephaly, 256, 258

angina pectoris, 165, 193, 199, 273
angiography
    contrast agents of, 42–3
    costs of, 243
    digital subtraction, 291–2
angioplasty, 277
*Annals of Internal Medicine*, 142
antisepsis, 8
aortic stenosis, 327, 328, 329
applied research, 58
arrhythmias, cardiac, 268, 272
"Art, The" (Hippocrates), 4
arteriography, coronary, 157–61, 273, 274,
    276, 277
arteriosclerosis, 44
artherosclerotic vascular disease, 287
artificial hearts, 32, 126, 247–50
    costs and benefits of, 249
    insurance coverage for, 249–50
    recipients selected for, 248–9
artificial intelligence, 163–7
artificial kidneys, 14–15, 50–1, 54
Atkinson Morley Hospital, 69, 74
auscultation
    of fetal heart rate, 303
    of lungs, 279

Babinski sign, 313
background radiation, 42
bacteria, 8
*Bailey v. Lally*, 122
balloon pumps, 97, 100
basic research, 57–8
Bayes, Thomas, 196
Bayes' theorem, 205–7, 273
BB isoenzymes, 270
Bear ventilators, 216, 219

355

bed control systems, 236
Beecher, Henry K., 129
Bell, Alexander Graham, 10
Bernard, Claude, 188
bias, in testing, 198
Bibring, G., 182–3
Bice, T., 80
biochemical analysis, 29, 30
biophysics, 50
biopsies, 123
birth defects, 255
blind testing, 198
blood pressure
    mistakes in measurement of, 280
    systolic, 154
Blue Cross/Blue Shield, 284, 289
bradyarrhythmia, 329
brain death, 13–14, 129–31
branching logic, of algorithms, 164, 167, 173
*Brown v. Hughes*, 121
burn intensive care units, 337–8
burns, 337–40
bypass surgery, *see* coronary artery bypass
    grafting

California
    computerized tomography scanners in, 80
    heart transplants in, 135–6
    paramedic program in, 106
    patients' rights decision in, 127–8
cancer
    cervical, 128
    pancreatic, 341–6
    radiation doses and, 41–2, 297–8
cannulation
    fistula, 350, 352
    intraarterial, 99
*Canterbury v. Spence*, 179
cardiac arrhythmias, 268, 272
cardiac care units (CCUs), 95–6, 268
cardiac defibrillators, 39
cardiopulmonary resuscitation (CPR), 280
case finding, 194
Cassell, E. J., 181
catheters, catheterization, 39, 40, 54, 158–62
    cardiac, 328, 329
    umbilical, 308
cathode ray tubes (CRTs), 28
cavitation, 37
cerebral palsy, 303, 304
certificate of need (CON) programs, 80–1
cesarean section, 304, 305, 306
chemotherapy, 33
chest pain, 267–78
cholecystitis, 287, 288, 289
chorion villus sampling (CVS), 255–6
Christensen-Szalanski, J. J., 174
chromatography, 29
chromosomal abnormalities, 255, 257

cimetidine, 140, 284
clinical assessment of tests, 201–2
cobalt therapy, 79–80
Coleman, R. E., 76
Collaborative Perinatal Study, 303–4
colon, diverticular disease of, 287, 288
color imaging, 294
combination testing, 202–4
communication, in technology diffusion, 75–7
co-morbid conditions, 199, 202
complete blood counts (CBCs), 156, 284
computerized tomography (CT) scanners, 55,
    56, 242, 309, 344
    competitors of, 84–6
    cost of, 74, 131
    description of, 69–70
    development of, 67–9
    diffusion of, 73–5, 77, 79, 80, 81, 84
    head injuries and, 311–19
    manufacturers of, 72–3
    number of, 70–3
    scientific literature on, 76
computers, 11–12, 13, 23–4, 29–30
    algorithms and, 174
    artificial intelligence and, 163–7
    hospital information systems and, 235–9
    outlook for, 113
conditional probability, 196
confirmation tests, 202
Cook County Hospital, 106
Cooley, Denton, 126–7
Cormack, A. M., 55–6, 69
*Corn v. French*, 123, 124
coronary arteries, narrowing of, 273–4, 276,
    277
coronary arteriography, 157–61, 273, 274,
    276, 277
coronary artery bypass grafting (CABG), 157–
    61, 273, 277
coronary artery disease, 158–9, 199, 202, 273,
    274, 276, 277
coronary artery stenosis, 277
Coronary Artery Surgery Study, 204
costs
    of adverse medical outcomes, 145
    of allergic reactions, 147
    analysis of, 139–48
    in cost–benefit analysis, 139–47
    in cost–effectiveness analysis, 139–42, 147–
        8
    escalation of, 15–16
    government regulation of, 80–1, 83, 131–2
    of intensive care, 221
    of respiratory care, 323–4
    of rheumatic fever, 145–6
creatine phosphokinase (CPK), 269–70
Creditor, M. C., 75
criteria maps, 171

Cromwell, J., 79–81
cryopreservation, 57
cryosurgery, 39
*Cunningham v. Charles Pfizer and Co.*, 129
cutoff values, 196–7
cyanosis, 222
cyclic peritoneal dialysis, 349, 351
cyclosporine, 352

Damadian, Raymond, 52
data banks, 163
data bases, in probability estimates, 187
death, definitions of, 13–14
debridement, 338, 339
Decadron, 314
decision analysis, 139–40
    patients' role in, 183–8
    probability assessment in, 185–6
    problem identification in, 157
    pros and cons of, 162, 187–8
    steps in, 157–62
    structuring options in, 185
    value assessment in, 186
    *see also* judgment, judgments
decision making, 153–76
    disclosure in, 179
    formal vs. informal approaches to, 177
    multivariate analysis in, 153–4
    patients involved in, 178–81
decision trees, 143, 148, 183
    bias toward technology in, 187
    clinical algorithms and, 168
    construction of, 158–9, 185
deconditioning, 334
*De corporis humani fabrica* (Vesalius), 4
decubitus ulcers, 333
defensive medicine, 123
defibrillators, cardiac, 39
deoxyribonucleic acid (DNA), 37, 40–1, 257
desperation–reaction model, 65, 67
diabetes mellitus, 33, 193
diagnosis, 7, 26–31
    dynamic mode of, 27, 29–30
    hospital information systems and, 236
    inaccurate, 112
    prenatal, 255, 257, 258
    static mode of, 26–9
diagnostic definition, of normal test results, 200
diagnostic protocols, 168
diagnostic related groups (DRGs), 83
diagnostic tests, 193–207
dialysis, *see* cyclic peritoneal dialysis; hemodialysis
differential calculus, 154
diffusion of technology, 65–86
digital radiography, 60, 291–2
digital subtraction angiography (DSA), 291–2
digital technology, 110, 294

disabled persons, and medical emergencies, 109
disclosure, in decision making, 179
discriminant functions, 155
disofenin scans, 344
disruption of membranes, 36–7
dissection, 4–5, 7
distribution, statistical, 199–200
diverticulitis, 288
doctor–patient relationship, 16–17, 180–1, 188
Donabedian, A., 167, 171
Doppler belts, 303
Doppler imaging, 29
drugs
    adoption of drugs, 76
    emergency-medical systems and, 110–11
    hospital information systems and, 235
    overdoses of, 155
    regulation of, 56, 131
Duke University Medical Center, 163

echocardiograms, 327
economics of health care, 135–51
*Economist*, 57
Eden, Murray, 54
Egeberg, Roger, 119
Einthoven, Willem, 10
elastomers, 43–4
electrical energy
    effects of, 39–40
    hazards of, 103
electrocardiograms (ECG), 23, 26, 30, 31, 110
    exercise, 273–4, 276
    Q wave of, 269
    ST segment of, 197, 200–1, 269, 274, 276
    T wave of, 269, 276
electroencephalograms (EEG), 23, 30, 79
electrolyte dysfunction, 111
electromagnetic energy, 40–2
electromyographs (EMG), 30
electronic fetal monitoring (EFM), 303–6
electronics, in health care technology, 50
electron spin resonance (ESR), 31
electrophoresis, 29
electrophysiology, 30
electroretinographs (ERG), 30
Elstein, A. S., 173
emergency departments (EDs), 105–15
    outlook for, 112–14
    recent history of, 105–7
    technology used in, 109–12
    triage in, 108
    types of patients in, 107–8
Emergency Medical Services System Act, 106
emotions, illness and, 181–2
emphysema, 213–20
endoscopic retrograde cholangiopancreatography (ERCP), 343–5
endoscopy, 283–5

endotracheal tubes, 308
energy exchange, 35–6
 electrical, 39–40
 electromagnetic, 40–2
 mechanical, 36–7
 thermal, 37–9
engineers, 55–6
enteroscopy, 28
ergonovine, 276, 277
ether, 7–8
ethics, 13–15, 18
 of cost analysis, 142, 335
 of genetic screening, 257–8
 of intensive care, 101–2, 309, 318–19
 of patient's choices, 178–9, 213–20, 322–3,
  330, 353
 of triage, 219
evoking strengths, in diagnostic programs,
 164–5
exercise electrocardiograms, 273–4, 276
exertional angina, 273
experimentation, clinical, 121–2
expert witnesses, 124
extraordinary measures, 130–1

false-positive rates, 194–200, 203, 204
family care, 12
fault tests, 120
federal hospitals, 119
fee-for-service delivery, 139
fetoscopy, 256
fistula cannulation, 350, 352
Fleiss, J. L., 172
flowcharts, 167
fluorescence-activated cell sorting (FACS),
 256–7
Foley catheters, 314
Food and Drug Administration (FDA), 56, 80,
 131, 259
 Bureau of Medical Devices, 80
forensic medicine, 119–33, 179
fractures, 112, 279

Galen, 4
gallstones, 155, 287, 288
Garrett, J. B., 75
gas–liquid chromatography (GLC), 29
gastritis, 284
gastroenterology, 283
gastrointestinal illness, 341–7
gastrointestinal (GI) x-ray series, 288, 297
*Gates v. Jensen*, 125
Gaussian distribution, 199–200
Geller, Irving, 59, 60, 61
General Electric, 60, 72, 77
genetic screening, 255–9
Georgetown University Medical Center, 69
Gittelsohn, A., 81

glaucoma, 124–5
glucose tolerance tests, 193, 194
Golding, A. L., 51
government
 health care costs regulated by, 80–1, 83,
  131–2
 technological development supported by,
  57–9
 *see also specific agencies*
*Grammar of Science, The* (Pearson), 8
Greenfield, S., 171–2
Greer, A. L., 78
group practices, 12, 79

Hand, Learned, 124
handicapped persons, and medical emergencies, 109
Harvard University Ad Hoc Committee on
 Brain Death, 129
Hastings Center, 257
Havens, L. L., 190
hay rakes, 338
head injuries, 311–19
head scans, 242–3
Health Care Financing Administration, 249
health insurance, *see* insurance programs
health maintenance organizations (HMOs), 79,
 82–3
Health Service Areas, 72
heart disease, 247, 249, 327–31
heart-lung machines, 129
hearts, artificial, *see* artificial hearts
heart transplants, 135–6
heat, biological effects of, 37–9
*Helling v. Carey and Laughlin*, 124–5
hematuria, 295
hemodialysis, 50–1, 100, 349–52
hemorrhage, intracranial, 309
hepatitis, 202, 261–3
heuristics, 164–5, 189, 190
high-frequency positive pressure ventilation
 (HFPPV), 97
high-performance liquid chromatography
 (HPLC), 29
*High Technology*, 59
Hippocrates, 3–4
holistic health movement, 178
Holter monitors, 327–8
home care, 10, 11, 325, 333, 350–2
Hooke, Robert, 5
Hooper, T. J., 124
hospital information systems (HIS)
 capabilities of, 235–6
 typical responses to, 236–8
hospitals
 acute care, 78
 administrators of, 78
 changing role of, 11
 federal, 119

growth of, 9–10
rate regulation effects on, 81
resource allocations in, 241–4
Hounsfield, G., 55, 69
humoral theory of illness, 3
Hutt, Peter, 63n1
hyaline membrane disease, 307
hydrocephalus, 257, 258
hyperalimentation, 346
hyperbaric chambers, 96
hypertension, 181, 185
hyperthermal treatments, 32, 38
hypothermal treatments, 38
hysterical personalities, 185, 186

iatrogenic illnesses, 98, 100
image intensifier video fluoroscopic systems,
    291–2
imaging, 26–9, 241–4, 291–6
    outlook for, 293–4
    real-time, 292
    specialists in, 294–5
    *see also specific techniques*
immune serum globulin (IG), 261–2
indeterminate test results, 200–1
*Industrial Research and Development*, 58
industry, in technological development, 56
infarction, myocardial, 153, 193, 268–72
informed consent, 122, 179, 284–5
innovation, 52–5, 61–2
    defined, 62–3n1
    forces behind, 53
    process of, 53–4
    profits and, 59–61
innovation–decision process, 76
insulin, 33
insurance programs, 9–10, 16, 79–80, 82–3
    for artificial hearts, 249–50
    Blue Cross/Blue Shield, 284, 289
    Medicaid, 15, 18, 84, 249–50
    Medicare, 15, 18, 79–80, 83, 84, 249
intensive care units (ICU), 16, 95–104, 214–
    16
    burn, 337–8
    as constrained resource, 221–5
    level of technology applied in, 98–100
    neonatal, 307–8
    organization of, 95–6, 214–15
    outlook for, 103
    personnel in, 227–30
    problems and effects of, 101–3
    therapeutic vs. diagnostic modes of, 100
    triage decisions in, 222
    types of patients in, 100–1
intermittent mandatory ventilation (IMV), 97,
    101
INTERNIST-1 program, 164–5
interventional radiography, 54
intraarterial cannulation, 99

intracranial hemorrhages, 309
intrapartum deaths, 303–4, 305
intrapartum hypoxia, 304
intravenous pyelograms (IVPs), 295
intubation, 214, 216–17, 218, 219
invasiveness, levels of, 98
ionization, 40–1
isoenzymes, 270, 272

Johns Hopkins University, 50–1
judgment, judgments
    influences on, 184–6
    limitations of, 168
    similarity vs. probability, 187
    *see also* decision analysis

Kahana, R., 182–3
Kaiser-Permanente health plan, 79
Karp, Haskell, 126–7
Kassirer, J. P., 173
Katz, E., 76
kidneys
    artificial, 14–15, 50–1, 54
    diseases of, 349–53
    *see also* hemodialysis
Koch, Robert, 8
Kolff, Willem J., 14, 51, 54
Komaroff, A. L., 169

laboratories
    automation and computerization of, 29–30
    emergency departments linked with, 110
    hospital information systems and, 235–6
    *see also* tests, testing
lactate dehydrogenase (LDH), 342
Laennec, René, 53
*Lane v. Candura*, 127
Langer, E., 178
laparotomies, 345
Lasersohn, Jack W., 60
laser technology, 38
Lauterbur, Paul, 52
law and medicine, 119–33, 179
leukotomy, 67
liability
    basis of, 120
    strict, 121
life cycle of technology, 67
lifesaving, 334–5
life support systems, 97, 129–31
linear regression, 154
Lister, Joseph, 8
living wills, 131
locality rule, 121
logistic regression, 155–6
"lottery method" of value assessment, 188
lumbar punctures, 309

lung scans, 202
lymphoma, 341

magnetism, in diagnostics, 31
malaria, 54
malpractice, 82, 119–24, 130
mannitol, 314
market system, 136–7
Massachusetts General Hospital, 76
Massell, B. F., 146
mass spectrometry, 29, 30
mastectomies, 123
Mayo, William, 9
Mayo Clinic, 69, 76
MB-CPK tests, 270, 272
MB isoenzymes, 270
mechanical energy, 36–7
mechanistic paradigm, 189
Medawar, Peter, 168
Medicaid, 15, 18, 84, 249–50
*Medical Devices Report*, 56
medical records, 10, 11–12
Medicare, 15, 18, 79–80, 83, 84, 249
mental retardation, 303, 304
Menzel, H., 76
metabolic tracers, 293
metabolites, 27, 29, 30
metallic materials, 43
microprocessors, 52
microscope, invention of, 5
microscopy, 28
microwave radiation, 37, 38, 40
Middle Ages, medicine in, 4
military medicine, 174
Miller, J. M., 146
Mitchell, S. Weir, 6
MM isoenzymes, 270
models, mathematical
    efficacy of, 156–7
    logistic regression, 155–6
    multiple regression, 154–5
molecular biology, 50
monitoring systems, 97
Morgagni, J. B., 6
morphologic imaging, 26–8
Morton, William, 7
multifactorial outcome measurement, 140, 143
multiple regression, 154–5
multivariate analysis, 30, 31, 153–4
    algorithms vs., 172
    pros and cons of, 156–7
    validation of, 157
MYCIN program, 164

National Academy of Sciences (NAS), 106
National Conference of Commissioners on
    Uniform State Laws, 129
National Heart, Lung, and Blood Institute
    (NHLBI), 247

National Highway Safety Act, 106
National Institute of Child Health and Human
    Development, 256
National Institutes of Health, 57, 131, 242,
    256
National Nursing Home Survey, 325
National Science Foundation, 57
negligence, 120
neonatal intensive care units, 307–8
neoplasia, 293
neural tube defects (NTD) screening, 258–9
neurological disorders, 311–19
Newton, Isaac, 5, 188–9
Nissenson, A. R., 51
nitrates, 273
nitroglycerin, 272
Nixon, Richard, 131
no-code orders, 322–3
nonbiological materials, effects of, 36, 42–4
normal distribution, 199–200
normal test results, 199–200
Norvitt, L., 51
nosologic characteristics, *see* sensitivity of
    tests; specificity of tests
nuclear magnetic resonance (NMR), 26, 28,
    30, 31, 52, 58, 60, 61, 84, 86, 243, 293
nuclear medicine, 292–3
Nuremberg code, 122
nurses
    clinical algorithms used by, 169
    in emergency departments, 108
    respiratory care and, 323
nursing homes, 325

obsessive personalities, 182, 185, 186
obstetrics
    prenatal diagnosis in, 255–9
    ulrasound techniques in, 292
occupational therapy, 338
Office of Technology Assessment, U.S., 59,
    74
Oldendorf, William, 69
*Opticks*, 5
optimism, and decision making, 185, 186
options, structuring of, 185
organ transplants
    heart, 135–6
    kidney, 349–53
overdoses, drug, 155

pacemakers, cardiac, 32, 39, 40
pancreatic tumors, 341–6
pancreatitis, 341
pap smears, 128
paradigms, probabilistic vs. mechanistic, 188–
    9
paramedics, 109
parenteral nutrition, 11

partitioning algorithms, 165
patents, 56
paternalism, 178, 180
patients
  ambulatory, 202
  in clinical choices, 177–91
  emotional health of, 181–2
  personality traits of, 182–3
  risks perceived by, 297–9
  *see also* doctor–patient relationship
patient's rights movement, 178
Pauker, S. G., 173
payoff values, 139, 145, 148
Pearson, Karl, 8
penicillin (PCN), 143, 146, 147, 148
peptic ulcers, 284, 285, 288
percentile method, 200
Perkin-Elmer, 59
personality, personalities
  hysterical, 185, 186
  obsessive, 185, 186
  of patients, 182–8
  of physicians, 182
pharmaceuticals, *see* drugs
pharmacy systems, 235
pharyngitis, 142–3
physical therapy, 323
physicians
  personality traits of, 182
  specialization of, 6, 9, 82, 182
  technology used by, 53–5, 78, 82–4
  traditional role of, 178
  *see also* doctor–patient relationship
physician's assistants, 169
Picker International, 58, 60
Pius XII (pope), 13
pneumonia, 321
pneumothorax, 280, 281
poisoning, 111
polio vaccine, 67, 129
Politser, P., 173
polymers, 43–4
polymyalgia rheumatica, 327
polypeptides, 270
polytetrafluoroethylene (PTFE), 51
positive end-expiratory pressure (PEEP), 97,
  101
positron emission transaxial tomography
  (PETT), 60–1, 85–6, 241–2, 293
poverty, health care and, 137
Pozen, M. W., 156
predictive value of tests, 195–6
prednisone, 287
preeclampsia, 305
pregnancy, 255–9, 303–6
premature infants, 307–10
primary care, 12
principled gambling, 190

probabilistic paradigm, 189–90
probability
  assessment of, 185–6
  conditional, 196
  in decision trees, 158–9
  subjective judgments and, 187
product development, 58
Professional Standards Review Organizations
  (PSROs), 84
profits, 59–61
prosthetic devices, 32
prototype development, 58
pulmonary embolisms, 202
pulmonary ventilation-perfusion scans, 202

quality assessment, 169–72
quality of life, 334–5
Quinlan, Joseph, 210
Quinlan, Karen Ann, 14, 219
Quinton, Wayne E., 51
Q waves, 269

radiation therapy, 32, 41–2
radiofrequency radiation, 37, 40
radiography
  digital, 60, 291–2
  image transmission, 113
  interventional, 54
radionuclide scanning, 85, 274, 276, 277
radionuclide tracers, 293
rads, 41
Raible, D., 51
real-time imaging, 292
receiver-operating characteristic (ROC)
  analysis, 196–7
  limitations of, 207
records, medical, 10, 11–12
referent values, 29
Regan, Louis, 121
Regional Medical Programs, 121
regression
  linear, 154
  logistic, 155–6
  multiple, 154–5
regulation
  of drugs, 56, 131
  of experimentation, 122
  of health care costs, 80–1, 83, 131–2
rehabilitation, 333–6
replication, cellular, 41
research and development, 57–8
*res ipsa loquitur* rule, 123
respirators, 14, 97, 308
respiratory illness, 321–6
  algorithms used with, 169
  cost of, 323–4
respiratory therapy, 323
"right to die" acts, 323

risk, patients' perceptions of, 297–9
Rodin, J., 178
Roentgen, Wilhelm Conrad, 291
Roundtree, Leonard G., 50–1
Royal Society of London, 5
Russell, L. B., 80

Salkever, D., 80
Sanctorius, 95
scans, scanning
    computerized tomography, *see* computerized
        tomography (CT) scanners
    disofenin, 344
    head, 242–3
    nuclear magnetic resonance (NMR), 84, 86,
        243
    positron emission transaxial tomography
        (PETT), 60–1, 85–6, 241–2, 293
    pulmonary ventilation-perfusion, 202
    radionuclide, 85, 274, 276, 277
scarcity of health care services, 137
science, conceptions of, 188–90
scintiscans, 276
screening, 194
Scribner, Belding H., 51
*Seats and Causes of Diseases Investigated by
    Anatomy, The* (Morgagni), 6
Seattle Artificial Kidney Center, 14
self-esteem, illness and, 181–2
sensitivity analysis, 147, 161–2
sensitivity of tests, 29, 194–200, 203, 204
serum creatinine phosphokinase (CPK) tests,
    178, 193, 269–70
serum sickness, 147
Shelling, Thomas, 142
Shortliffe, E. H., 164
Shumway, Norman, 135
sickle cell disease, 256
sigmoidoscopy, 288
similarity judgments, 187
skin grafts, 338, 339
SMA-12 tests, 342
Social Security Act, 51
Sox, H. C., 167–8, 169, 172, 174
specialization, 6, 9, 82
    physicians' personalities and, 182
    technological, 96
specificity of tests, 29, 194–200, 203, 204
spectrometry, mass, 29, 30
spina bifida, 258
Stancer, S. L., 146
standard deviations, 200
standards of medical practice, 120–1
Stanford University, 135–6, 164, 213
statistics, in assessment of diagnostic tests,
    194–6
steerable catheters, 54–5
Steins, A. M., 51
stenosis, 277, 287, 292

aortic, 327, 328, 329
stethoscope, invention of, 7, 53
stillbirths, 303
stress tests, 193, 202, 203, 204
strict liability, 121
stroke, 333–6
surgery, 7–8, 32
    for artificial heart implementation, 247–8
    frequency of, 81, 82
    ophthalmological, 38
surrogate tests, 194–205
Sweden, health care in, 135
symbolic reasoning, 164
sympathy, in doctor–patient relationship, 182
syncope, 327–8
synergistic effects, 36
    ignored by algorithms, 173
systolic blood pressure, 154
Szilard, Leo, 55

Technicon Corporation, 52
technology
    adoption of, 75–81
    diagnostic needs met by, 26–31
    diffusion of, 65–86
    digital, 110, 294
    doctor–patient relationship and, 180–1
    economic considerations in, 135–51
    in emergency departments, 109–12
    engineers and, 55–6
    evolution of, 24–6
    examples of, 50–3, 65–75
    excessive use of, 111–12, 183–4
    factors affecting use of, 81–4
    government and, 57–9
    historical overview of, 3–19
    inappropriate use of, 280–1
    industry and, 56–7
    in intensive care units, 98–100
    legal obligation to use, 123
    life cycle of, 67
    malpractice and, 82
    modern role of, 23–4
    patients' needs met by, 32–3
    physicians and, 53–5, 78, 82–4
    profit motive and, 59–61
    in rehabilitation, 335
    as response to uncertainty, 183–4
    side effects of, 35–45
    specialization in, 96
tests, testing, 193–207
    bias in, 198
    clinical assignment of, 201–2
    complete blood count (CBC), 156, 284
    confirmation, 202
    glucose tolerance, 193, 194
    indeterminate, 200–1
    limitations of, 267–78
    MB-CPK, 270, 272

multiple, 202–4
nosologic assessment of, 194–200, 203, 204
predictive value of, 195–6
ROC analysis of, 196–7, 207
serum creatinine phosphokinase, 178, 193, 269–70
SMA-12, 342
stress, 193, 202, 203, 204
surrogate, 194–205
thallium-201, 274, 276
upper gastrointestinal (UGI) series, 284
*see also* laboratories
thallium-201, 274, 276
therapy, technology and, 32–3
thermal energy, 37–9
threshold analysis, 161
Tompkins, R. K., 142, 143, 145
tonsillectomies, 67
total body surface area (TBSA), 337
transhepatic cholangiography, 344
Transportation Department, U.S., 106
trauma units, 106, 112
triage, 99, 100, 221–6
    in emergency departments, 108
    in intensive care units, 222
true-positive rates, 194–200, 203, 204
*Truman v. Thomas*, 127–8
Turner, B. B., 50–1
T waves, 269, 276

ulcers
    decubitus, 333
    peptic, 284, 285, 288
ultrasonic radiation, 243–4, 292
    in alpha fetoprotein testing, 259
    effects of, 36–7
    growth of, 60, 85, 113
    as imaging technique, 28, 31
    in obstetrical care, 256
umbilical artery catheters, 308
uncertainty
    acceptance of, 190
    denial of, 178–9
    personality factors and, 182–3
    sharing of, 188–90

situational factors and, 181–2
    stress caused by, 177
    technology as response to, 183–4
unifactorial outcome measurement, 140
upper gastrointestinal (UGI) series, 284
upper respiratory infections (URIs), 143
    cost–effectiveness models and, 147–8
uric acid levels, 111–12
urticaria, 147
utility analysis, 141
utility assessment, 159
utility theory, 318–19

vaccines, 137
    polio, 67, 129
validation, of multivariate models, 157
value
    assessment of, 186, 188
    in cost analysis, 140–1
vegetative state, 318–19
ventilators, 213–19, 322–5
verapamil, 287
Vesalius, Andreas, 4, 7

wedge procedures, 126
Wennberg, J., 81
wheelchairs, 333–6
Wirtschafter, D., 172
Wood, R. W., 168–9, 172
World Medical Association, 135

x-rays
    in angiography, 42–3, 243
    appropriate use of, 280–1
    cancer risk of, 41–2, 297–8
    discovery of, 291
    gastrointestinal, 288, 297
    as imaging technique, 26, 28
    as legal evidence, 123
XYY condition, 257

Yale University Medical School, 106

zeugmatography, 28